Housing and Health in Europe

Based on the World Health Organization's pan-European study on the state of housing across Europe, the research presented in this book provides fresh evidence for links between housing conditions and the health of inhabitants in a time of change and growing membership of the EU.

Explanation of the nature and development of this unique study is followed by focused analysis of survey results by experts from a range of disciplines and countries. This cross-disciplinary approach enables a thorough introduction and analysis of the topics covered which include:

- Indoor air quality, dampness and thermal comfort
- Mental health and the housing environment
- Quality of life and housing
- Noise and morbidity
- Domestic accidents.

With both methodological and analytical appeal, *Housing and Health in Europe* will be of interest to built environment and medical academics as well as policymakers in housing and public health.

David Ormandy is Professor in the School of Law at the University of Warwick.

Housing and society series
Edited by Ray Forrest
School for Policy Studies, University of Bristol

This series aims to situate housing within its wider social, political and economic context at both national and international level. In doing so it will draw on the full range of social science disciplines and on mainstream debate on the nature of contemporary social change. The books are intended to appeal to an international academic audience as well as to practitioners and policymaker – to be theoretically informed and policy relevant.

Housing and Health in Europe
Edited by David Ormandy

The Hidden Millions
Graham Tipple and Suzanne Speak

Housing, Care and Inheritance
Misa Izuhara

Housing and Social Transition in Japan
Edited by Yosuke Hirayama and Richard Ronald

Housing Transformations
Shaping the space of 21st century living
Bridget Franklin

Housing and Social Policy
Contemporary themes and critical perspectives
Edited by Peter Somerville with Nigel Sprigings

Housing and Social Change
East–West perspectives
Edited by Ray Forrest and James Lee

Urban Poverty, Housing and Social Change in China
Ya Ping Wang

Gentrification in a Global Context
Edited by Rowland Atkinson and Gary Bridge

Housing and Health in Europe

The WHO LARES Project

Edited by David Ormandy

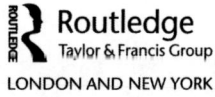

LONDON AND NEW YORK

First published 2009
by Routledge
2 Park Square, Milton Park, Abingdon, Oxon OX14 4RN

Simultaneously published in the USA and Canada
by Routledge
270 Madison Avenue, New York, NY 10016

Routledge is an imprint of the Taylor & Francis Group, an informa business

© 2009 David Ormandy for selection and editorial matter; individual chapters, the contributors

Typeset in Times New Roman by
Keyword Group Ltd
Printed and bound in Great Britain by
CPI Antony Rowe, Chippenham, Wiltshire

All rights reserved. No part of this book may be reprinted or reproduced or utilised in any form or by any electronic, mechanical, or other means, now known or hereafter invented, including photocopying and recording, or in any information storage or retrieval system, without permission in writing from the publishers.

The publisher makes no representation, express or implied, with regard to the accuracy of the information contained in this book and cannot accept any legal responsibility or liability for any errors or omissions that may be made.

British Library Cataloguing in Publication Data
A catalogue record for this book is available from the British Library

Library of Congress Cataloging in Publication Data
 Housing and health in Europe: the WHO LARES Project/edited by David Ormandy.
  p.; cm. – (Housing and society series)
 Includes bibliographical references.
  1. Housing and Health – Europe. 2. WHO LARES Project. I. Ormandy, David. II. Series.
 [DNLM: 1. WHO LARES Project. 2. Housing – Europe. 3. Cross-sectional Studies – Europe. 4. Health Priorities – Europe. 5. Health Status – Europe. 6. Health Surveys – Europe. 7. Urban Health – Europe. WA 795 H8395 2009]
 RA770.H644 2009
 362.1094–dc22   2008046971

ISBN10: 0-415-47735-2 (hbk)
ISBN10: 0-203-88523-6 (ebk)

ISBN13: 978-0-415-47735-2 (hbk)
ISBN13: 978-0-203-88523-9 (ebk)

Contents

Preface	vii
Dedication	viii
Contributors	ix
The LARES Project Network	xi
Figures and tables	xiii

Part I: The LARES survey		**1**
1	Background and introduction	3
	Xavier Bonnefoy, Matthias Braubach, Nathalie Röbbel,	
	Brigitte Moissonnier and David Ormandy	
	Appendix 1.1 – The survey form and questionnaires	17
	Appendix 1.2 – Distribution of the population by city quarters	74
	Appendix 1.3 – Distribution of the households by city quarters	76
	Appendix 1.4 – Distribution of the housing types	78
2	The cities	79
3	The surveys	94
	Nathalie Röbbel	

Part II: The results of the analyses of the LARES data		**103**
4	Introduction	105
5	Scores and conventions	107
6	Potential sources of indoor air pollution and asthma and allergic diseases	111
	Isabella Annesi-Maesano and David Moreau	
7	Damp, mould and health	125
	Peter Rudnai, Mihaly J. Varro, Tibor Malnasi,	
	Anna Páldy, Simon Nicol and Alan O'Dell	
8	The effect of cold homes on health: evidence from the LARES study	142
	Ben Croxford	

Contents

9	Residential energy systems: links with socio-economic status and health in the LARES study *Véronique Ezratty, Anne Duburcq, Corinne Emery and Jacques Lambrozo*	155
10	Perception of safety and fear of crime *Maggie Davidson*	168
11	Housing and mental health *Jérmone Fredouille, E. Laporte and Mounir Mesbah*	184
12	Building Quality of Life-related Housing scores using the LARES study *Mounir Mesbah*	200
	Appendix 12.1 Quality of Life scoring	216
	Appendix 12.2 Anxiety scoring	217
	Appendix 12.3 Depression scoring (SALSA)	218
	Appendix 12.4 How to analyse these scores as response variables	219
13	Residential environmental quality and quality of life *Irene van Kamp, Annemarie Ruysbroek and Rebecca Stellato*	220
14	The health relevance of the immediate housing environment *Matthias Braubach*	247
15	Noise effects and morbidity *Hildegard Niemann and Christian Maschke*	275
16	Domestic accidents *Richard Moore*	295
17	A brief résumé of recommendations *David Ormandy*	319

Index 323

Preface

During 2002/2003, the World Health Organisation (WHO) European Centre for Environment and Health (Bonn Office) organised and supervised housing and health surveys in eight cities in eight European countries. The initial analysis of the data collected from each city provided information on the potential relationship between the housing conditions and the health of the residents for local policymakers.

The methodology and instruments used in each survey were identical, making it possible not only to analyse the data for each city but also to combine the data and compare findings from all eight. This in itself was a unique opportunity. To make the most of this, WHO took a novel approach. It brought together experts from a range of disciplines and from several different countries, some with no particular background in housing-related matters, and invited them to interrogate the combined database from their own particular perspective. Meetings were held that brought together the experts at various stages and provided opportunities for cross-discipline interaction and gave insights into the different approaches adopted.

The result is this unique book. The first part describes the background to the surveys, the development of the survey forms, and the organisation of the surveys themselves. The second part contains contributions from experts involved in the analyses, introducing the subject area they concentrated on, explaining their individual approach, and detailing their findings and conclusions.

This book will be of particular interest to policymakers, to housing professionals, to medical professionals and to academics. It also provides a template for those wishing to organise their own survey, and a benchmark for comparison of results.

Dedication

This book is dedicated to Xavier Bonnefoy who sadly died in November 2007. Xavier was a committed advocate of environmental health and an enthusiastic campaigner for the recognition of the importance of the links between housing conditions and health.

Neither the LARES study, nor this book, would have been possible without the vision and hard work of Xavier. As Regional Advisor at WHO ECEH, Xavier and his team steered the LARES study from concept to completion.

Contributors

Isabella Annesi-Maesano, Epidemiology of Allergic and Respiratory Diseases (EPAR), UMRS-S 707, Pierre et Marie Curie University, Medical School St Antoine, 75571 Paris CEDEX 12

Xavier Bonnefoy (deceased), former Regional Adviser, WHO European Centre for Environment and Health, WHO Regional Office for Europe

Matthias Braubach, Technical Officer, WHO European Centre for Environment and Health, WHO Regional Office for Europe

Ben Croxford, Bartlett School of Graduate Studies, University College London, UK

Maggie Davidson, Building Research Establishment, United Kingdom

Anne Duburcq, Cemka-Eval, Bourg-la-Reine, France

Corinne Emery, Cemka-Eval, Bourg-la-Reine, France

Véronique Ezratty, Service des Etudes Médicales d'EDF et de Gaz de France

Jémone Fredouille, MD, Hôpital Le Vinatier, Lyon, France

Jacques Lambrozo, Service des Etudes Médicales d'EDF et de Gaz de France

E. Laporte, Hôpital Le Vinatier, Lyon, France

Tibor Malnasi, National Institute of Environmental Health, Fodor József National Center for Public Health, Hungary

Christian Maschke, Interdisciplinary Research Network Noise & Health, Berlin, Germany

Mounir Mesbah, PhD, Université Pierre et Marie Curie, Paris, France

Brigitte Moissonnier, Ministry of Health, France

Richard Moore, Independent housing consultant, London, United Kingdom

Contributors

David Moreau, Epidemiology of Allergic and Respiratory Diseases (EPAR), UMRS-S 707, Pierre et Marie Curie University, Medical School St Antoine, 75571 Paris CEDEX 12

Simon Nicol, Building Research Establishment, United Kingdom

Hildegard Niemann, Interdisciplinary Research Network Noise & Health, Berlin, Germany

Alan O'Dell, Building Research Establishment, United Kingdom

David Ormandy, Professor and principal reserach fellow, Safe and Healthy Housing Unit, Law School, University of Warwick, UK

Anna Páldy, National Institute of Environmental Health, Fodor József National Center for Public Health, Hungary

Nathalie Röbbel, WHO European Centre for Environment and Health, WHO Regional Office for Europe

Peter Rudnai, National Institute of Environmental Health, Fodor József National Center for Public Health, Hungary

Annemarie Ruysbroek, Centre for Environmental Health Research/National Institute of Public Health and the Environment, the Netherlands (RIVM)

Rebecca Stellato, Centre for Environmental Health Research/National Institute of Public Health and the Environment, the Netherlands (RIVM)

Irene van Kamp, Centre for Environmental Health Research/National Institute of Public Health and the Environment, the Netherlands (RIVM)

Mihaly J. Varro, National Institute of Environmental Health, Fodor József National Center for Public Health, Hungary

The LARES Project Network

The LARES Project Network

The personnel listed here were all, to a greater or lesser extent, involved with the analyses of the LARES data and in the preparation of this work.

Dr Isabella Annesi-Maesano Epidemiology of Allergic and Respiratory Diseases (EPAR), Pierre et Marie Curie University, Medical School St Antoine, France

Dr Ben Croxford, Bartlett Graduate School, University College London, United Kingdom

Dr Anne Ellaway, MRC Social and Public Health Services Unit, Scotland

Dr Jérôme Fredouille, Médecin Psychiatre, Hôpital du Vinatier, France

Dr Ulla Haverinen-Shaughnessy National Public Health Institute (KTL), Finland

Prof. Kevin Leyden, West Virginia University, USA

Prof. Mounir Masbah, Université Pierre et Marie Curie, France

Dr Richard Moore, Independent housing consultant, United Kingdom

Prof Tim Blackman, University of Durham, United Kingdom

Mrs Maggie Davidson, Building Research Establishment, United Kingdom

Dr Véronique Ezratty, Service des Etudes Médicales, EDF and Gaz de France, France

Dr Maria João Freitas, Laboratório Nacional de Engenharia Civil Grupo Ecologia Social, France

Dr Christa Kliemke, Institut für Gesundheitswissenschaften, Germany

Dr Christian Maschke Forschungs- und Beratungsbüro Maschke, Germany

Prof Rebecca Miles, Florida State University, USA

Dr David Moreau, INSERM U 472, France

The LARES Project Network

Mr Simon Nicol, Building Research Establishment, United Kingdom

Dr Carita Nygren University of Lund, Sweden

Ms Rita Pazdrazdyte, Ministry of Health, Lithuania.

Prof David Ormandy, University of Warwick, United Kingdom

Dr Annemarie Ruysbroek National Institute for Public Health and the Environment (RIVM), Netherlands

Dr Manfred Schmitz Bundesministerium für Gesundheit und Soziale Sicherung, Germany

Dr Irene van Kamp, National Institute for Public Health and the Environment (RIVM), Netherlands

Dr Paul Wilkinson, London School of Hygiene and Tropical Medicine, United Kingdom

Dr Hildegard Nieman, Berliner Zentrum Public Health, Germany

Dr Mark Petticrew, MRC Social and Public Health Sciences Unit, Scotland

Dr Julius Ptashekas, Advisor to Ministry of Health, Lithuania

Dr Peter Rudnai, National Institute of Environmental Health, Hungary

Dr Romualdas Sabaliauskas Ministry of Health, Lithuania

Dr Edmond Shenassa, Brown Medical School, USA

Dr Mihály János Varró, National Institute of Environmental Health, Hungary

WHO Personnel involved in the LARES project

Mr Xavier Bonnefoy, WHO ECEH (Bonn Office), Germany

Mr Rokho Kim, WHO ECEH (Bonn Office), Germany

Mr Kubanychbek Monolbaev WHO Liaison Office, Kyrgyzstan

Ms Célia Rodrigues, WHO ECEH (Bonn Office), Germany

Mr Matthias Braubach, WHO ECEH (Bonn Office), Germany

Ms Brigitte Moissonnier, WHO ECEH (Bonn Office), Germany

Ms Nathalie Röbbel, WHO ECEH (Bonn Office), Germany

Figures and tables

Figures

1.1	The general structure of the surveyor training	10
1.2	Local survey implementation time frame	12
2.1	Geographical location of the survey cities	79
6.1	Prevalence of asthma and allergies in the past year	116
7.1	LARES – distribution of homes by mould indicator	134
7.2	LARES – prevalence of some chronic diseases by mould indicator	134
7.3	LARES – prevalence of some chronic diseases by mould indicator	135
7.4	LARES – prevalence of people with some acute illnesses in the last 12 months by mould indicator	135
7.5	LARES – prevalence of some symptoms during the last 12 months by mould indicator	136
7.6	LARES – adjusted odds ratios of some chronic and acute diseases among people living in homes with much mould/dampness	136
7.7	LARES-adjusted odds ratios of the prevalence of some symptoms in the last 12 months among people living in homes with much mould/dampness	137
10.1	Percentage of respondents indicating whether they feel safe returning home when it is dark by city	172
12.1	Overview	201
12.2	Health explained by Housing Conditions, after adjustment on individual profile	202
12.3	Health explained by Housing Conditions, without adjustment on individual profile	202
12.4	Causal relationship between Housing Conditions and Health	202
12.5	Quality of Housing scores	203
12.6	Cronbach alpha curve for defaults	209

xiii

Figures and tables

12.7	Analysis of Housing Conditions on Quality of Life as a sufficient outcome for Health	210
13.1	Model showing the relationships between residential domain satisfactions and quality of life	223
13.2	Measurement model concerning environmental quality, residential satisfaction and quality of life	226
13.3	Difference of means between cities on dissatisfaction dwelling, area and unwell-being	229
13.4	Selected aspects of environmental quality per city	231–232
13.5	Difference of means by level of urbanisation on dissatisfaction dwelling, area and unwell-being	233
13.6	Selected aspects of environmental quality by level of urbanisation	233–234
13.7	Difference of means by neighbourhood type on dissatisfaction dwelling, area and unwell-being	234
13.8	Selected aspects of environmental quality by neighbourhood type	235–236
13.9	Difference of means by building age on dissatisfaction house, area and unwell-being	236
13.10	Selected aspects of environmental quality by building age	237–238
13.11	Outcome model concerning environmental quality and satisfaction with the living area	242
13.12	Outcome model concerning environmental quality, dissatisfaction with the dwelling and unwell-being	242
15.1	Frequency of occurrence of annoyance in the LARES study for six selected sources of noise – adults, children and elderly	276
15.2	Frequency of occurrence of sleep disturbances in the LARES study for six selected sources of noise – adults, children and elderly	278
15.3	A comparison of the prevalence of selected medically diagnosed illnesses in adults, elderly and children in the LARES study	278
15.4	Relative disease risks for adults who indicated noise-induced annoyance by general traffic noise within the last 12 months, compared to adults without traffic noise-induced annoyance	281
15.5	Relative disease risks for adults who indicated noise-induced annoyance by general neighbourhood noise within the last 12 months, in comparison with adults without neighbourhood noise-induced annoyance	282

Figures and tables

15.6	Relative disease risks for children who indicated noise-induced annoyance by general traffic noise within the last 12 months, compared to children without traffic noise-induced annoyance	283
15.7	Relative disease risks for children who indicated noise-induced annoyance by general neighbourhood noise within the last 12 months, compared to children without neighbourhood noise-induced annoyance	284
15.8	Relative disease risks for elderly people who indicated noise-induced annoyance by traffic noise within the last 12 months, in comparison with elderly people without traffic noise-induced annoyance	285
15.9	Relative disease risks for elderly people who indicated noise-induced annoyance by neighbourhood noise within the last 12 months, in comparison with elderly people without neighbourhood noise-induced annoyance	285
15.10	Relative disease risks for adults who indicated noise-induced sleep disturbances within the last 12 months, in comparison with adults without noise-induced sleep disturbances	287
15.11	Relative disease risks for children who indicated noise-induced sleep disturbances within the last 12 months, in comparison with children without noise-induced sleep disturbances	288
15.12	Relative disease risks for elderly people who indicated noise-induced sleep disturbances within the last 12 months, in comparison with elderly people without noise-induced sleep disturbances	289
16.1	Sample proportions of number and types of accident reported.	297
16.2	Accident rates for cuts and burns by age group and gender	301
16.3	Main accident rates by body weight for persons aged 20–80 years old	303
16.4	Accident rate by sleep disturbance from noise	308
16.5	Number of accidents reported where hazard(s) were identified, by surveyor	312
16.6	Odds ratios for significant psycho-social predictors for an accident of any type	316
16.7	Odds ratios for significant housing predictors for an accident of any type	316

Figures and tables

Tables

1.1	Housing and health aspects covered in the survey instruments	8
1.2	Dwelling and inhabitant samples in the LARES project	13
2.1	Average temperature in Angers	80
2.2	Population by age group in Angers	80
2.3	Household size in Angers	81
2.4	Housing stock in 1999	81
2.5	The climate of Bonn	82
2.6	Population by age group in Bonn	82
2.7	Household structure of Bonn	82
2.8	Age of the housing stock in Bonn	83
2.9	The climate of Bratislava	84
2.10	Population by age group in Bratislava	84
2.11	Household size in Bratislava	84
2.12	Age of the housing stock in Bratislava	85
2.13	The housing market in Bratislava	85
2.14	Population by age group in Budapest	86
2.15	Household size in Budapest	86
2.16	Age of the housing stock in Budapest	87
2.17	Population by age group in Ferreira do Alentejo	88
2.18	Household size in Ferreira do Alentejo	88
2.19	The climate of Forlì	89
2.20	Population by age group in Forlì	90
2.21	Household size in Forlì	90
2.22	The climate of Geneva	91
2.23	Population by age group in Geneva	91
2.24	Age of the housing stock in Geneva	92
2.25	The climate of Vilnius	92
2.26	Household size in Vilnius	93
2.27	Age of the housing stock in Vilnius	93
5.1	Age bands	108
6.1	Evidence of indoor pollutants	112
6.2	Prevalence of doctor-diagnosed asthma and allergies in the past year by age and by sex	116
6.3	Percentage prevalence of doctor-diagnosed asthma and allergies in the past year by city	117
6.4	Percentage prevalence of indoor air pollutants according to percentiles of the socio-economic index	118
6.5	Prevalence of doctor-diagnosed asthma and allergies in the past year according to exposure to indoor air pollutants	119–120

Figures and tables

6.6	Odds ratios between doctor-diagnosed asthma and allergies in the past year and indoor air pollutants – logistic regression models including all the air pollutants and the confounders at the same time	121
7.1	Summary of basic data on mould growth	129
7.2	Per cent of dwellings with dampness and mould by city	130
7.3	CHAID models of dampness and humidity indices	131
7.4	Predictions of one of the CHAID models	133
8.1	Variables related to cold homes from the LARES survey	144
8.2	Variables used in the logistic regression model	146
8.3	Summary of all statistical analyses	148–149
8.4	Prevalence of respiratory symptoms	150
8.5	Prevalence of CVD symptoms	151
8.6	Prevalence of arthritis symptoms	152
9.1	Variables used in the analyses models	160
9.2	Health variables and adjustments	161
10.1	Simple analysis of LARES data on per cent of households feeling unsafe returning home after dark – respondent characteristics	173
10.2	Simple analysis of LARES data on per cent of households feeling unsafe returning home after dark – building design and condition aspects	174
10.3	Simple analysis of LARES data on per cent of households feeling unsafe returning home after dark – management of blocks and common areas	175
10.4	Simple analysis of LARES data on per cent of households feeling unsafe returning home after dark – immediate environment facilities, design and problems in the area	176
10.5	Simple analysis of LARES data on per cent of households feeling unsafe returning home after dark – area characteristics	177
10.6	Results of stages of regression analyses	178
10.7	Percentage of households in each 'feeling safe returning home after dark' category having other problems	181
11.1	Direct mental health effects of housing factors	185
11.2	Recent mental health studies in Europe	186
11.3A	Individual risk factors of a good Quality of Life	191
11.3B	Housing risk factors of a good Quality of Life	192–193
11.4A	Individual risk factors of Anxiety	194
11.4B	Housing risk factors of Anxiety	195
11.5A	Individual risk factors of Depression	196
11.5B	Housing risk factors of Depression	197

Figures and tables

12.1	Scores of Quality of Life and declaration of anxiety and depression	210
12.2	Score of Quality of Life and chronic illnesses	211
12.3	Score of Quality of Life and acute illnesses	211
12.4	Score of Quality of Life and symptoms in last 12 months	211
12.5	Score of Quality of Life and accidents in dwelling	212
12.6	Score of Quality of Life and other health variables	212
12.7	Score of Quality of Life and significant Housing Condition factors	213–214
13.1	Types of indicator ordered by importance	221
13.2	Review of instruments used to measure environmental quality and quality of life	225
13.3	Review of instruments to measure environmental quality and quality of life	227
13.4	Pearson correlations between outcome variables	228
13.5	Pearson correlations between environmental quality and outcome variables	228
13.6	The regression models for dissatisfaction with area on observed and perceived environmental quality	239
13.7	The multilevel models for dissatisfaction with the dwelling on observed and perceived environmental quality	240
13.8	The multilevel models for unwell-being on observed and perceived environmental quality	241
14.1	Variables used for analysis	250
14.2A	Bivariate analysis for neighbourhood types and problems with the housing environment	252–253
14.2B	Bivariate analysis for self-rated health	254
14.3	Overview of models	256
14.4A	Logistic regression results – examining the impact of the neighbourhood on health outcomes for self-rated health and sleep disturbance	257–259
14.4B	Logistic regression results – examining the impact of the neighbourhood on four health outcomes	260–261
14.5	Overview of significant associations	267
15.1	Control variables divided into five analysis blocks	279
15.2	Relative risks for illnesses/disease symptoms in children experiencing chronic annoyance through traffic noise and neighbourhood noise	291
16.1	The 20 most frequently recorded accident combinations	298
16.2	Percentage of persons reporting accidents by degree of tiredness	302

16.3	Percentage of adults reporting accidents by hours in the home	305
16.4	Percentage of persons reporting accidents by satisfaction with dwelling size	305
16.5	Percentage of persons reporting accidents by satisfaction with kitchen	306
16.6	Number of types of accident reported by whether or not sleep was disturbed by noise	308
16.7	Percentage of persons reporting falls by floor fault index	310
16.8	Odds ratios for psycho-social and housing variable for each accident type	314

Part I
The LARES survey

1 Background and introduction

Xavier Bonnefoy, Matthias Braubach, Nathalie Röbbel, Brigitte Moissonnier and David Ormandy

The aims of the LARES project

In recognition that, internationally, there were limited data on the link between housing conditions and health effects, the first recommendation made by a housing and health expert meeting convened by WHO in Paris in 2000 (WHO 2000) was the designing and carrying out of a large, exploratory pan-European housing survey. The intention of this survey was to try to identify and compare the health risks associated with housing conditions in several European cities and to identify action priorities.

At the centre of the study design was the WHO definition of housing as a broad concept involving four interrelated elements – the home, the dwelling, the community and the immediate environment (or neighbourhood).

For each of these individual domains, there is an array of potential influences that can have a direct or indirect effect on physical, social and/or mental health, or an effect on the quality of life. It is also important to recognise that the four elements are interlinked.

The **home** is the social, cultural and economic structure created by the household. It represents a refuge from the outside world, enables the development of a sense of identity and attachment – as an individual or as a part of a household – and it provides a space to be oneself. Any intrusion of external factors or stressors strongly limits the strong psychosocial feeling of safety, intimacy and control, so inhibiting the mental and social function of the home.

The **dwelling** is the physical structure providing shelter and the necessary space, facilities and amenities for the household. Any unsatisfactory condition of the dwelling may lead to one or more direct health effects. Mould growth, poor

Background and introduction

indoor air quality and emissions from building materials are as relevant as the infestations of pests, energy inefficiency, inadequate sound attenuation and the lack of hygiene and sanitation amenities. Equally, the quality and the design of the dwelling can result in potential threats of physical injury, interfere with the social functionality of the dwelling and be the cause of barriers for residents with physical limitations. The dwelling should also be affordable and of adequate size and design for the household.

Like the home, the **community** is the social, cultural and economic structure built by those within a neighbourhood. There is evidence to suggest that the social cohesion of the community, and the sense of trust and collective worth, depends to some extent on the quality of a neighbourhood and the **immediate environment**, which can have an impact on social, mental and physical health through the quality of urban design. Poorly planned or badly maintained residential areas, often lacking public services, greenery, parks, playgrounds and walking areas, have been associated with a lack of physical exercise, increased prevalence of obesity, cognitive problems in children and a loss of the ability to socialise. Symptoms of neighbourhood decline affect residents through both visual mechanisms (litter, pollution, etc.) and social mechanisms (segregation, loitering, increased insecurity). The urban planning and layout may lead to an increased dependence on individual transportation, triggering increased pollution and noise exposure, and endangering or isolating the more vulnerable groups such as the very young, the elderly and those with functional limitations.

The specific objectives of the project

The specific objectives of the project were to:

- assess the quality and condition of the housing stock
- identify indications of potential priorities to address problems related to housing and health
- design and test an instrument that could be used by local authorities to investigate housing and health conditions within their cities or regions
- produce a comprehensive database
- suggest guidelines and recommendations to inform policy-makers.

The Large Analysis and Review of European housing and health Status (**LARES**) was carried out during 2002 and 2003 in eight European cities – Angers (France), Bonn (Germany), Bratislava (Slovakia), Budapest (Hungary), Ferreira do Alentejo (Portugal), Forlì (Italy), Geneva (Switzerland) and Vilnius (Lithuania). In total, data was obtained from 8,519 individual residents in 3,373 dwellings.

The survey design

LARES was designed to be an exploratory cross-sectional study. For many of the housing characteristics and the health statuses, there were no functional or targeted hypotheses or they seemed to be limited, so an exploratory design seemed the best option. This method was chosen to give an indication of the prevalence of some key health conditions in a population (Rushton and Elliott 2003). However, it was recognised that such a design would limit any causal analyses (Bonaiuto et al 1999; Diez Roux 2001, 2002).

The approach adopted focused on subjective data and the perception of the residents collected through face-to-face interviews in the homes of the sampled households, but included objective information gathered by an independent survey of the dwelling.

No recording of physical measurements such as temperature, humidity and noise were taken. Primarily this was for reasons of the cost of equipment and staff, but also because of the logistical challenge of taking measurements in private households in various countries over at least 1 week (to provide useful and reliable data).

To devise common survey instruments for use in different countries involved a number of challenges:

1. **Differences in dwelling design and construction**
   So that the data collected from each city could be compared, the same survey instruments were to be used in each city. Therefore, the instruments focused on global housing issues that would be relevant to a majority of the cities and ignored potential regional differences. But, even for general questions about conditions, the variety of housing and building types posed many challenges: for example, the design, choice of materials and amenities in the dwelling. Portuguese village houses may have no heating systems but thick stone walls with few windows, whereas Lithuanian multi-family houses may have large double-glazed windows, central heating and pre-cast concrete walls.
2. **Practical and legal issues relating to confidentiality and the use of public records**
   Conducting interviews and surveys in people's homes necessarily requires consideration of privacy and protection of anonymity; the development of guidelines for the use of addresses and personal data as well as the general rule that it would not be possible to identify an individual or household from the collected data. It was also necessary to check and follow the different national rules and guidelines for privacy and ethical requirements in each country.

Background and introduction

The development of the survey instruments

The development of the survey tools drew on an extensive review of the literature and the advice of a multidisciplinary network of urban planners, epidemiologists, architects, sociologists and public health specialists from WHO and other institutions. In addition, expert meetings were organised by WHO to discuss methods and approaches (WHO 2000). To provide ongoing advice, WHO used its European Housing and Health Task Force, which served as a steering committee for the WHO programme on housing and health from 2001 until the completion of the preliminary analyses of the data.

The survey instruments integrated topics, elements and questions from existing validated questionnaires such as the English House Condition Survey[1] (EHCS), the Scottish Health, Housing and Regeneration Research Project[2] (SHARP), the Eurobarometer,[3] the Medical Outcome Short Form (SF36), the depression screening tool SALSA[4] (Brody *et al* 1998) and EQ5D (The EuroQol Group 1990). This approach enabled not only the use of validated question sets but also a better comparison and benchmarking of the results with other relevant studies.

Three related survey instruments were developed – an Inhabitant Questionnaire, a Housing Inspection Survey Sheet and a Housing and Health Questionnaire. These were based on a pilot study carried out in 2000/2001 in Vilnius (Lithuania), Bratislava (Slovakia) and Schwedt-Oder (Germany) (Bonnefoy *et al* 2003).

1. **Inhabitant Questionnaire**
   This was for recording the responses from a face-to-face interview with one of the inhabitants on his/her perception of and satisfaction with a variety of characteristics of the home.
2. **Housing Inspection Survey Sheet**
   This recorded the findings from a visual inspection, covering data on the state and physical condition of the dwelling and the associated facilities and amenities.
3. **Housing and Health Questionnaire**
   This was a self-completion health status questionnaire to be filled out by all inhabitants of the dwelling.

The survey instruments were translated from English into Italian, German and Lithuanian and then piloted in 20 dwellings in each country. This piloting showed that a full survey and interview visit should take around 1 hour.

---

[1] www.communities.gov.uk/housing/housingresearch/housingsurveys/englishhousecondition/ (accessed 4 April 2008).
[2] www.sphsu.mrc.ac.uk/studies/sharp/index.php?Page=25&mitem25=1 (accessed 4 April 2008).
[3] http://ec.europa.eu/public_opinion/index_en.htm (accessed 4 April 2008).
[4] See Chapter 11 for an explanation of SALSA.

Background and introduction

Once finalised, the instruments were translated into the local languages where the surveys were to be carried out. The translation was carried out by WHO staff or by local counterparts and survey coordinators in the countries. Clearly, this had to be done with care to try to ensure that the meaning of questions and answers was not changed. Because of time and financial constraints, a back-translation into English was not done for any language. However, all translations were tested for understanding in each country in five to six households with different age and education groups.

As often as possible a 5-point Likert scale for ranking and assessment questions was used. Such a scale seemed the most general and acceptable choice for all the countries and cultures involved. The final scales that were used in the survey tools can be categorized into three types:

1. Five-point ranking scales using smiley faces (so-called Kunin scales) were used to assess subjective satisfaction. This avoided both numerical values (1–5) and expressions ('bad' to 'good'), which could be interpreted differently depending on cultural background.
2. Five-point Likert scales with written assessment only for option 1 (e.g. 'highly dissatisfied') and 5 (e.g. 'highly satisfied') were used. These so-called 'anchored' ranking scales only define the ends of the scale, but do not limit the individual's assessment of the intermediate ranking options.
3. Five-point Likert scales with continuous ranking values were used for frequency (for example, 'never, seldom, sometimes, often, permanent').

The final versions of the survey instruments contained 290 questions, 13% of which used the Likert scale format, 11% allowed for open answers and the remaining 76% were closed questions.

The finalised survey instruments[5] covered the range of housing and health aspects shown in Table 1.1.

Survey methodology

City selection

The selection of cities was based on WHO networks, on the resources of the cities and on their interest in being involved in the project. Consequently, the survey cities cannot be said to be representative of their country, although each full survey was representative of that city.

---

[5]The survey instruments are included as Appendix 1 to this chapter.

Background and introduction

Table 1.1 Housing and health aspects covered in the survey instruments

Housing aspects
Household size and composition
Temperature, heating and insulation
Air quality, air pollution and ventilation
Damp, humidity and moulds
Natural light and artificial lighting
Sanitary and hygiene installations
Safety and risk of accidents
Pests, insects and infestations
Environmental tobacco smoke (ETS)
Noise exposure conditions
Density and overcrowding
Accessibility and barriers
Building characteristics and equipment
Dwelling satisfaction and mobility
Housing environment conditions
Socioeconomic characteristics

Health aspects
Personal characteristics
Lifestyle / health behaviour (alcohol consumption, smoking behaviour, physical activity)
Self-rated health status
Functional / physical limitations
Problems to use dwelling
Mental condition / quality of life
Depression screening tool
Sleep disturbance / noise annoyance
Dwelling satisfaction
Psychosocial benefits of the home
Accidents / injuries
Chronic and acute illnesses and symptoms (reported and diagnosed)
Use of medicines

Sampling methods

For six of the cities, the city population register was used as the sampling frame to produce a representative sample of residents in each city. The selected person from the register provided the link to a full household and the dwelling. The sampling frames used all residential addresses, excluding:

- secondary residential addresses (except in Budapest and Bratislava)
- nursing homes, military barracks and dormitories.

For the other two cities, because of specific national privacy laws, alternative sources had to be used. In Angers the database of built properties provided by the local tax

Background and introduction

registry was used as the sampling frame. In Ferreira do Alentejo the sample was drawn from the SINUS database, which includes all health service users of the city.

The sample in each city was randomly generated, the sample size of between 600 (Ferreira do Alentejo) and 1,700 (Budapest) reflecting the size of the city and the expected participation rate. A response rate of between 40% and 60%, and a non-contact rate of around 20% was expected.

To meet the requirements of the national privacy laws, addresses were only kept for the time of the survey, and the information was destroyed after data entry was completed. However, with the permission of the household, some addresses were kept to allow further contact if it was necessary during the analysis.

Local base set-up

The practical arrangements for managing the surveys were similar in all cities. The control centre was located in a large room, or in an office with several rooms to allow an easy exchange of information and management of the work. These rooms were provided by the local counterparts of WHO and the collaborating bodies (usually the local authorities/municipalities, or health services). They were equipped with tables, phones, PCs, printing and copying facilities, etc. A WHO representative, assisted by a local person, coordinated the work.

In each city, 16–26 surveyors, working in pairs, would be spending 17–18 days full time on the survey. The surveyors were either students in their 4th or 5th year of university (from relevant backgrounds, such as medicine, sociology, architecture, or geography) or young professionals registered as unemployed. They were supported by additional staff to help collect the Housing and Health Questionnaires (which were left by the surveyors for self-completion by the residents) and to enter data. All staff were recruited locally by the local municipalities or their national counterparts.

Surveyor training

The surveyors were given a standardised training programme over 3 days, led in the local language by a WHO representative (Figure 1.1). The programme included general guidelines and theoretical background intended to ensure that the surveyors would have:

- a good understanding of each individual survey instrument
- the ability to explain the objective of the questionnaires and the purpose of the survey project
- the ability to explain the individual questions and pre-coded answers
- a similar standard of evaluation and assessment of conditions (to reduce surveyor variability)

Background and introduction

Training schedule

Day 1

- Introduction to project and survey, background, methods used
- General information on survey work, interviewers' manual
- Explanation of inspection sheet (and definitions)
- Desktop exercise (photographs and descriptions of conditions)

Day 2

- Feedback and discussion on Desktop exercise
- Housing questionnaire (and definitions): explanation
- Practical exercise: making contact by telephone
- Test on technical definitions and terminology
- Practical exercise: full inspection in dwelling and follow-up

Day 3

- Housing and Health questionnaire explanation
- Practical exercise: door contact situation
- Survey team selection, sample distribution, general information on coordination of survey
- Start of survey work: phone calls under supervision

1.1   The general structure of the surveyor training.

- the capacity to conduct interviews and lead a conversation
- a good overview of their daily tasks and duties as surveyors.

Training consisted of lectures and practical exercises such as assessment tests, followed by feedback and discussion, and simulation of the interview situation. To try to ensure that each surveyor had a similar interpretation and understanding, clear definitions were given and they were provided with a glossary of the technical terms.

To overcome the complexity of visually assessing building elements systematically, the surveyors assessed the conditions described and shown in photographs. Differences in the assessments were then discussed to develop a common understanding of what conditions should be labelled as good, average, or bad. The surveyors were then asked to inspect a dwelling and complete the full inspection sheet. This exercise highlighted any problem areas for discussion to try to reduce

---

[6]Such methods were developed from those used in House Condition Surveys throughout the UK to improve consistency of surveyors' assessments of housing conditions. However, it should be emphasised that these surveys use professional surveyors and involve a 5- or 6-day training course covering the physical inspection alone.

Background and introduction

surveyor variability. The discussions triggered by this practical exercise were probably the most decisive and important component of the training.[6]

Contact with households

Three steps were taken to maximise the response rate:

1. A week before the start of the survey, a local press conference was held to explain the purpose behind the survey and the information that would be collected. The role of the local authority was also explained, and assurances given about confidentiality.
2. Each selected household was sent a letter signed by both WHO and the mayor of the city.[7] The letter explained the study and gave details of a contact point where further information could be obtained.
3. If a household's telephone number was traced (in around 50–70% of cases), a call was made to obtain cooperation and to arrange a date for the survey and interview. Where no telephone number could be traced, the surveyors 'cold-called'. If there was no answer, they left an information card with a telephone number to call for an appointment. This strategic choice is likely to have resulted in an overselection of those households with a telephone. However it can be assumed that using only 'cold-visiting' methods would probably have resulted in lower response rates, especially given the short duration of the fieldwork.

Data collection

The interview for the Inhabitant Questionnaire was conducted by one surveyor with one member of the household (normally the head of household or partner) while the second surveyor inspected the dwelling and the immediate environment and completed the Housing Inspection Survey Sheet.

To provide an incentive and to maximise completed surveys and interviews, surveyors were paid according to results rather than a flat rate per day. They had preset objectives, with added incentives in case of particularly good performance or severe difficulties.

At the end of the survey and interview, sufficient copies of the Housing and Health Questionnaire were left for each member of the household. It was

---

[7] Introductory letters have proved to be a useful method for increasing participation rates among those receiving them (Smith *et al* 1995).

[8] This age was a guideline – in some cases younger children wanted to fill out the health questionnaire by themselves, whereas in other cases parents filled out the questionnaires of older children.

Background and introduction

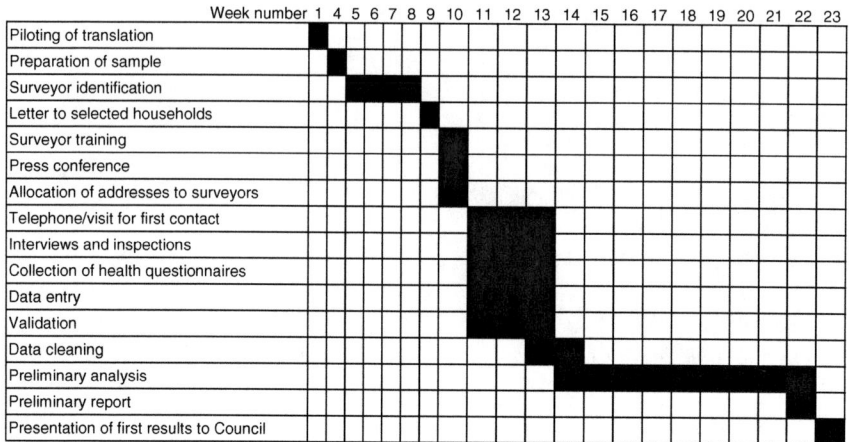

1.2 Local survey implementation time frame.

explained that each occupant should complete it themselves, although an adult should give the information for children under 12.[8] To maximise the response rate for this Housing and Health Questionnaire, the surveyors arranged to collect the completed forms rather than simply relying on the respondents to mail them.

Quality controls

1. **Allocation of addresses**
   The training methods and use of objective questions described above helped to reduce the surveyor variability. However, it was possible that one team would be stricter than another. To minimise the chances of bias and further reduce variability, surveyor teams were randomly allocated addresses throughout all neighbourhoods from the sample.
2. **Visual checking of completed questionnaires**
   All completed questionnaires were checked as soon as they were returned. Where information was missing or unclear, the surveyor was asked to resolve the query. This checking proved to be particularly useful in filling gaps and reconciling inconsistencies. It also identified surveyors who were repeatedly making the same mistakes so they could be provided with the necessary help or feedback to improve their work in the future.
3. **Checks of interviews**
   A random selection of between 8% and 10% of households were called or visited to confirm that the surveyors had carried out the survey and interview, and to check some key data collected.

Background and introduction

Table 1.2 Dwelling and inhabitant samples in the LARES project

Location	Dwelling sample	Dwellings surveyed		Inhabitants covered
		No.	AR*	
Angers (France)	800	427	56.0	880
Bonn (Germany)	1,100	390	43.4	946
Bratislava (Slovakia)	1,314	338	32.7	892
Budapest (Hungary)	1,768	447	27.9	1,086
Ferreira do Alentejo (Portugal)	600	357	77.3	1,055
Forlì (Italy)	800	397	50.8	1,157
Geneva (Switzerland)	1,200	333	34.0	710
Vilnius (Lithuania)	1,100	684	63.3	1,793
Totals	**8,682**	**3373**	**385.4**	**8,519**

*AR = Adjusted response rate – ratio of the number of interviews to the number of eligible households selected where attempts had been made to contact the household.

4. **Date entry validation and cleaning**

    After data entry, a random 10% were checked for quality. Once all the data from the city had been entered, a representative of that city 'cleaned' that database. Any missing information was added by going back to the questionnaires. This process ensured that the database was as complete as possible, and helped eliminate any inconsistencies not detected during the first quality checks.

Representativeness of the sample for each city

The distribution of the characteristics of the respondents for each city was compared with data supplied by the cities. While this official data were of uneven quality and sometimes used different categorisations and definitions, it did give some indication of the representativeness, and of any bias in the sample.

Population database: age, gender and neighbourhood distribution

There are no indications of any significant gender bias in the data for any of the cities. However, there is some bias in the age distribution of the population in six cities, although that bias is not consistent between the cities. In Vilnius, for example, those aged less than 20 were under-represented, but were over-represented in Bonn, Budapest and Geneva. In Angers those aged ≥80 were slightly over-represented. Those aged 40–59 were over-represented in Ferreira do Alentejo, while those between 60 and 79 were under-represented. In Bratislava and Forlì there was no significant difference in the age distribution from the city data and from the sample.

---

[9] The exceptions to this were Angers and Ferreira do Alentejo where the samples were drawn from another source.

Background and introduction

For Budapest, Forlì, Ferreira do Alentejo and Vilnius there were some significant differences between the proportions of inhabitants living in each quarter for the sample and the city data. Bonn, Bratislava and Geneva show no significant differences (see Appendix 2).

Housing database: household size and house type

As a consequence of the sampling methodology, the average household size in the database was larger than the average household size for each city.[9] Although the most reliable method to guarantee the comparability of the data was to take the sample from population registers, as these registers included all children, it increased the probability of selection of larger households.

The geographical distribution of the sample households showed some significant differences from the city data for Angers, Budapest and Forlì, but not for the other cities (see Appendix 3). The distribution of the housing types showed no major deviations, with the exceptions of Geneva, where multi-family houses were over-represented, and Angers, where multi-family houses were under-represented (see Appendix 4).

Overall representativeness of the samples

The results suggested that there were some biases and that some adjustments were needed before analysis of the data to try to ensure that estimates were reliable. While, ideally, additional comparisons could have been made, the data from the cities was limited. For the analysis of the combined data set for relationships between personal characteristics, housing and health problems, there was no need to create correction factors.

References

Bonaiuto M., Aiello A., Perugini M., Bonnes M., Ercolani A.P. (1999) Multidimensional perception of residential environmental quality and neighbourhood attachment in the urban environment. *Journal of Environmental Psychology* 19 (4): 331–52.

Bonnefoy X.R. *et al* (2003) Housing and health in Europe: preliminary results of a pan-European study. *American Journal of Public Health* 93 (9): 1559–63.

Brody D.S., Hahn S.R., Spitzer R.L. *et al* (1998) Identifying patients with depression in the primary care setting: a more efficient method. *Archives of Internal Medicine* 158: 2469–75.

Diez Roux A.V. (2001) Investigating neighborhood and area effects on health. *American Journal of Public Health* 91 (11): 1783–9.

Diez Roux A.V. (2002) Places, people and health. *American Journal of Epidemiology* 155 (6): 516–19.

Background and introduction

Rushton L., Elliott P. (2003) Evaluating evidence on environmental health risks. *British Medical Bulletin* 68: 113–28.
Smith W., Chey T., Jalaludin B. *et al* (1995) Increasing response rates in telephone surveys: a randomized trail. *Journal of Public Health Medicine* 17 (1): 33–8.
The EuroQol Group (1990) EuroQol: a new facility for the measurement of health-related quality of life. *Health Policy* 16 (3): 199–208.
WHO (2000) Integrated Approaches to Housing and Health: Report on a WHO Expert Meeting. Paris 12–13 July 2000. WHO Regional Office for Europe, Copenhagen.

Further reading

2nd HABITAT Conference in Istanbul (1996) *Declaration on Human Settlements and Adequate Shelter for All*. UN Habitat, Istanbul.
Altgeld T. (2004) *Gesundheitsfördernde Settingansätze in benachteiligten städtischen Quartieren*. Expertise E&C: Entwicklung und Chancen junger Menschen in sozialen Brennpunkten. Available at: www.eundc.de.
Basolo V., Strong D. (2002) Understanding the neighbourhood: from residents' perceptions and needs to action. *Housing Policy Debate* 13 (1): 83–105.
Burridge R., Ormandy D. (eds) (1993) Unhealthy Housing: Research, Remedies and Reform. London: E & FN Spon.
Cattell V. (2001) Poor people, poor places, and poor health: the mediating role of social networks and social capital. *Social Science and Medicine* 52: 1501–16.
Cohen D.A. *et al* (2003) Neighborhood physical conditions and health. *American Journal of Public Health* (93) 3: 467–71.
Dunn J.R., Hayes M.V. (2000) Social inequality, population health, and housing: a study of two Vancouver neighborhoods. *Social Science and Medicine* 51: 563–87.
Ellaway A. *et al* (2001) Perceptions of place and health in socially contrasting neighbourhoods. *Urban Studies* 38 (12): 2299–316.
Evans G.W. (2003) The built environment and mental health. *Journal of Urban Health* 80 (4): 536–55.
Fiedler K. (1997) Alles über gesundes Wohnen. Wohnmedizin im Alltag. München: Beck.
Fiedler K. (1998) Wohnen und Gesundheit. *Gesundheitswesen* 60: 656–60.
Foster H.D. (1992) Health, Disease and the Environment. London: Belhaven Press.
Fuller-Thomson E. *et al* (2000) The Housing/health relationship: what do we know? *Reviews on Environmental Health* 15 (1–2): 109–33.
Hiscock R. *et al* (2001) Ontological security and psycho-social benefits from the home: qualitative evidence on issues of tenure. *Housing, Theory and Society* 18: 50–66.
Ineichen B. (1993) Homes and Health: How Housing And Health Interact. London: E & FN Spon.

Background and introduction

Kearns A. *et al* (2000) 'Beyond four walls'. The psycho-social benefits of home: evidence from West Central Scotland. *Housing Studies* 15 (3): 387–410.

Latkin C.A., Curry A.D. (2003) Stressful neighbourhoods and depression: a prospective study of the impact of neighbourhood disorder. *Journal of Health and Social Behaviour* 44: 34–44.

Lawrence R.J. (2000) Urban health: a new agenda? *Reviews on Environmental Health* 15 (1–2): 1–12.

Lowry S. (1991) Housing and Health. London: British Medical Journal.

Mackenbach J.P., Howden-Chapman P. (2002) Houses, neighbourhoods and health. *European Journal of Public Health* 12: 161–2.

Morrow V. (2001) Networks and Neighbourhoods: Children and Young People's Perspectives. London: Health Development Agency.

Petrovitch A. (1996) Begriffsabgrenzungen und Einflussfaktoren. [Sick building syndrome]. *Umweltmedizin in Forschung und Praxis* (3): 143–50.

Ranson R. (1991) Healthy Housing – A Practical Guide. London: E & FN Spon.

Raw G.J., Hamilton R.M. (eds) (1995) Building Regulation and Health. *Building Research Establishment Report* 289, BRE, Watford.

Relph E. (1976) Place and Placelessness. London: Pion.

Shaw M. (2004) Housing and public health. *Annual Reviews of Public Health* 25:08. 1-08.22.

Stafford M., Marmot M. (2003) Neighbourhood deprivation and health: does it affect us all equally? *International Journal of Epidemiology* 32: 357–66.

Thomson H. *et al* (2001) Health effects of housing improvement: systematic review of intervention studies. *British Medical Journal* 323: 187–90.

Van Poll R. (1997) The Perceived Quality of the Urban Residential Environment. A Multi-Attribute Evaluation. Roermond: Westrom.

WHO (1995a) Sick Building Syndrome. Health and environment briefing pamphlet series 2. WHO Regional Office for Europe, Copenhagen.

WHO (1995b) Lead and Health. Health and environment briefing pamphlet series 1. WHO Regional Office for Europe, Copenhagen.

WHO (1996) Radon. Health and environment briefing pamphlet series 10. WHO Regional Office for Europe, Copenhagen.

WHO (1999) Healthy Cities and the City Planning Process. WHO Regional Office for Europe, Copenhagen.

WHO (2004) Housing and Health. Health and environment briefing pamphlet series 41. WHO Regional Office for Europe, Copenhagen.

Appendix 1.1 The survey form and questionnaires

Housing and Health Questionnaire

Date:_____   ID: |__|__|__||__|__|__|__||__|

This questionnaire is about your health condition. It will help us to find out if any health problems you have might be related to the dwelling you are living in. The questionnaire will take around 10 minutes to fill out, and all information given will be handled confidentially.
Please circle the number or tick the boxes that are correct for you or write the figures.

General Information

HH_1 What is your gender?

    1 Male
    2 Female

HH_2	What is your age?	|__|__|__| years
HH_3	How tall are you?	|__|__|__| cm
HH_4	What is your weight?	|__|__|__| kg

HH_5 Are you covered by a health insurance ?

    1 Yes – public insurance
    2 Yes – private insurance
    3 Yes – both insurances
    4 No
    99 Don't know

Background and introduction

HH_6 **What is your marital status?**

1 Married, living together with spouse
2 Married, separated from spouse
3 Single
4 Divorced
5 Widowed
6 You live together with a steady partner

HH_7 **Which school leaving certificate do you have?**

1 Primary/elementary
2 Secondary first stage
3 Secondary second stage
4 Post-secondary (university or similar)
5 No education at all
99 Don't know

HH_8 **What is your current employment status?**

1 Full-time work
2 Part-time work
3 Student / pupil
4 Pensioner
5 Unemployed or laid off
6 Taking care of your household or a family member
7 Recruit or non-military service
8 Other

HH_9 **What is or was the main profession of your father?**

✎ _____

HH_9a **Were you born in** *name of respective country*?

1 Yes *(please go to HH_10)*
2 No

HH_9b **For how many years have you been living in** *name of respective country*?

|__|__| years

Background and introduction

HH_10	**Which statement do you think best describes your smoking behaviour?** 1 I have never smoked 2 I used to smoke 3 I now smoke occasionally 4 I smoke daily less than 5 cigarettes 5 I smoke daily 5–15 cigarettes 6 I smoke daily more than 15 cigarettes 7 I smoke daily other tobacco products than cigarettes
HH_11	**Which statement do you think best describes your alcohol consumption?** 1 I have never been drinking 2 I used to drink 3 I now drink occasionally 4 I drink daily 1 or 2 glasses of alcoholic beverages 5 I drink daily 3–4 glasses of alcoholic beverages 6 I drink daily more than 4 glasses of alcoholic beverages
HH_12	**Which statement do you think best describes your amount of sport or physical exercise (both at work and during leisure time)?** 1 I have never done sport / physical exercise 2 I used to do sport / physical exercise 3 I now occasionally do sport / physical exercise 4 I frequently do sport / physical exercise on moderate level 5 I frequently do sport / physical exercise on intense level
HH_13	**How many hours per day do you on average spend *out of your dwelling* ?** *(Please write number from 0 to 24 hours)* (workdays) |__|__| hours (weekends) |__|__| hours

Background and introduction

General health and constraints

Now we come to questions that are about your health.
Please circle the number or tick the boxes that are correct for you:

H_1 How is your health in general?

1	2	3	4	5
Very good	Good	Fair	Bad	Very bad

H_2 Do you have some kind of physical constraint or handicap?

1 Yes
2 No

H_2a Can you distinctly hear what is said in a conversation with one other person?

1 Yes, without a problem
2 No
3 Yes, but only with hearing aids or devices

H_3 Can you without difficulty go up and down a flight of stairs?

1 Yes
2 No

H_4 Can you without difficulty use your fingers to grasp or handle a small object (like a pen)?

1 Yes
2 No

H_5 Can you without difficulty turn a tap on?

1 Yes
2 No

H_6 Can you without difficulty bend down and kneel down?

1 Yes
2 No

H_7 Do you feel that due to your age or general fitness, you have some problems to make a normal use of the dwelling as it is now?

1 Yes
2 No

Background and introduction

H_8	Due to age, low fitness or any physical constraint / handicap, are there any specific adaptations of the dwelling (e.g. lift, broader doors, no doorsteps, specific installations, walk-in shower . . .) that you need in order to make the best-possible use of your dwelling? 1 Yes 2 No *(please go to H_11)*
H_9	Please, give the three most important adaptations needed (under 9_1), and mark those adaptations already realized in the dwelling (under 9_2). If they have not yet been realized, please indicate if a realization is possible at all (under 9_3)

H_9_1	Adaptation needed	9_2 Adaptation realized	9_3 Adaptation possible
	_____	☐	☐
	_____	☐	☐
	_____	☐	☐

H_10	If the required adaptation/s are not possible in your dwelling, would this be a reason to consider moving into another dwelling? 1 Yes 2 No 99 Don't know

Background and introduction

Quality of life

H_11 **During the past month, have you felt particularly nervous?**

    1 All of the time
    2 Most of the time
    3 A good bit of the time
    4 Some of the time
    5 A little of the time
    6 None of the time

H_12 **During the past month, have you felt so down in the dumps nothing could cheer you up?**

    1 All of the time
    2 Most of the time
    3 A good bit of the time
    4 Some of the time
    5 A little of the time
    6 None of the time

H_13 **During the past month, have you felt calm and peaceful?**

    1 All of the time
    2 Most of the time
    3 A good bit of the time
    4 Some of the time
    5 A little of the time
    6 None of the time

H_14 **During the past month, have you felt downhearted and miserable?**

    1 All of the time
    2 Most of the time
    3 A good bit of the time
    4 Some of the time
    5 A little of the time
    6 None of the time

H_15 **During the past month, have you been happy?**

1 All of the time
2 Most of the time
3 A good bit of the time
4 Some of the time
5 A little of the time
6 None of the time

H_16 **During the past month, did you have lots of energy?**

1 All of the time
2 Most of the time
3 A good bit of the time
4 Some of the time
5 A little of the time
6 None of the time

H_17 **During the past month, did you feel worn out?**

1 All of the time
2 Most of the time
3 A good bit of the time
4 Some of the time
5 A little of the time
6 None of the time

H_18 **During the past month, did you feel full of life?**

1 All of the time
2 Most of the time
3 A good bit of the time
4 Some of the time
5 A little of the time
6 None of the time

H_19 **During the past month, did you feel tired?**

1 All of the time
2 Most of the time
3 A good bit of the time
4 Some of the time
5 A little of the time
6 None of the time

Background and introduction

H_20	Did you have sleep disturbance every day for a period of 2 weeks or more? 1 Yes 2 No
H_21	Did you have loss or decreasing of interest in activities every day for a period of 2 weeks or more? 1 Yes 2 No
H_22	Did you have low self-esteem every day for a period of 2 weeks or more? 1 Yes 2 No
H_23	Did you have decreased appetite every day for a period of 2 weeks or more? 1 Yes 2 No
H_24	If you answered 'Yes' to any of H_20, H_21, H_22 or H_23, do you think that at least one of those is related to your dwelling? 1 Yes 2 No

Background and introduction

Sleep disturbance

H_25	How long did it usually take for you to fall asleep during the past 4 weeks? *(Circle one)*
	1 0–15 minutes
	2 16–30 minutes
	3 31–45 minutes
	4 46–60 minutes
	5 More than 60 minutes

H_26	On average, how many hours did you sleep each night during the past 4 weeks?
	Write in numbers of hours per night |__|__|

H_27	Has your sleep been disturbed by noise during the past 4 weeks?
	1 Yes
	2 No *(please go to H_29)*

H_28	If 'Yes', what was/were the source/s of noise? *(please tick all appropriate boxes)*
	☐ Noise from surrounding area (bars, disco, events)
	☐ Playgrounds, schools, recreational facilities
	☐ Traffic noise
	☐ Airplane noise
	☐ Train noise
	☐ Parking and parking lots
	☐ Neighbour's flat (talking, music, TV, repairs, animals, etc.)
	☐ Animals/birds (from outside)
	☐ Noise from commercial, industrial or construction sites
	☐ Staircase use
	☐ Playing children in building
	☐ Ventilation, heating or installation system, waste chute
	☐ Lift
	☐ Noise sources within own dwelling
	☐ Other, please specify_____

Background and introduction

H_29 Thinking about the last 12 months, when you are here at home, how much would you say that noise from the following sources bothers or annoys you?

Please circle the appropriate number for all noise sources!

	Not at all	Slightly	Moderately	Strongly	Extremely
Surrounding area (bars, disco, events)	1	2	3	4	5
Playgrounds, schools, recreational facilities	1	2	3	4	5
Traffic noise	1	2	3	4	5
Airplane noise	1	2	3	4	5
Train noise	1	2	3	4	5
Parking and parking lots	1	2	3	4	5
Neighbour's flat (talking, music, TV, repairs, animals, etc.)	1	2	3	4	5
Animals/birds (outside)	1	2	3	4	5
Commercial, industrial or construction sites	1	2	3	4	5
Staircase use	1	2	3	4	5
Playing children in building	1	2	3	4	5
Ventilation, heating or installation system, waste chute	1	2	3	4	5
Lift	1	2	3	4	5
Noise sources in own dwelling	1	2	3	4	5
Other source of noise, please specify below ✎	1	2	3	4	5

Background and introduction

Flat satisfaction					
H_30 How would you evaluate your dwelling on a scale from 1 (very good) to 5 (very bad)?					
	1 Very good	2 Good	3 Fair	4 Bad	5 Very bad

H_31 How strongly do you agree or disagree with each of the following opinions that people might have about their home?
(Please circle or tick one box for each statement)

	Strongly agree	Agree	Neither agree or disagree	Disagree	Strongly disagree
I feel I have privacy in my home	1	2	3	4	5
I can get away from it all in my home	1	2	3	4	5
I can do what I want when I want in my home	1	2	3	4	5
Most people would like a home like mine	1	2	3	4	5
I feel in control of my home	1	2	3	4	5
My home makes me feel that I'm doing well in my life	1	2	3	4	5
I worry about losing my home	1	2	3	4	5
My home life has a sense of routine	1	2	3	4	5
My home feels safe	1	2	3	4	5
My home expresses my personality and values	1	2	3	4	5

Background and introduction

> *Accidents/injuries*
>
> For the following questions, we would like you to think of both the dwelling and the commonly used building spaces (corridor, staircase, basement / utility rooms), and tell us about all the – small and big – accidents, injuries or mishaps that you experienced in the following cases:
>
> - a first aid kit was used
> - a doctor / hospital / ambulance car was contacted
> - pain or any kind of physical limitation still existed the day after the event.

H_32 **What kind of accidents did you experience in this dwelling (during the last 12 months)?** *(please tick all appropriate boxes)*

☐ Falls
☐ Burns
☐ Cuts
☐ Choking/suffocating/drowning
☐ Collision/striking
☐ Poisoning/chemical agents
☐ Gas intoxication
☐ Electric accident
☐ Other, please specify_____
☐ No accident at all *(go to H_36)*

H_33 **What items were involved in these accidents?** *(please tick all appropriate boxes)*

☐ Construction features
  (walls, floor, doors, windows, indoor stairs, lift)
☐ Electric equipment
☐ Water/sanitary system
☐ Heating/cooling equipment
☐ Kitchen equipment
☐ Knives and silverware
☐ Furniture/furnishing (carpets, curtains, etc.)
☐ Washing/cleaning products, detergents, liquids, etc.
☐ Gases and fumes
☐ Food items
☐ Animals and pets
☐ Toys
☐ Other, please specify _____

H_34 **Which part of your body was injured?** *(please tick all appropriate boxes)*

☐ Head
☐ Neck/throat
☐ Thorax/chest/upper back
☐ Lower trunk
☐ Arm/upper limb
☐ Leg/lower limb
☐ Surface area
☐ Whole body affected
☐ Other, please specify _____

H_35 **What was the outcome?** *(Please tick all appropriate boxes)*

☐ Self-help, bandaging
☐ Visit to a doctor, examination only
☐ Visit to a doctor, prescribed treatment
☐ Hospitalization
☐ Other outcome, please specify _____

Background and introduction

Disease prevalence

For the following questions, please look at the following example, which shows you how to fill out the questions.

If you circled
① Yes → please go to the boxes on the right and fill in the answers

If you circled
② No ↓ please go to the next disease or symptom below

H_36 Do you have or have ever had any of the following chronic illnesses or conditions? *(reply to each of the illnesses)*

	Did you have it during the last 12 months?	If YES → If NO ↓	Was it diagnosed by a physician?	Have you taken prescribed medicine for this?	Would you think it is related to your flat?
Diabetes	1 Yes 2 No	→ ↓	1 Yes 2 No	1 Yes 2 No	1 Yes 2 No
Hypertension (high blood pressure)	1 Yes 2 No	→ ↓	1 Yes 2 No	1 Yes 2 No	1 Yes 2 No
Heart attack (myocardial infarction)	1 Yes 2 No	→ ↓	1 Yes 2 No	1 Yes 2 No	1 Yes 2 No
Stroke, cerebral haemorrhage	1 Yes 2 No	→ ↓	1 Yes 2 No	1 Yes 2 No	1 Yes 2 No
Malignant tumour (including leukaemia and lymphoma)	1 Yes 2 No	→ ↓	1 Yes 2 No	1 Yes 2 No	1 Yes 2 No
Asthma	Yes 2 No	→ ↓	1 Yes 2 No	1 Yes 2 No	1 Yes 2 No
Chronic bronchitis, emphysema	1 Yes 2 No	→ ↓	1 Yes 2 No	1 Yes 2 No	1 Yes 2 No
Arthrosis (rheumatic) arthritis	1 Yes 2 No	→ ↓	1 Yes 2 No	1 Yes 2 No	1 Yes 2 No
Chronic anxiety and depression	1 Yes 2 No	→ ↓	1 Yes 2 No	1 Yes 2 No	1 Yes 2 No
Migraine and frequent headache	1 Yes 2 No	→ ↓	1 Yes 2 No	1 Yes 2 No	1 Yes 2 No
Serious skin diseases	1 Yes 2 No	→ ↓	1 Yes 2 No	1 Yes 2 No	1 Yes 2 No

Background and introduction

(continuation)	Did you have it during the last 12 months?	If YES → If NO ↓	Was it diagnosed by a physician?	Have you taken prescribed medicine for this?	Would you think it is related to your flat?
Allergy (excluding allergic asthma)	1 Yes 2 No	→ ↓	1 Yes 2 No	1 Yes 2 No	1 Yes 2 No
Osteoporosis	1 Yes 2 No	→ ↓	1 Yes 2 No	1 Yes 2 No	1 Yes 2 No
Cataract	1 Yes 2 No	→ ↓	1 Yes 2 No	1 Yes 2 No	1 Yes 2 No
Gastric or duodenal ulcer	1 Yes 2 No	→ ↓	1 Yes 2 No	1 Yes 2 No	1 Yes 2 No
Tuberculosis	1 Yes 2 No	→ ↓	1 Yes 2 No	1 Yes 2 No	1 Yes 2 No
Other, please, specify below					
✎	1 Yes 2 No	→ ↓	1 Yes 2 No	1 Yes 2 No	1 Yes 2 No
✎	1 Yes 2 No	→ ↓	1 Yes 2 No	1 Yes 2 No	1 Yes 2 No

Background and introduction

H_37 Do you have or in the last 12 months have you had any of the following acute illnesses or conditions? (reply to each of the *illnesses*)

	Did you have it during the last 12 months?	If YES → If NO ↓	Was it diagnosed by a physician?	Have you taken prescribed medicine for this?	Would you think it is related to your flat?
Cold or a throat illness	1 Yes 2 No	→ ↓	1 Yes 2 No	1 Yes 2 No	1 Yes 2 No
Acute bronchitis or pneumonia	1 Yes 2 No	→ ↓	1 Yes 2 No	1 Yes 2 No	1 Yes 2 No
Diarrhoeal diseases	1 Yes 2 No	→ ↓	1 Yes 2 No	1 Yes 2 No	1 Yes 2 No
Other, please specify below					
✎	1 Yes 2 No	→ ↓	1 Yes 2 No	1 Yes 2 No	1 Yes 2 No
✎	1 Yes 2 No	→ ↓	1 Yes 2 No	1 Yes 2 No	1 Yes 2 No

H_38 Do you have or in the last 12 months have you had any of the following symptoms and conditions? *(reply to each of the illnesses)*

	Did you have it during the last 12 months?	If YES → If NO ↓	Was it diagnosed by a physician?	Have you taken prescribed medicine for this?	Would you think it is related to your flat?
Wheezing or whistling in your chest	1 Yes 2 No	→ ↓	1 Yes 2 No	1 Yes 2 No	1 Yes 2 No
Attack of asthma	1 Yes 2 No	→ ↓	1 Yes 2 No	1 Yes 2 No	1 Yes 2 No
Any nasal allergies, including hay fever	1 Yes 2 No	→ ↓	1 Yes 2 No	1 Yes 2 No	1 Yes 2 No
Problem with sneezing, or runny or a blocked nose when you did not have a cold or the flu	1 Yes 2 No	→ ↓	1 Yes 2 No	1 Yes 2 No	1 Yes 2 No

Background and introduction

(continuation)	Did you have it during the last 12 months?	If YES → If NO ↓	Was it diagnosed by a physician?	Have you taken prescribed medicine for this?	Would you think it is related to your flat?
Eczema or any kind of skin allergy	1 Yes 2 No	→ ↓	1 Yes 2 No	1 Yes 2 No	1 Yes 2 No
Fatigue	1 Yes 2 No	→ ↓	1 Yes 2 No	1 Yes 2 No	1 Yes 2 No
Headache	1 Yes 2 No	→ ↓	1 Yes 2 No	1 Yes 2 No	1 Yes 2 No
Watery eyes or eye inflammation	1 Yes 2 No	→ ↓	1 Yes 2 No	1 Yes 2 No	1 Yes 2 No
Other, please specify below					
✎	1 Yes 2 No	→ ↓	1 Yes 2 No	1 Yes 2 No	1 Yes 2 No
✎	1 Yes 2 No	→ ↓	1 Yes 2 No	1 Yes 2 No	1 Yes 2 No

H_39 Have you taken any medicines without a prescription from a doctor during the last 2 weeks?
1 Yes
2 No

H_40 If 'Yes', what types of medicines did you take? Were they medicines for ... *(please mark all options that apply)*

☐ Pain
☐ Cold, flu or sore throat
☐ Allergic symptoms
☐ Stomach trouble
☐ Vitamins, minerals or tonic
☐ Sleep
☐ Some other medicines not prescribed by a doctor?
☐ If 'Yes' – what type?
✎ _____

Background and introduction

Thank you very much for your help!

> Please give the questionnaire to the surveyor while he's still in your home, or put the questionnaire into the envelope, close it and send it back when everyone has filled out one questionnaire.

Housing Inspection Survey Sheet

ID: |__|__|__|__|__|__|__|__|

City quarter:_____   Time of survey:_____
Street:_____   Date of survey:_____

Housing information

HI_1	**Neighbourhood type** *(see definition)*	Panel block housing estate	1
		Mainly detached houses	2
		Mainly semi-detached houses	3
		Mainly terraced houses	4
		Mainly apartment-block-dominated	
		- Up to four floors	5
		- Five or more floors	6
		Mixed neighbourhood	7
HI_2	**Housing type** *(see definition)*	Panel block	1
		Brick house	2
		Detached one-family house	3
		Semi-detached housing unit	4
		Terraced housing unit	5
		Multi-family apartment block	
		- Up to 6 residential units	6
		- More than 6 residential units	7

HI_3 **Which of the following housing circumstances / locations comes closest to the surveyed property / dwelling?** *(see definition)*

in an urban centre close to a busy street	1
in an urban centre at a less busy street	2
in a (sub)urban neighbourhood close to a busy street	3
in a (sub)urban neighbourhood at a less busy street	4
in a rural area close to a busy street	5
in a rural area at a less busy street	6

Background and introduction

HI_4 **Dwelling located on floor number** *(ground / entrance floor on street level counted as the 1st floor, basement counted as 0)*:

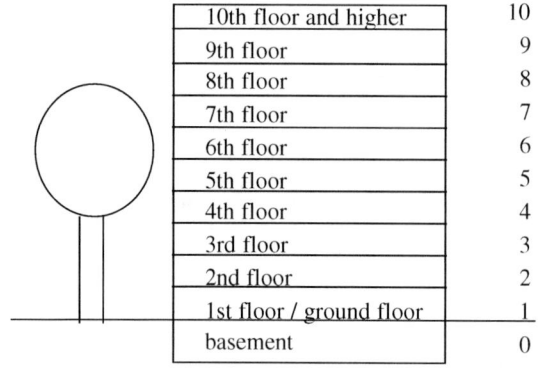

10th floor and higher	10
9th floor	9
8th floor	8
7th floor	7
6th floor	6
5th floor	5
4th floor	4
3rd floor	3
2nd floor	2
1st floor / ground floor	1
basement	0

If dwelling is a house, or located on several floor levels, mark the lowest floor of the dwelling!

For one-family houses, put '1' even if they have rooms in the basement

HI_5 **Is any inhabitable part of the dwelling (or the dwelling as such) located right under the roof?** *(see definition)*

Yes 1
No 2

HI_6 **Building age (year of construction)** *(ask residents if they know)*

Before 1900	1
1900–1920	2
1921–1945	3
1946–1960	4
1961–1970	5
1971–1980	6
1981–1990	7
1991–2000	8
2001 and after	9
Don't know	99

General aspects in all parts of the flat *(see definition for rooms and room selection)*

The following matrix asks about the existence of rooms, their functions and their conditions. In each room, go through the list from top to bottom and fill out the different questions.

Fill in WC only if there is a single detached toilet outside the bathroom. The toilet in the bathroom is considered part of the bathroom.

		Kitchen	Bathroom	WC	Corridor	Room 1	Room 2	Room 3	Room 4		FLAT
GA_1	Room exists (please tick off):	( )	( )	( )	( )	( )	( )	( )	( )		
GA_2	Function / second function (def.)	⌐⌐	⌐⌐	⌐⌐	⌐⌐	⌐⌐	⌐⌐	⌐⌐	⌐⌐		
GA_3	Window in room	( )	( )	( )	( )	( )	( )	( )	( )		
GA_4	Window can be opened (def.)	( )	( )	( )	( )	( )	( )	( )	( )	GA_14 (def.)	( )
GA_5	Window(s) can be closed (please circle)(see definition)										
	Tight	1	1	1	1	1	1	1	1	GA_15 (def.)	1
	Not tight: draught	2	2	2	2	2	2	2	2		2
	Not tight: draught + visible gap	3	3	3	3	3	3	3	3		3
GA_6	Window quality										
	Single-glazed windows	1	1	1	1	1	1	1	1	GA_16 (def.)	1
	Double-glazed windows	2	2	2	2	2	2	2	2		2
GA_7	Installed heating system (see definition)										
	Yes – with thermostat	1	1	1	1	1	1	1	1	GA_17 (def.)	1
	Yes – without thermostat	2	2	2	2	2	2	2	2		2
	No heating	3	3	3	3	3	3	3	3		3
GA_8	Additional heating devices (def.)	( )	( )	( )	( )	( )	( )	( )	( )	GA_18 (def.)	( )
GA_9	Visual mould growth (total area) (see definition)										
	No mould growth visible	1	1	1	1	1	1	1	1	GA_19 (def.)	1
	One or two small spots	2	2	2	2	2	2	2	2		2
	Bigger than a postcard (A6)	3	3	3	3	3	3	3	3		3
	Bigger than an A3 sheet	4	4	4	4	4	4	4	4		4
	Bigger than a square metre	5	5	5	5	5	5	5	5		5
GA_10	Smell of dampness / mould	( )	( )	( )	( )	( )	( )	( )	( )	GA_20 (def.)	( )
GA_11	Condensation signs at windows (def.)	( )	( )	( )	( )	( )	( )	( )	( )	GA_21 (def.)	( )
GA_12	Wallpaper, paint, etc., gets off wall	( )	( )	( )	( )	( )	( )	( )	( )	GA_22 (def.)	( )
GA_13	Lighting equipment										
	Exists and is operational	1	1	1	1	1	1	1	1	GA_23 (def.)	1
	Exists but is not operational	2	2	2	2	2	2	2	2		2
	Not existing	3	3	3	3	3	3	3	3		3

GA_2 coding: Living room: 1 Bed room: 2 Children's room: 3 Dining room: 4 Utility room: 5 Office: 6 Other: 7

Background and introduction

Faults, disrepair or deterioration symptoms (see definitions for coding)

CODING:
- 0   not relevant / not existing
- 1   no faults / deterioration symptoms
- 2   small faults or deterioration symptoms at specific places only
- 3   faults at several places of the same element
- 4   faulty element or deterioration of the whole elements

Visible faults, disrepair or deterioration symptoms of . . .
(WC only if detached room and not in bathroom)

	Kitchen	Bathroom	WC	Corridor	Room 1	Room 2	Room 3	Room 4	FLAT
D_1 Ceilings	|_|	|_|	|_|	|_|	|_|	|_|	|_|	|_|	D_8|_|
D_2 Floors	|_|	|_|	|_|	|_|	|_|	|_|	|_|	|_|	D_9|_|
D_3 Walls to outside	|_|	|_|	|_|	|_|	|_|	|_|	|_|	|_|	D_10|_|
D_4 Walls to inside	|_|	|_|	|_|	|_|	|_|	|_|	|_|	|_|	D_11|_|
D_5 Doors	|_|	|_|	|_|	|_|	|_|	|_|	|_|	|_|	D_12|_|
D_6 Windows	|_|	|_|	|_|	|_|	|_|	|_|	|_|	|_|	D_13|_|
D_7 Room assessment	|_|	|_|	|_|	|_|	|_|	|_|	|_|	|_|	D_14|_|

Kitchen

K_1   **Is there a ventilation system in the kitchen?** *(see definition)*
(*Not the exhaust system above cooking place!*)

Yes – free ventilation	1
Yes – forced ventilation	2
Yes – don't know which	3
Not existing	4

K_2   **Water access is available in the kitchen**

Yes	1
No	2

K_3   **Hot water is available in the kitchen**

Yes	1
No	2

K_4   **Is there a gas water heater in the kitchen?** *(see definition)*

Yes – connected to the outside	1
Yes – not connected to the outside	2
No	3

Background and introduction

K_5   Fridge   Yes   1
                                                         No   2

K_6   Deepfreezer   Yes   1
                                                         No   2

K_7   Kitchen sink   Yes – one sink   1
                                                         Yes – two sinks 2
                                                         No   3

K_8   Kitchen workspace next to the sink   Yes   1
          (see definition)   No   2

K_9   Separate solid waste disposal facility / waste bin *(see definition)*

          Yes – in a cupboard   1
          Yes – bin without lid   2
          Yes – bin with lid   3
          Yes – on balcony or terrace   4
          No   5

K_10 Is there an exhaust system above the cooking place? *(see definition)*

          Yes – connected to the outside   1
          Yes – not connected to the outside   2
          No   3

K_11+12 Energy source in the kitchen

K_11		K_12	
Cooking place		**Oven**	
1	No cooking place	1	No oven
2	Solid fuel (coal, wood)	2	Solid fuel (coal, wood)
3	Gas	3	Gas
4	Electricity	4	Electricity
5	Oil	5	Oil
6	Other:_____	6	Other:_____

Bathroom / toilet

BT_1 Is there a ventilation system in the bathroom? *(see definition)*

          Yes – free ventilation   1
          Yes – forced ventilation   2
          Yes – don't know   3
          No   4

BT_2 Water access is available in the bathroom

          Yes   1
          No   2

Background and introduction

BT_3 **Hot water is available in the bathroom**

Yes   1
No   2

BT_4 **Is there a gas water heater in the bathroom?** *(see definition)*

Yes – connected to the outside	1
Yes – not connected to the outside	2
No	3

BT_5 **What type of floor does the bathroom have?**

Tiles	1
Carpet	2
PVC / plastic	3
Concrete	4
Wood	5
Other:_____	6 _____

BT_6 *(if there is a detached toilet)* **Is there a ventilation system in the toilet?**

No toilet:	99
Yes – free ventilation	1
Yes – forced ventilation	2
Yes – don't know	3
No	4

BT_7 *(if there is a detached toilet)* **Is there a wash-hand basin in the toilet?**

No toilet:	99
Yes – cold and warm water	1
Yes – cold water only	2
No	3

BT_8 **Total number of flush / water toilets in dwelling** |___|

BT_9 **Total number of showers and / or bath tubes** |___|

BT_10 **Total number of hand-wash basins** |___|
(not including kitchen sink)

Background and introduction

Safety / accessibility

SA_1 **Are there any doorsteps in the door frames (*Multicode*)?** *(see definition)*

    ( )   No doorsteps
    ( )   Dwelling entrance door
    ( )   Between rooms
    ( )   To the bathroom
    ( )   To balcony / terrace / garden
    ( )   Other:_____ _____

SA_2 **Are there any installations / locations in the flat that you see as potentially harmful?** *If yes, please fill in keywords! (see definition)*

_____ _____
_____ _____
_____ _____

SA_3+4 Are there any rooms in the dwelling with loose carpets, or slippery or unfixed floor materials? *(see definition)*

    SA_3   SA_4
    Yes   1 => Which ones: _____ _____
    No   2   _____ _____
                                        _____ _____

SA_5 **Can most streets or pathways be overlooked from the dwelling through windows?**

    Yes   1
    No   2

SA_6 **Can most open spaces and play areas be overlooked from the dwelling through windows?**

    Yes   1
    No   2
    Not relevant   3   *(if no spaces / play areas)*

Steps and staircase

SC_1 **Does the *dwelling* have steps or a staircase inside the dwelling?** *(NOT general staircase in building!!)*

    Yes   1
    No   2 *(go to SC_5)*

SC_2 **Do the steps or the staircase have handrails?**

    Yes   1
    No   2

Background and introduction

SC_3 **Are there any loose or broken steps, damaged or uneven surfaces, disrepair or other safety threats?** *(see definition)*

Stairs are perfect and safe	1
Stairs are slightly damaged or loose	2
Stairs are heavily damaged and unsafe	3

SC_4 **Are there many height differences where people can stumble?**

Yes	1
No	2

SC_5 **Are there any steps or height differences in front of the building entrance?**

Yes	1
No	2

> *The following questions SC_6 to SC_14 apply only to multi-family houses. In case of one-family houses, go to HE_1*

SC_6 **Does the *building* have steps or a staircase?**

Yes	1
No	2

SC_7 **Does the staircase have adequate, working light equipment?**

Yes – operational and sufficient	1
Yes – operational but not sufficient	2
Yes – but not operational	3
No light equipment	4

SC_8 **Do the steps or the staircase have handrails?**

Yes	1
No	2

SC_9 **Are there any loose or broken steps, damaged or uneven surfaces, disrepair or other safety threats?** *(see definition)*

Stairs are perfect and safe	1
Stairs are slightly damaged or loose	2
Stairs are heavily damaged and unsafe	3

SC_10 **Are there many height differences where people can stumble?**

Yes	1
No	2

Background and introduction

SC_11 Are there any signs of decoration or appropriation in the staircase (flowers, pictures, carpets, furniture, etc.)? *(see definition)*

    Yes   1
    No   2

SC_12 Are there any signs of vandalism in the staircase (graffiti, destroyed wallpaper, broken handrails, etc.)

    Yes   1
    No   2

SC_13 Lift / elevator in the building? *(see definition)*

    Yes – operational   1
    Yes – not operational   2
    No   3 *(go to HE_1)*

SC_14 Does the lift serve all floors in the building?

    Yes   1
    No   2

Housing environment

HE_1 Is there any open or green space that belongs to the building, which can be used by the household residents (except streets, parking, etc.)? *(see definition)*

    Yes, private garden   1
    Yes, commonly shared area   2
    No 3   *(go to HE_3)*

HE_2 How would you evaluate the general condition / impression of these spaces?

    Well maintained / taken care of   1
    Not well maintained but also not run-down   2
    Not maintained and run-down   3
    Mix of all above   4

HE_3 Is there any graffiti on the respective building or the buildings you can see around?

    No graffiti at all   1
    One or two   2
    Three to five   3
    Six or more   4

Background and introduction

HE_4 **How would you evaluate the amount of litter on the ground in the immediate housing environment?**

Very dirty / littered area	1
	2
↕	3
	4
Not at all dirty / littered	5

HE_5 **How would you evaluate the amount of dog droppings / animal excrement in the immediate housing environment?**

Extreme amount	1
	2
↕	3
	4
No excrement at all	5

HE_6 **Is any kind of vegetation / greenery visible in the immediate housing environment? (Multicode)**

No	( )
Yes, along streets	( )
Yes, on public grounds	( )
Yes, on private grounds / gardens	( )
Yes, on facades / windows / balconies	( )

HE_7 **Is there a park or green open space close to the dwelling (up to 100 m), which is accessible to the public?**

| Yes | 1 |
| No | 2 |

HE_8 **Are parking sites close to the buildings?** *(maximum distance = 50 m)*

| Yes | 1 |
| No | 2 |

COMMENTS:

Inhabitant Questionnaire

ID-code: |__| |__|__| |__|__|__|__|

Date of survey:_____ City quarter:_____ Time:_____
Health questionnaires left behind   **Questionnaire pick-up:**
in the flat to be filled out: |__|__| Date:_____ Time:_____

For the selection of the interview partner, ask which person deals most with the day-to-day-questions of the household and has the best overview about the inhabitants and the things happening at home. If this person is available, we want to talk to him / her. Otherwise, ask who would be the best person now available for answering questions about the household and dwelling. If only one person is at home, the choice is clear.

Inhabitant information

Person to be interviewed

    I_1   **Gender**:   female 1
                                  male   2

I_2   **How many people live permanently in this dwelling (in total)?** |__|__|
        (see definition)

I_3   **How old are the inhabitants?** ... *(ask for each resident, less than 1 year = 1, don't know = 99, 99 years = 98)*

Interviewed person: |__|__|__| Person 5: |__|__|__|
Person 2: |__|__|__| Person 6: |__|__|__|
Person 3: |__|__|__| Person 7: |__|__|__|
Person 4: |__|__|__|

I_4   **For how many years have you been living in this dwelling?**

|__|__| years   *(less than 1 year = 0; 2,5 years = 2; don't know = 99)*

I_5   **How satisfied are you with the dwelling?** *(use showcard)*

    ☹ 1   🙁 2   😐 3   🙂 4   😊 5

Background and introduction

Building structure and equipment

Temperature and heating

T_1   Do you perceive the temperature in the dwelling during the summer season as a problem? *(if yes: read options 2–5) (if no: go to question T_3)* **(use showcard)**

T_2   If you have a problem with the temperature in your dwelling in summer, is it because it is too warm or too cold?

T_3   Do you perceive the temperature in the dwelling during the transient season as a problem ? *(if yes: read options 2–5) (if no: go to question T_5)* **(use showcard)**

T_4   If you have a problem with the temperature in your dwelling in the transient season, is it because it is too warm or too cold?

T_5   Do you perceive the temperature in the dwelling during the winter season as a problem (with heating in use) ? *(if yes: read options 2–5) (if no: go to question T_7)* **(use showcard)**

T_6   If you have a problem with the temperature in your dwelling in winter, is it because it is too warm or too cold?

	T_1 In summer	T_3 In transient season	T_5 In winter
Never / No	1	1	1
Seldom	2	2	2
Sometimes	3	3	3
Often	4	4	4
Permanent	5	5	5
Don't know	99	99	99

	T_2 In summer	T_4 In transient season	T_6 In winter
Too warm	1	1	1
Too cold	2	2	2
Both too warm and cold	3	3	3

Background and introduction

T_7* **If it is cold in winter or transient season, what are the reasons?** *(Read options. If not cold: mark first option)* *(Multicode)*

No such problem	( )
Household cannot afford it	( )
Flat is too big for efficient heating	( )
Low efficiency / standard of heating system	( )
Lack of heating system in some rooms	( )
Lack of control of heating	( )
Non-functional heating	( )
Wrong placement of heating devices	( )
Insufficient thermal insulation of the building	( )
Windows not tight or single-glazed	( )
No obvious reason	( )
Other *(please specify)* _____	( ) _____

T_8 **How would you evaluate the quality of the heating system in your dwelling on a scale from 1 (highly dissatisfied) to 5 (highly satisfied)?** *(use showcard)*

Highly dissatisfied	1
↕	2
	3
	4
Highly satisfied	5

T_9 **Does this dwelling have a heating system in all inhabitable rooms (except corridor, bathroom, utility rooms and kitchenettes under 4 sqm)?** *(see definition for 'inhabitable')*

Yes	1 *(go to T_11)*
No	2
Don't know	99

T_10 **Which of the following rooms do not have a heating system** *(read options)*? **(Multicode)** *(see definition for heating system)*

Kitchen	( )	All rooms have heating systems: ☐
Bathroom	( )	
Separate toilet	( )	
Living room	( )	
Bedroom/s, children room/s	( )	
Other:_____	( ) _____	

Background and introduction

T_11 **Is there any room with a heating system that can NOT be regulated by the inhabitants?** *(Multicode) (see definition)*

Kitchen	( )	
Bathroom	( )	All heating systems can be regulated: ☐
Separate toilet	( )	
Living room	( )	
Bedroom/s, children room/s	( )	
Other:_____	( ) _____	

Energy consumption and heating

E_1 **Are you connected to a central heating scheme that provides warmth for the dwelling?** *(read options) (see definition)*

Yes – heating source for dwelling	1 *(go to E_3)*
Yes – heating source for building	2 *(go to E_3)*
Yes – heating source for district / neighbourhood	3 *(go to E_3)*
No	4
Don't know	99

E_2 **If you don't have central heating supply, what is the major heating material used to heat the dwelling (Multicode)?**

Don't know	( )
Solid fuel (coal, wood)	( )
Gas	( )
Electricity	( )
Oil	( )
Kerosene	( )
Other:_____	( ) _____

E_3 **Do you use additional heating devices or heat sources during the cold or transient season?** *(if yes, read options 2–5) (see definition)*

No use of additional heating devices	1 *(go to question E_5)*
Yes – but less than once per week	2
Yes – once or twice a week	3
Yes – three times and more per week	4
Yes – everyday	5
Don't know	99

Background and introduction

E_4 If you use any additional heating devices in the dwelling, what energy source do they need? *(Multicode)*

Don't know	( )
Solid fuel (coal, wood)	( )
Gas	( )
Electricity	( )
Oil stove	( )
Kerosene	( )
Other:_____	( ) _____

E_5* What interventions and housing improvements could contribute to reduce your energy consumption (heating, electricity, hot water)? *(Multicode)*

Don't know	( )
None	( )
Better standard / efficiency of heating equipment	( )
Better control / regulation of heating	( )
More / better thermal insulation	( )
Tight windows / double glazing	( )
Less window surface	( )
Better placement of heating devices	( )
Other:_____	( ) _____

E_6* How would you evaluate the thermal insulation in your dwelling on a scale from 1 (highly dissatisfied) to 5 (highly satisfied)? *(use showcard)*

Highly dissatisfied	1
↕	2
	3
	4
Highly satisfied	5

E_7* What proportion of the disposable annual household net income after taxes is spent on heating expenses? *(read options) (see definition)*

Up to 5%	1
From more than 5 to 10%	2
From more than 10% to 20%	3
More than 20%	4
Don't know	99

Background and introduction

E_8* How would you rate the expenditure for heating in your dwelling?
(read options) (see definition)

Expensive	1
Rather expensive	2
Moderate	3
Rather cheap	4
Cheap	5

Lighting / window view

Li_1 On a clear day, do you sometimes need to turn on the lights during the daylight hours because the natural lighting of the dwelling is not sufficient?

Yes	1
No	2
Don't know	99

Li_2 Are you satisfied with the amount of natural lighting that you get through the windows, or do you sometimes miss the daylight?

Miss daylight	1
Satisfied with amount of natural light	2
Too much light / glare	3
Don't know	99

Li_3 Is there at least one window in the following rooms? If yes, what is its orientation (south, north, west, east) *(Multicode)? (see definition)*

	No window	South	North	West	East	Don't know
Living room	( )	( )	( )	( )	( )	( )
Bedroom	( )	( )	( )	( )	( )	( )
Bathroom	( )	( )	( )	( )	( )	( )
Kitchen	( )	( )	( )	( )	( )	( )
_____	( )	( )	( )	( )	( )	( )
_____	( )	( )	( )	( )	( )	( )
_____	( )	( )	( )	( )	( )	( )
_____	( )	( )	( )	( )	( )	( )

Background and introduction

Li_4 **How do you like the view or outlook from the building / windows on a scale from 1 (highly dissatisfied) to 5 (highly satisfied)?** *(use showcard)*

Highly dissatisfied	1
↕	2
	3
	4
Highly satisfied	5

Air humidity

AH_1 **Do you have problems with dampness or condensation in your dwelling (including attic rooms and basement rooms)** *(if yes, read options 2–5)? (use showcard)*

Never / No	1 *(go to AH_3)*
Seldom	2
Sometimes	3
Often	4
Permanent	5
Don't know	99

AH_2 **In which rooms do you often find problems with dampness or condensation (Multicode)?** *(see definition)*

Don't know	( )
No specific problem rooms	( )
Kitchen	( )
Bathroom	( )
Separate toilet	( )
Corridor	( )
Living room	( )
Bedroom/s, children room/s	( )
Utility room in dwelling	( )
Non-inhabitable rooms in basement	( )
Non-inhabitable attic / rooms right under roof	( )
Other:_____	( ) _____

AH_3 **Do you have problems with visible mould growth in your dwelling** *(if yes, read options 2–5)? (use showcard)*

Never / No	1 *(go to AH_5)*
Seldom	2
Sometimes	3
Often	4
Permanent	5
Don't know	99

Background and introduction

AH_4 **In which rooms did you already find visible mould growth** *(Multicode)*?
Ask for each room with mould: **Where exactly** *(e.g. wall, under window, behind furniture, corner of rooms, ceiling . .)?*

Don't know	( )	**Location:**
No specific problem rooms	( )	
Kitchen	( )	_____
Bathroom	( )	_____
Separate toilet	( )	_____
Corridor	( )	_____
Living room	( )	_____
Bedroom(s), children room(s)	( )	_____
Utility room in dwelling	( )	_____
Other:_____	( )	_____

AH_5 **Where do you dry your laundry most of the year** *(Multicode)*?

Don't know	( )
Kitchen	( )
Bathroom	( )
Corridor	( )
Living room	( )
Bedroom(s), children room(s)	( )
Utility room in dwelling	( )
Cellar / utility room / laundry room in building	( )
Outside of building / balcony	( )
Other:_____	( ) _____

If answer is 'outside of building / balcony', ask in which room drying is done if outside / balcony is not possible (winter, rain, etc.)

'Dryer' is not an answer! In which room is the dryer?

Air quality

AQ_1 **How would you evaluate the air quality in your dwelling on a scale from 1 (highly dissatisfied) to 5 (highly satisfied)?** *(use showcard) (definition)*

Highly dissatisfied   1
↕   2
                         3
                         4 *(go to AQ_4)*
Highly satisfied   5 *(go to AQ_4)*

Background and introduction

AQ_2 *If AQ_1 was answered with 1–3:* **What are the reasons for the dissatisfaction with the air quality in your dwelling ?** *(read options – Multicode)*

Dampness	( )
Dryness	( )
Dust and particles	( )
Smell	( )
Smoke	( )
Not enough air exchange, stale air	( )
Too much air exchange, draught	( )
Outside air pollution	( )
Other:_____	( ) _____

AQ_3 Why do you think the problem(s) mentioned in AQ_2 occur? *(ask for causes such as not tight windows, access of humidity, insufficient insulation, etc.)*

_____   _____

_____   _____

AQ_4 Do you think that dust represents a particularly large problem in your dwelling?

Yes	1
No	2
Don't know	99

Ventilation / air exchange

V_1 **Do you have a ventilation system in your dwelling in at least one room?** *(if yes – what kind of system?) (see definition for ventilation systems)*

Yes – free ventilation	1
Yes – forced ventilation	2
No	3 *(go to V_4)*
Don't know	99

V_2 **Can the ventilation be regulated by the residents?** *(if yes, mark box) (see definition)*

Ventilation system can be regulated   ☐

V_3* **How satisfied are you with the ventilation system(s) in your dwelling on a scale from 1 (highly dissatisfied) to 5 (highly satisfied)?** *(showcard)*

Highly dissatisfied	1
↕	2
	3
	4
Highly satisfied	5

Background and introduction

V_4 Do you – especially in winter time – have problems with moving air and draught in your dwelling because doors / windows cannot be closed tightly or have insufficient quality *(if yes, read options 2–5)*? *(showcard)*

Never / No	1
Seldom	2
Sometimes	3
Often	4
Permanent	5
Don't know	99

Environmental tobacco smoke

ETS_1 How many cigarettes (or other tobacco products) are smoked in the dwelling per day by all residents? *(not including balcony)*

|__|__|__| None = 0,   Don't know = 99   *(if none, go to P_1)*

ETS_2 Are people sleeping in the rooms where people have smoked? *(if yes: read options 2 and 3)*

Never	1
Sometimes	2
Always	3

ETS_3 Are children sleeping in the rooms where people have smoked? *(if yes, read options 2 and 3)*

Never	1
Sometimes	2
Always	3

Background and introduction

Pests and insects

P_1–5 In the last 12 months until now, which of the following pests are – or were – present in *your dwelling?* (*Multicode*) *(read options)*

	P_1 Never	**P_2** Past	**P_3** Present	**P_4** Past and Present	**P_5** Don't know
Mice	( )	( )	( )	( )	( )
Rats	( )	( )	( )	( )	( )
Cockroaches	( )	( )	( )	( )	( )
Mites	( )	( )	( )	( )	( )
Fleas	( )	( )	( )	( )	( )
Bedbugs	( )	( )	( )	( )	( )
Ants	( )	( )	( )	( )	( )
Flies	( )	( )	( )	( )	( )
Other:_____	( )	( )	( )	( )	( )_____

P_6 No infestations: ( ) *(go to P_8)*
(see definition)

P_7 How do you think the pests come into your dwelling?

_____
_____

P_8 *(P_8 only for buildings with more than one dwelling):* **Do you have or have you had any pests, infestations or rats and mice in this building in the last 12 months?** *(If yes, read options 1–3. In case of one–family house, mark option 98)*

Yes – in the past	1	*In case of one-family house, where dwelling and building are the same, mark '98'*
Yes – right now	2	
Yes – in the past and right now	3	
No, so far never	4	
One-family house	98	
Don't know	99	

P_9 **In the last 12 months, has there been any pest control treatment carried out in order to control pest infestations in your dwelling?** *(If yes, read options 1–3)* (*Multicode*)

Yes – non-chemical physical traps with or without bait	( )
Yes – bait for ingestion by pest (poisoned or not)	( )
Yes – insecticidal spray or contact poison	( )
No	( )
Don't know	( )

Background and introduction

P_10 **Do you have any pets / animals in *your dwelling*?**
(If yes: **Which pets** *(Multicode)*?)*

No pets	( )
Cat	( )
Dog	( )
Bird	( )
Fish	( )
Hamster / guinea-pig	( )
Other:_____	( ) _____

Layout and structure

L_1+2 **How big is your dwelling in square meters (dwelling in total)?** *(Write in the exact size and circle the according size group. If not known, leave L_1 empty and estimate dwelling size for L_2)*

L_1 |__|__|__| m²   L_2
1   under 30 sqm   2   30–39 sqm
3   40–49 sqm   4   50–59 sqm
5   60–79 sqm   6   80–99 sqm
7   100–119 sqm   8   120 sqm and more

L_3+4 **How many inhabitable rooms does this dwelling have?**
(see definition 'inhabitable room')

L_3 |__|__| rooms

L_5 **How satisfied are you – on a scale from 1 (highly dissatisfied) to 5 (highly satisfied) – with the dwelling size?** *(use showcard)*

Highly dissatisfied	1
↑	2
↕	3
↓	4
Highly satisfied	5

L_6 **How satisfied are you – on a scale from 1 (highly dissatisfied) to 5 (highly satisfied) – with the layout of the dwelling?** *(use showcard)*

Highly dissatisfied	1
↑	2
↕	3
↓	4
Highly satisfied	5

Background and introduction

L_7 Would you need more or less rooms in your dwelling?

Number of rooms is sufficient	1
More rooms needed	2
Less rooms needed	3
Don't know	99

L_8 What is the maximum number of adult residents sleeping in the same room?

|__| adults

L_9 What is the maximum number of children sleeping in the same room?

|__| children

L_10 Is there a place in your dwelling where you can go when you want to be by yourself?

Never want to be alone	1
Yes – always	2
Yes – but not always	3
No	4

Noise

N_1 Do you ever feel disturbed by noise in your dwelling (with closed windows) *(if yes, read options 2–5)*?

Never	1
Seldom	2
Sometimes	3
Often	4
Permanently	5

Background and introduction

N_2–5 **Considering the following noise sources, is there any disturbance by one or more of them?** *(Multicode)(read all options)*? *(mark 'No' if no noise disturbance. For chosen sources, ask for noise intensity from 1 (weak) to 3 (strong) and frequency from 1 (rare) to 3 (often))*

	N_2 NO	N_3 INTENSITY	N_4 FREQUENCY
Noise from surrounding area (bars, disco, events)	( )	1 2 3	1 2 3
Playgrounds, schools, recreational facilities	( )	1 2 3	1 2 3
Traffic noise	( )	1 2 3	1 2 3
Airplane noise	( )	1 2 3	1 2 3
Train noise	( )	1 2 3	1 2 3
Parking & parking lots	( )	1 2 3	1 2 3
Neighbour's flat (talking, music, TV, repairs, animals)	( )	1 2 3	1 2 3
Animals/birds (from outside)	( )	1 2 3	1 2 3
Noise from commercial, industrial or construction sites	( )	1 2 3	1 2 3
Staircase use	( )	1 2 3	1 2 3
Playing children in building	( )	1 2 3	1 2 3
Ventilation, heating or installation system, waste chute	( )	1 2 3	1 2 3
Lift	( )	1 2 3	1 2 3
Noise sources within own dwelling	( )	1 2 3	1 2 3
Other:_____ _____	( )	1 2 3	1 2 3

N_6 **Where in your dwelling do you think the sound insulation is a problem** *(Multicode)*?

No problem with insulation	( )
Ceiling	( )
Floor	( )
Walls inside the dwelling	( )
Walls to the outside	( )
Walls to other dwellings / staircase	( )
Windows	( )
Roof	( )
Door to outside / staircase	( )
Other:_____	( ) _____

N_7 **Do you think that the noise annoyance may be due to an insufficient sound insulation?**

Yes	1
No	2
Don't know	99

> If no noise exposure, mark option 2: 'No'

Background and introduction

N_8 Has noise already been discussed / mentioned as a reason for sleeping problems or regular disturbance of sleep of any household resident?

    Yes   1
    No   2
    Don't know 99

N_9 Has there ever been any frustration and anger of any household resident due to the noise conditions?

    Yes   1
    No   2
    Don't know 99

N_10 Do you in general feel vibrations, associated or not with noise, in your dwelling (caused by traffic, construction sites, subway, airplanes, etc.)?

    Never   1
    Seldom   2
    Sometimes 3
    Often   4
    Permanent   5
    Don't know 99

> Earthquakes are NOT included!

N_11 *(Ask only for people that have a noise problem in their flat: N_1 = 3, 4 or 5)* **You said that you were disturbed by noise in your dwelling. If you could have the same dwelling, but without the noise, how much money per month would you be ready to pay (either in addition to the rent you pay now, or as a general payment) for having this quiet dwelling?**

    _____ *(name of currency)*   Don't know: write '99'

N_12 *(Ask only for people that do not have a noise problem: N_1 = 1 or 2)* **You said that you were not disturbed by noise in your dwelling. Imagine that from tomorrow on, there will be a new situation and noise (e.g. from new traffic, outdoor restaurants or playgrounds close to your house) will be perceptible in your dwelling. How much would you expect the monthly rent to go down (or which monthly compensation payment would be acceptable) so that you would be satisfied by the financial compensation for the new noise exposure?**

    _____ *(name of currency)*   Don't know: write '99'
                                                      Would move out: write '−1'

Background and introduction

Hygiene and sanitation

HS_1 Did you ever experience any trouble with the quantity of the water supply during the last year? *(if yes, read options 2–5) (see definition)*

HS_2 Did you ever experience any trouble with the quantity of the hot water supply during the last year? *(if yes, read options 2–5) (see definition)*

HS_3 Did you ever experience any trouble with the quality of the water supply (coloured water, bad smell, bad taste, etc.)? *(if yes, read options 2–5)*

HS_4 Did you ever experience any trouble with the water drainage system? *(if yes, read options 2–5)*

	HS_1	HS_2	HS_3	HS_4
Never	1	1	1	1
Seldom	2	2	2	2
Sometimes	3	3	3	3
Often	4	4	4	4
Permanent	5	5	5	5
Don't know	99	99	99	99

HS_5 Is it necessary to treat the water that is provided to your dwelling before drinking? *(e.g. boiling, cleaning, filtering, etc.)*

Yes	1
No	2
Don't drink the water	3
Don't know	99

HS_6 How satisfied are you – on a scale from 1 (highly dissatisfied) to 5 (highly satisfied) – with the equipment and the installations in the bathroom? *(use showcard)*

Highly dissatisfied	1
	2
	3
	4
Highly satisfied	5

Background and introduction

HS_7 How satisfied are you – on a scale from 1 (highly dissatisfied) to 5 (highly satisfied) – with the equipment and the installations in the kitchen? *(showcard)*

Highly dissatisfied	1
↕	2
	3
	4
Highly satisfied	5

HS_8 *If in questions HS_6 and HS_7, the options 1,2 or 3 were chosen at least once, ask following question:* **What are the reasons for dissatisfaction with equipment and installations?**

_____   _____
_____   _____
_____   _____

HS_9 **Is there enough workspace in the kitchen in order to prepare food?** *(see definition for 'enough')*

Yes	1
No	2
Don't know	99

HS_10 **Is there a waste chute inside the dwelling or in the staircase?** *(If yes, read options 1 and 2) (see definition)*

In staircase	1
In dwelling	2 *(go to A_1)*
No	3 *(go to A_1)*

HS_11 **Is the waste chute in the staircase rather clean or rather dirty?**

Rather clean	1
Rather dirty	2
Don't know	99

Background and introduction

Safety and accidents

Please read aloud for the interviewed person to understand what we are looking for in this section:
Every day, many accidents and injuries occur in homes which do not require medical treatment by a doctor, but still limit the quality of life and provide small-term handicaps and pain.
For the following questions, we would like you to think of both the dwelling and the commonly used building spaces (corridor, staircase, basement / utility rooms), and tell us about all the – small and big – accidents and injuries that happened to you and the other household members in the following cases:
- a first aid kit was used
- a doctor / hospital / ambulance car was contacted
- pain or any kind of physical limitation was still existing the day after the event.

A_1–4 Which of the following accidents or injuries – big or small – have already occurred in the building in the last 12 months?
(read list starting with 'Falls / stumbling' – one by one, then ask for person suffering this type of accident) (Multicode) (see definition for accident types)

	A_1	A_2 Child	A_3 Adult	A_4 above 65
Don't know	( ) *go to A_6*			
None	( ) *go to A_6*			
Falls / stumbling	( )	( )	( )	( )
Burns	( )	( )	( )	( )
Cuts / puncture wounds	( )	( )	( )	( )
Choking / suffocating / drowning	( )	( )	( )	( )
Collisions / striking	( )	( )	( )	( )
Poisoning / chemical agents	( )	( )	( )	( )
Gas intoxication	( )	( )	( )	( )
Electric shock / accident	( )	( )	( )	( )
Other:_____	( )	( )	( )	( )

Background and introduction

A_5 Which items have been involved in these accidents and injuries that have occurred *(Multicode)?*

Don't know	( )
Construction features (walls, floor, doors, windows, stairs)	( )
Electrical equipment / installations	( )
Water / sanitary system	( )
Heating / cooling equipment, stove, oven	( )
Stairs, staircase	( )
Kitchen equipment	( )
Knives and silverware	( )
Furniture / furnishings (carpets, curtains, etc.)	( )
Washing / cleaning products, detergents, liquids, etc.	( )
Gases and fumes	( )
Food items	( )
Animals and pets	( )
Toys	( )
Other:_____ _____	( )

A_6 Which places or equipment items do you assess as dangerous for the residents in general *(Multicode)?*

Don't know	( )
Stove / oven	( )
Kitchen equipment / water heater	( )
Bathroom	( )
Windows / window frames	( )
Doors / door frames, doorsteps	( )
Corridor	( )
Heating equipment	( )
Staircase	( )
Stairs and steps in dwelling	( )
Electrical equipment / installations	( )
Cables on floor / walls / from ceiling	( )
Balcony / terrace	( )
Lift / elevator	( )
Floor coverings (carpet, etc.)	( )
Furniture items	( )
Other:_____	( ) _____
No dangerous places / items	☐

Background and introduction

A_7+8 Is there a place / item in the dwelling which is especially dangerous for children? *(if yes, which?)*

	A_7	A_8
Yes	1 => *Which place / item:*	_____
No	2	_____
Don't know	99	

A_9+10 Is there a place / item in the dwelling, where / with which at least two accidents / injuries have already occurred? *(if yes, which?)*

	A_9	A_10
Yes	1 => *Which place / item:*	_____
No	2	_____
Don't know	99	

A_11 Are your electrical installations earthed? *(see definition)*

Yes, all of them	1
Yes, but not all	2
No	3
Don't know	99

A_12 Can the household members easily escape from the house in case of fire in the building?

Yes	1
No	2
Don't know	99

A_13 Is there any fire detection equipment in the building or in the dwelling?

Yes	1
No	2
Don't know	99

Building quality & maintenance

B_1 *(For multi-family houses only)* **How many dwellings in this building are not inhabited and empty?** *(read options 1–5)*

All dwellings are inhabited	1
Under 10% are empty	2
11–20% are empty	3
21–30% are empty	4
More than 30% are empty	5
Don't know	99

Background and introduction

B_2 **Do you know whether the roof is waterproof?**

    Roof is waterproof   1
    Roof is not waterproof / is leaking   2
    Don't know   99

B_3 **Has there ever been a renovation of the *building* (= outside envelope and/or indoor common spaces such as staircase, basement, roof) since you have been living here?** *(see definition)*

    Yes   1
    No   2
    Don't know   99

B_4 **Has there ever been a renovation of the *dwelling* since you have been living here (except minor do-it-yourself activities)?** *(see definition)*

    Yes   1
    No   2
    Don't know   99

B_5 **Did your household – in the last year – do any do-it-yourself activities (repairs, new paint, etc.) or bring in new furniture *(Multicode)*?**

    Don't know   ( )
    No such work done   ( )
    Yes – new furniture   ( )
    Yes – do-it-yourself work   ( )
    Yes – due to moving in   ( )

B_6 **Is there a housekeeper who takes care of the maintenance and daily business?**

    Yes   1
    No   2
    Don't know   99

B_7 **Who is responsible for the cleaning of the building and the staircases *(Multicode)*?** *(Read options) (see definition)*

    Don't know   ( )
    Private owner   ( )
    Housing agency as owner   ( )
    Municipality as owner   ( )
    Cooperatives   ( )
    Rental households themselves   ( )
    Service company contracted   ( )
    Combination of options above   ( )
    Housekeeper / caretaker   ( )
    Administrator   ( )

Background and introduction

B_8 **Who is responsible for the maintenance of the building and the staircases in case of repairs** *(Multicode)? (Read options) (see definition)*

Don't know	( )
Private owner	( )
Housing agency as owner	( )
Municipality as owner	( )
Cooperatives	( )
Rental households themselves	( )
Service company contracted	( )
Combination of options above	( )
Housekeeper / caretaker	( )
Administrator	( )

Housing adaptability

Ha_1 **Is the *building* easily accessible for handicapped people with wheelchair, walking aids like canes or any other physical constraints (blind, deaf . . .)?** *(see definition)*

Yes	1
No	2
Don't know	99

Ha_2 *(Ha_2 only for multi-family houses)* **Is your *dwelling* easily accessible for handicapped people with wheelchair, walking aids like canes or any other physical constraints (blind, deaf . . .)?** *(see definition)*

Yes	1
No	2
Don't know	99

Ha_3 **Does anyone in the household have any kind of physical constraint or handicap?**

Yes	1
No	2 *(go to DS_1)*
Don't know	99 *(go to DS_1)*

Ha_4 **Do you feel that the building / dwelling is well equipped and adapted for the specific needs that may arise from the existing physical constraint of this person?**

Yes	1 *(go to DS_1)*
No	2
Don't know	99

Background and introduction

Ha_5 What are the specific needs of this person that are not being fulfilled by the dwelling? *(ask for max. keywords such as bigger doors, no doorsteps, lift . . .)*

_____ _____
_____ _____
_____ _____

Ha_6 Is it possible at all to realize the required adaptations in the dwelling?

    Yes   1 *(go to DS_1)*
    No   2
    Don't know   99

Ha_7 If not, why is it not possible? *(keywords only, maximum of three)*

_____ _____
_____ _____
_____ _____

Dwelling satisfaction

DS_1 For how long would you like to live in this dwelling, on a scale from 1 (as short as possible) to 5 (forever)? *(use showcard)*

1	2	3	4	5
As short as possible				Forever

For DS_2 and DS_3:
Ask people for building-related answers only. The immediate environment section comes later!

DS_2 There may be some aspects or characteristics for which you are not satisfied with your dwelling / building. What are the main reasons for dissatisfaction with your dwelling / building? Please give up to three keywords! *(see definition)*

    1)_____ _____
    2)_____ _____
    3)_____ _____

DS_3 On the other hand, there may be some aspects or characteristics for which you are satisfied with your dwelling / building. What are the main reasons for satisfaction with the dwelling / building? Please give up to three keywords! *(see definition)*

    1)_____ _____
    2)_____ _____
    3)_____ _____

Background and introduction

DS_4 **Did you already discuss moving into another dwelling because you are not happy with the current living conditions?**

> Yes 1
> No 2
> Don't know 99

DS_5 **If moving – would you prefer to move to . . .** *(read options)*

> Another dwelling in this building – higher floor level 1
> Another dwelling in this building – lower floor level 2
> Another dwelling in this area / neighbourhood 3
> Another housing area / neighbourhood 4
> Another city

> Please have DS_5 answered even if they don't want to move – it is a hypothetical question!
>
> => **If you had to move – would you prefer to ...**

Immediate environment

Please read out:
Now, I will ask you some questions on the immediate housing environment, which is the area around your dwelling that you pass through or see every day. This comprises both the space closely around your residential building (be it private or not) and the surrounding area with neighbouring streets, buildings, gardens, playgrounds, parks, etc.

IE_1 **Overall, how would you rate this area as a place to live on a scale from 1 (very bad) to 5 (very good)?** *(showcard)*

> Very bad 1
> ↕ 2
> 3
> 4 *(go to IE_3)*
> Very good 5 *(go to IE_3)*

IE_2 **What are the major reasons for your dissatisfaction?** *(max. 3)*

> 1) _____ _____
> 2) _____ _____
> 3) _____ _____

Background and introduction

IE_3 What are characteristics of the immediate housing environment that you do like? *(max. 3)*

1) _____ _____
2) _____ _____
3) _____ _____

IE_4 How do you think this residential area is evaluated by other people who are not living in this area? *(use showcard)*

　　1　　2　　3　　4　　5

IE_5 Is this living place well connected to the city centre so that all household members can get there without problems (using the available transport means)? *(read options)*

Yes, for all inhabitants	1
Yes, for some inhabitants	2
No	3
Don't know	99

IE_6 With which of the following means of transport can you easily reach the city centre of *Name of Survey City*? (**Multicode**)

By public transport	( )
Walking	( )
By bicycle	( )
By private car	( )

If they live in the city centre: Cross option 'Walking'

IE_7 If there is public transportation to the city centre, at what time in the evening is the last ride back? *(please write time: 23.30; 0.45, etc.,* (Coding: Living in city centre: 97, No public transport connection: 98, Don't know: 99)

_____

IE_8 How satisfied are you with the parking arrangements on a scale from 1 (highly dissatisfied) to 5 (highly satisfied)? *(showcard)*

Highly dissatisfied	1
	2
	3
	4
Highly satisfied	5

Only parking arrangements at living place are meant, not in city centre

Background and introduction

IE_9 How annoyed are you by litter and trash in the immediate environment on a scale from 1 (very annoyed) to 5 (not annoyed at all)? *(showcard)*

Very annoyed	1
↑	2
↕	3
↓	4
Not annoyed at all	5

IE_10–12 In your immediate housing environment (including private and public spaces), are there enough recreational areas for ... *(read three population groups)*? **(see definition)**

		Yes	To some extent	Not really	Don't know
IE_10	Children	1	2	3	99
IE_11	Teenagers	1	2	3	99
IE_12	Elderly	1	2	3	99

IE_13 Would you encourage your children to play on the local playgrounds?

Yes	1
Only on some	2
No, not at all	3
No playgrounds	98
Don't know	99

Or: If you had children, would you encourage ..

IE_14 Are there some places in the immediate housing environment (including private and public spaces) where you can sit and relax, or talk peacefully to neighbours and friends?

Yes	1
No	2
Don't know	99

IE_15 Do you feel safe when returning to your home when it is dark?

Yes	1 (go to IE_17)
To some extent	2
No, not at all	3
Don't know	99

IE_16 What are the major reasons why you don't feel safe in your immediate housing environment? (max. 3)

1) _____ _____
2) _____ _____
3) _____ _____

Background and introduction

IE_17 What is the first thing you would change in your immediate housing environment? *'Nothing' is a valid answer option!*

Socioeconomic information

Finance, housing and households

Fi_1 Is the dwelling owned or rented?

    Owned   1
    Rented   2
    Don't know   99

Fi_2+3 How many household members have an income that contributes to the total household income? *(see definition)*

    Fi_2 |__|__| residents

Fi_4 How many people in the household are currently unemployed (except children, teenagers, students, elderly and people unable to work)? *(see definition)*

    |__|__| Don't know 99

Fi_5 The next question would be important for us in order to find out whether income really has an impact on the housing conditions: What disposable income (after deduction of taxes, etc.) does the household have per month? Please use one of the following income groups: *(read options 1–6) (see definition)*

EU cities (in Euro)	Vilnius (in Litas)	Bratislava (in SK)
1 Under 500	1 Under 250	1 Under 5,500
2 501–1,000	2 251–500	2 5,501–10,000
3 1.001–1,500	3 501–750	3 10,001–20,000
4 1,501–2,000	4 751–1,000	4 20,001–40,000
5 2,001–2,500	5 1,001–1,250	5 40,001–60,000
6 Above 2,500	6 Above 1,250	6 Above 60,000
7 No answer	7 No answer	7 No answer
99 Don't know	99 Don't know	8 Don't know

Background and introduction

Fi_6 How many per cent of the disposable household net income after taxes are roughly spent for housing-related expenses as an average per month (including rent, loan, water, energy, maintenance, insurance, etc.)? *(see definition)*

|_|_|_| Don't know 99

Fi_7 Is it a problem for the household to pay the total housing expenditure?

    Yes   1
    No   2
    Don't know 99

Fi_8 Does this household receive a housing allowance? *(see definition)*

    Yes   1
    No   2
    Don't know 99

Fi_9 Could you afford to move to a better dwelling – if you wanted to do so?

    Yes   1
    No   2
    Don't know 99

Time of interview end: _____

It may be that after a first data analysis, several questions arise about specific issues that remain unclear or need a more detailed explanation. In order to follow up on such new or still open questions, or in case we would need to explore a specific issue in detail, would you agree that we contact you or your household again?

If yes, we would need your street address and your phone number. Both will be kept confidential and will only be used for contacting you in case we have a specific information deficit.

Background and introduction

Name: _____

Street address: _____

Zip code / city: _____

Phone: _____ **Signature:** _____

Thank the interviewee for their time and attention.
Go to inspection part of survey visit.

Background and introduction

Appendix 1.2 Distribution of the population by city quarters

	Survey estimate % (95% confidence limits)	City information %	Comments
Bratislava			
Bratislava I	11.2 (9.2; 13.2)	10.5	
Bratislava II	23.8 (21.1; 26.5)	25.2	
Bratislava III	15.6 (13.3; 17.9)	14.3	
Bratislava IV	23.1 (20.4; 25.8)	21.7	
Bratislava V	26.3 (23.5; 29.1)	28.3	
Bonn			
Bonn	46.2 (43.1; 49.3)	46.5	
Bad Godesberg	21.1 (18.5; 23.7)	22.2	
Beuel	22.1 (19.5; 24.7)	20.9	
Hardtberg	10.6 (8.7; 12.5)	10	
Forlì			
Forlì C1	11 (9.2; 12.8)	15.3	Under-represented
Forlì C2	13.4 (11.5; 15.3)	11.3	Over-represented
Forlì C3	22.7 (20.3; 25.1)	18.2	Over-represented
Forlì C4	29.9 (27.3; 32.5)	28.5	
Forlì C5	22.7 (20.3; 25.1)	26.6	Under-represented
Geneva			
Geneve	87.5 (85.1; 89.9)	86.7	
Onex	7.4 (5.5; 9.3)	8	
Versoix	5.2 (3.6; 6.8)	5.3	
Vilnius			
Antakalnis	7.7 (6.5; 8.9)	7.2	
Fabijoniskes	6 (5; 7)	6.7	
Justiniskes	6 (5; 7)	5.7	
Karoliniskes	6.6 (5.5; 7.7)	5.7	
Lazdynai	6.7 (5.6; 7.8)	5.9	
Naujamiestis	5.1 (4.1; 6.1)	5.1	
Naujininkai	5.7 (4.7; 6.7)	6.1	
Naujoji Vilnia	5.4 (4.4; 6.4)	6	
Paneriai	0.9 (0.5; 1.3)	1.5	Under-represented
Pasilaiciai	4.1 (3.2; 5)	4.7	
Pilaite	2.6 (1.9; 3.3)	2.9	
Rasos	1.9 (1.3; 2.5)	2.3	
Senamiestis	3.5 (2.7; 4.3)	3.8	
Verkiai	4.2 (3.3; 5.1)	5.6	Under-represented
Vilkpede	6 (5; 7)	5.5	
Virsuliskes	3.5 (2.7; 4.3)	3	
Seskine	8 (6.7; 9.3)	6.7	
Snipiskes	3.9 (3.1; 4.7)	3.5	
Zirmunai	10.4 (9; 10.1)	8.7	
Zverynas	1.8 (1.2; 2.4)	2.2	

Background and introduction

Ferreira
Ferreira	49 (46; 52)	53.5	Under-represented
Alfundao	11.6 (9.7; 13.5)	10.8	
Canhestros	6 (4.6; 7.4)	5.8	
Fig. Cavaleiros	19.5 (17.2; 21.8)	17.6	
Ovidelas	9.8 (8.1; 11.5)	7.7	Over-represented
Peroguarda	4.2 (3; 5.4)	4.7	

Budapest
I	0.8 (0.3; 1.3)	1.5	Under-represented
II	4.6 (3.4; 5.8)	5.2	
III	6.7 (5.3; 8.1)	7.4	
IV	6.1 (4.7; 7.5)	5.8	
V	2 (1.2; 2.8)	1.6	
VI	3 (2; 4)	2.4	
VII	4.1 (3; 5.2)	3.6	
VIII	5.2 (3.9; 6.5)	4.7	
IX	4.8 (3.6; 6)	3.5	
X	5.7 (4.4; 7)	4.5	
XI	4.7 (3.5; 5.9)	8	Under-represented
XII	1.6 (0.9; 2.3)	3.4	Under-represented
XIII	4.2 (3.1; 5.3)	6.3	Under-represented
XIV	6.3 (4.9; 7.7)	6.8	
XV	5.6 (4.3; 6.9)	4.8	
XVI	4.3 (3.1; 5.5)	4	
XVII	5.3 (4; 6.6)	4.6	
XVIII	8.8 (7.2; 10.4)	5.5	
XIX	5.3 (4; 6.6)	3.6	
XX	1.1 (0.5; 1.7)	3.7	
XXI	5.1 (3.8; 6.4)	4.6	
XXII	3.9 (2.8; 5)	3	
XXIII	0.6 (0.2; 1)	1.2	

Background and introduction

Appendix 1.3 Distribution of households by city quarters

	Survey estimate % (95% confidence limits)	City information %	Comments
Bratislava			
Bratislava I	10.1 (6.9; 13.3)	12.1	
Bratislava II	28.4 (23.6; 33.2)	26.7	
Bratislava III	16.3 (12.4; 20.2)	15.9	
Bratislava IV	22.5 (18; 26.9)	21.2	
Bratislava V	22.8 (18.4; 27.2)	23.94	
Bonn			
Bonn	45.4 (40.4; 50.3)	46.6	
Bad Godesberg	21 (17; 25)	22.7	
Beuel	21.8 (17.7; 25.9)	20.7	
Hardtberg	11.8 (8.6; 15)	10	
Angers			
Centre ville	29.5 (25.1; 33.8)	22	Over-represented
Saint-Serge/ Ney-Chalouère	2.8 (1.2; 4.4)	7.2	Under-represented
Madeleine/ Saint-Lèonard	10.1 (7.3; 12.9)	8.2	
La Fayette/ Éblé	6.3 (4; 8.6)	12.6	Under-represented
Belle-Beille	9.4 (6.7; 12.1)	7.5	
Saint-Jacques/ Nazareth	4.7 (2.7; 6.7)	5.4	
Capucins/ Verneau	4.2 (2.3; 6.1)	4.9	
Monplaisir	5.9 (3.7; 8.1)	6.1	
Deux-Croix/ Banchais	5.6 (3.4; 7.8)	7	
Justices	4.7 (2.7; 6.7)	5.3	
Roseraie/ Orgemont	12.4 (9.3; 15.5)	10.8	
Lac-de-maine/ Mollière	2.6 (1.1; 4.1)	2.9	
Forlì			
Forlì C1	12.6 (9.3; 15.8)	18	Under-represented
Forlì C2	13.6 (10.2; 17)	10.7	
Forlì C3	22.2 (18.1; 26.3)	17.2	Over-represented
Forlì C4	30.2 (25.7; 34.7)	28.3	Over-represented
Forlì C5	21.2 (17.2; 25.2)	25.7	Under-represented
Budapest			
I	0.9 (0.1; 1.7)	2	Under-represented
II	5.4 (3.4; 7.4)	5.6	
III	7.4 (5; 9.4)	6.9	
IV	5.8 (3.7; 7.9)	5.2	
V	1.8 (0.6; 3)	2.3	
VI	2.9 (1.4; 4.5)	3	

VII	3.4 (1.8; 5)	4.2	
VIII	6.3 (4.1; 8.5)	4.8	
IX	3.8 (2.1; 5.5)	4	
X	5.6 (3.5; 7.7)	4.2	
XI	5.8 (3.7; 7.9)	8.5	Under-represented
XII	2.2 (0.9; 3.5)	4	Under-represented
XIII	5.8 (3.7; 7.9)	7.2	
XIV	7.2 (4.9; 9.5)	7.7	
XV	4.9 (2.9; 6.9)	4.5	
XVI	3.6 (1.9; 5.3)	3.3	
XVII	4.3 (2.5; 6.1)	3.5	
XVIII	7.6 (5.2; 10)	4.7	Over-represented
XIX	5.1 (3.1; 7.1)	3.2	
XX	1.6 (0.5; 2.7)	3.5	Under-represented
XXI	4.5 (2.6; 6.4)	3.9	
XXII	3.6 (1.9; 5.3)	2.5	
XXIII	0.7 (0; 1.5)	1	

Appendix 1.4 Distribution of housing types

	Survey estimate % (95% confidence limits)	City information %	Comments
Angers			
One-family house	30.4 (26.1; 34)	22.0	
Multi-family house	69.6 (65.3; 73.9)	78.0	Under-represented
Bonn			
One-family house	33.4	n.a.	
Multi-family house	66.6	n.a.	
Bratislava			
One-family house	12.1 (8.6; 15.6)	10	
Multi-family house	87.9 (84.4; 91.4)	90	
Budapest			
One-family house	28.9	n.a.	
Multi-family house	71.1	n.a.	
Ferreira			
One-family house	95.8 (93.8; 97.8)	96	
Multi-family house	4.2 (2.2; 6.2)	4	
Forlì			
One-family house	38.3 (33.5; 43.1)	40.0	
Multi-family house	61.7 (56.9; 66.5)	60.0	
Geneva			
One-family house	4.6 (2.3; 6.9)	19.6	Under-represented
Multi-family house	95.4 (93.1; 97.7)	80.4	Over-represented
Vilnius			
One-family house	8.8 (5.8; 10.2)	8.0	
Multi-family house	91.2 (89.8; 94.4)	92.0	

2   The cities

Description of the cities

The LARES project involved surveys carried out in eight cities in eight European countries (see Figure 2.1). While the survey was intended to be identical in terms of the process and the information collected, the cities themselves are very different. The following descriptions and information are given to provide some background to the findings from the project.[1]

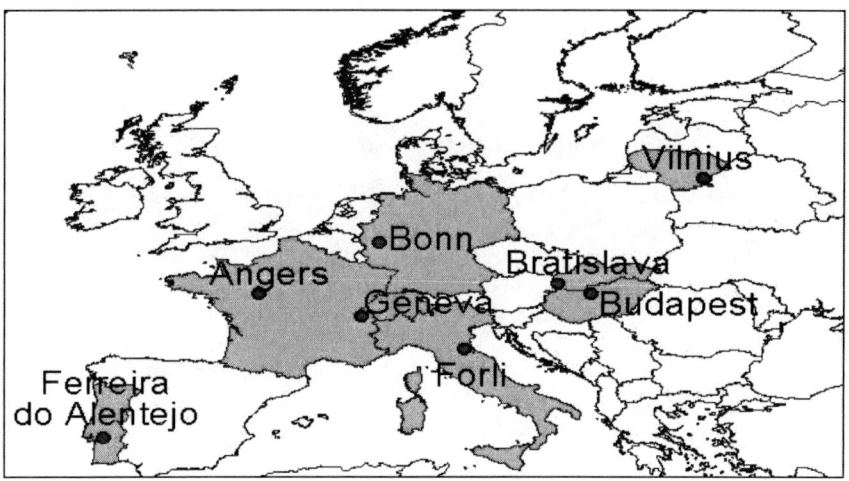

2.1   Geographical location of the survey cities.

---

[1]The information is based on that provided by each city and the amount and content available varies.

The cities

Angers (France)

Angers, a city of Western France, is the capital of the Maine-et-Loire Département. It is a trade centre for vegetables, fruits and flowers from the region, and produces electronic devices, machines and textiles.

Angers is the capital of the ancient Anjou region and claims to be one of the most beautiful cities of France. The cathedral of Saint Maurice (12th to 13th century) with its two towers, and the Saint Jean Hospital built in the 12th century by Henry II of England have now been transformed into a museum.

It is located at latitude 47° 50' north and longitude 0°32' west and is approximately 45 m above sea level.

Climate

The climate is temperate oceanic, the average temperature ranging from 4°C in December and January to 19°C in July and August (Table 2.1). The average annual precipitation is 667 mm, with an average sunshine hours per year of 1,874.

Table 2.1 Average temperature in Angers

	J	F	M	A	M	J	J	A	S	O	N	D
Ave. temp.	4	5	7	11	14	17	19	19	16	12	7	4

Population and household structure

The population by age group of Angers in 1999 is given in Table 2.2. The household sizes are given in Table 2.3.

Description of the housing stock

The city was built progressively from the Middle Ages to the 20th century, starting from the old city centre located next to the river Maine. The old building stock

Table 2.2 Population by age group in Angers

Age	Total	Per cent
0–4	7,599	5.06
5–15	16,183	10.78
16–29	48,697	32.44
30–64	55,792	37.16
65+	21,855	14.56
Total	**150,126**	**100.00**

The cities

Table 2.3 Household size in Angers

Household size (persons)	Number	Per cent
1	32,949	46.53
2	19,425	27.43
3	7,971	11.26
4	6,230	8.80
5 or more	4,235	5.98
Total	**70,810**	**100.00**

is still part of the city centre. In the 1950s the expansion of the city on the periphery with social housing began in response to the industrialisation and urbanisation process (Table 2.4). The city quarters of Angers are part of the urban renewal programmes.

Table 2.4 Housing stock in 1999

Principal residences	70,810
Occasional dwellings	816
Secondary residence	491
Empty dwellings	4,406
House owners	20,791
Lettings	48,522
Gratis housing	1,497
Individual houses or farms	17,484
Flat in apartment blocks	51,078
Other	2,248

Source: INSEE.

Bonn (Germany)

For the new Federal Republic that succeeded the three western zones of occupation in 1949, Bonn became provisional capital of West Germany. In 1969, nine surrounding towns, including Bad Godesberg, Duisdorf and Beuel, were incorporated into the city. After German unification in 1990, the German Parliament decided that Berlin should again be the German capital and seat of government, although Bonn retains some government functions as Bundesstadt. The move to the new capital was mostly completed in 1999.

Bonn is the 19th biggest city in Germany and covers an area of approximately 141 square kilometres. It is located at latitude 50°43' north and Longitude 7°7' east, and lies between 45 m and 191 m above sea level (average 60 m).

The cities

Climate

The average temperature ranges from 1°C in December to 19°C in July and August, with an average annual precipitation of 633 mm (Table 2.5).

Population (2003)

The population of about 313,000 was made up as shown in Table 2.6.

Household structure

In 2002, the population of 311,000 formed a total of 165,206 households. The structure of these households was as given in Table 2.7.

Table 2.5 The climate of Bonn

	J	F	M	A	M	J	J	A	S	O	N	D
Ave. temp.	1	3	6	10	15	17	19	19	15	11	6	3
Ave. max. temp.	3	5	8	13	17	20	22	23	18	13	7	5
Ave. min. temp.	0	1	2	5	10	13	15	14	11	7	4	2
Ave. rain days	1	1	2	1	2	1	2	1	2	1	2	2
Ave. snow days	0	1	0	0	0	0	0	0	0	0	0	0

Table 2.6 Population by age group in Bonn

Age	Total	Per cent
0–5	17,988	5.76
6–17	34,895	11.17
18–29	55,579	17.78
30–64	151,810	48.58
65+	52,255	16.72
Total	**312,527**	**100.00**

Table 2.7 Household structure of Bonn

Single-person households	Multi-person households						Total households
	Households with children				Single parent		
	Number of children			<18	Total		
	1	2	3+				
88,708	15,073	10,500	4,027	49,643	7,569	6,631	**165,206**

The cities

Description of housing stock

Today Bonn is a polycentric city with four main city districts. Having its origin in the Roman time, the oldest part of the city is the city centre. Due to the Second World War only a few old buildings are left.

The city centre is surrounded by well-maintained houses built in Wilhelminian style (1875–1910). When Bonn became the capital in 1949, the need for new houses increased and new city quarters such as Tannenbusch, Heiderhof and Venusberg were built. These new city districts integrated 21 independent villages surrounding Bonn. Today nearly 40% of the city surface is urbanised. In 1950, each citizen of Bonn was living in an average of 13.5 m^2. In 2003, the living surface per inhabitant was 40.2 m^2. In 1987, just over three-quarters (76%) of households rented their accommodation.

The age of the housing stock is given in Table 2.8.

Table 2.8 Age of the housing stock in Bonn

Age range	Number	Per cent
Pre 1900	5,012	10.81
1901–1918	4,107	8.86
1919–1948	5,867	12.66
1949–1957	8,460	18.25
1958–1968	11,514	24.84
1969–1978	5,983	12.91
Post 1978	5,402	11.66
Total	**46,345**	**100.00**

Bratislava (Slovakia)

Bratislava is the capital of the Slovakia. The Slovak republic was created on 1 January 1993, after the dissolution of the Czech and Slovak Federative Republics. The city covers an area of approximately 370 square kilometres, and has a population of nearly 447,000.

It is located at latitude 48°20' north and longitude 17°20' east, and is approximately 133 m above sea level.

Climate

Bratislava has a temperate, continental climate, the average temperature ranging from 0°C in December and January to 20°C in July and August. The average annual precipitation is 527 mm (Table 2.9).

The cities

Table 2.9 The climate of Bratislava

	J	F	M	A	M	J	J	A	S	O	N	D
Ave. temp.	0	2	5	10	15	18	20	20	15	10	4	0
Ave. max. temp.	2	6	10	16	21	24	26	26	20	15	7	2
Ave. min. temp.	−3	−1	1	5	10	12	15	15	10	6	1	−2
Ave. rain days	8	7	11	9	9	9	10	7	9	8	10	7
Ave. snow says	6	4	4	1	0	0	0	0	0	0	2	4

Table 2.10 Population by age group in Bratislava

Age	Total	Per cent
0–4	16,492	3.69
5–14	50,066	11.19
15–29	107,186	23.96
30–64	218,591	48.86
65+	55,010	12.30
Total	**447,345**	**100.00**

Table 2.11 Household size in Bratislava

Household size (persons)	Number	Per cent
1	69,405	36.71
2	47,860	25.31
3	34,080	18.02
4	30,256	16.00
5	5,897	3.12
6 or more	1,587	0.84
Total	**189,085**	**100.00**

Population

In 2000, there was a total population of about 447,000 (Table 2.10).

Household structure

The population formed 189,100 households, the structure of which was as shown in Table 2.11.

Description of housing stock

Bratislava has a diverse housing stock (Table 2.12). The city centre has the old town (Stare Mesto) and the new town (Nove Mesto), both of which were built a long time ago and consist of old urban buildings with several floor levels.

The cities

Table 2.12 Age of the housing stock in Bratislava

Age range	Number	Per cent
Pre 1900	3,980	2.40
1900–1919	2,606	1.57
1920–1945	13,132	7.93
1946–1970	47,184	28.49
1971–1980	46,945	28.35
1981–1990	40,855	24.67
1991–2001	10,885	6.57
Total	**165,587**	**100.00**

Other, newer areas of the city, Dubravka, Karlova Ves, Petrzalka, Ruzinov and Vrakuna, are dominated by panel-block apartment buildings, the largest and newest being Petrzalka (with more than 120,000 inhabitants), which was built in the 1970s.

Bratislava also has an open urban fringe to the surrounding area, and therefore also some rural-type settlements and villages (Jarovce, Rusovce, Cunovo), although these account for less than 1% of the population.

Tenure (2001)

The housing market in Bratislava is very tight since the government has mostly privatised the formerly state-owned housing stock. Houses and flats (apartments) of adequate quality have high prices and finding a flat to rent is difficult (Table 2.13).

Table 2.13 The housing market in Bratislava

Total number of dwellings:	181,021
permanently occupied	165,587 (91.5%)
in cooperative ownership	26,670 (16.1%)
in inhabitants' ownership	99,522 (60.1%)
others (municipality, legal entities, etc.)	39,395 (23.8%)

Budapest (Hungary)

Budapest, capital and by far the largest city of Hungary, is located in northern Hungary on both banks of the Danube River. Home to about 17% of Hungary's population, Budapest is the country's cultural and industrial centre. Three towns – Pest, Buda and Obuda – were combined in 1873 to form the capital of newly autonomous Hungary. It is located at latitude 47° north and longitude 20° east, and is approximately 102 m above sea level. It covers an area of approximately 525 square kilometres.

The cities

Table 2.14 Population by age group in Budapest

Age	Total	Per cent
0–14	216,533	12.59
15–29	379,718	22.09
30–49	462,440	26.90
50–59	251,358	14.62
60+	409,293	23.81
Total	**1,719,342**	**100.00**

Climate

Budapest has a temperate climate. Spring usually arrives in early April, followed by hot, humid summers. The temperature in July averages 22°C. It is often cloudy and damp during the short and cold winters; the average January temperature is −2°C. Snowfall can be heavy.

Population

In 2003, the population of Budapest was just over 1,719,000 (Table 2.14).

Household structure

The household sizes were structured as shown in Table 2.15.

Description of housing stock

Budapest has a diverse housing stock. The city centre includes District 5 and some neighbouring streets, and consists of mainly old urban buildings of several floor levels. Offices, banks, hotels and governmental buildings dominate this part of the city.

Table 2.15 Household size in Budapest

Household size (persons)	Numbers	Per cent
1	212,257	29.55
2	218,860	30.47
3	138,022	19.22
4–5	133,516	18.59
6–7	12,897	1.80
8+	2,674	0.37
Total	**718,226**	**100.00**

The cities

The Districts 1, 6–9 and 13 form the inner residential area, which consists primarily of multi-family houses, most of them built before 1920. The elite suburb quarter (mainly one-family houses of the upper class and not many institutional buildings) is located in Districts 2 and 12 and part of the Districts 3 and 11. Districts 9, 10, 13 and 14 and the southern part of the District 11 are a mixed, transitional zone. This is a heterogeneous zone, originally with industrial function, although that function is decreasing, and there are one-family houses, apartment blocks and panel block housing estates in this area.

The outskirts, Districts 4, 15, 16, 18, 19, 20, 21, 22 and 23, consist of rural areas and the largest panel block estates.

The age of the housing stock is given in Table 2.16.

The housing market is very tight since the privatisation of the formerly state-owned housing stock. Adequate quality housing has a high price and finding accommodation is difficult. The vast majority of housing (about 85%) is owner-occupied.

Table 2.16   Age of the housing stock in Budapest

Age range	Number	Per cent
Pre 1944	330,583	40.27
1945–1969	153,495	18.70
1970–1979	161,459	19.67
1980–1989	131,000	15.96
1990–2001	44,440	5.41
Total	**820,977**	**100.00**

Ferreira do Alentejo (Portugal)

Ferreira do Alentejo has been a municipality since 1516. It is located in the southern half of Portugal in the province of Alentejo. It has six districts, covers an area of approximately 652 square kilometres, and has a population of just over 9,000. The main district is the town itself, which has 50% of the population. The main economic activities are agriculture and services.

In spite of the small population, Ferreira do Alentejo is well equipped with public structures such as the high school, the court of law, public library, archaeological museum, summer swimming pool, winter swimming pool, sports pavilion, public gardens, bus station and cultural centre.

It is located at latitude 38°04' north and longitude 8°06' west, and is approximately 136 m above sea level.

The cities

Table 2.17 Population by age group in Ferreira do Alentejo

Age	Total	Per cent
0–4	354	3.93
5–14	802	8.90
15–29	1,740	19.31
30–64	3,869	42.94
65+	2,245	24.91
Total	**9,010**	**100.00**

Climate

Ferreira do Alentejo has a temperate climate. The average temperature is 16.2°C and the average annual precipitation is 586 mm.

Population

In 2001, the population was just over 9,000 (Table 2.17).

Household structure

The household sizes were structured as shown in Table 2.18.

Description of housing stock

There are 3,368 dwellings in the city, of which 3,333 are individual houses. The houses are of one or two floors with a small yard behind. There are few apartment blocks. Nearly 50% of the housing is over 50 years old and less than 1% is less than 10 years old.

Table 2.18 Household size in Ferreira do Alentejo

Dwelling size (persons)	Number	Per cent
1	656	19.48
2	1,070	31.77
3	807	23.96
4	596	17.70
5	159	4.72
6	55	1.63
7	20	0.59
8	1	0.03
9 or more	4	0.12
Total	**3,368**	**100.00**

The cities

Tenure

There are no data on tenure status in Ferreira do Alentejo. But, as for the rest of Portugal, in general only the older houses are rented, and the houses built over the last 30 years are owned by the residents.

Forlì (Italy)

Built along the layout of the Via Emilia, on settlements dating back to the first half of the Iron Age and located between the Montone and Rabbi rivers, the town acquired an organic appearance towards the second century BC with the building of the first Roman centre called Forum Livi. A transit place and crossroads of Romagna between the sea and hills along the consular road, the town developed as a commercial knot of the centurated plain and during the Augustan Age it became a municipium. It kept its strategically pre-eminent role also during the Gothic, Byzantine and Lombardic periods. Between the 10th and 11th century AD the town proclaimed itself a free city, and later became the Ghibelline pole of clerical Romagna. In the 16th century Cesare Borgia delivered up the town to the Pope, who kept it under his control until the time of Napoleon. During the 17th and 18th centuries, the buildings of Forlì were submitted to imposing renewal interventions. The abolition of the religious orders and the church properties (1797 and 1811) contributed to the town's transformation. During the Neoclassical Age, many buildings were restored under the banner of the new values of the emerging bourgeoisie: the house became an intimate and functional place. The last milestone of the city was the town planning undertaken during the 1920s and 1930s: the designing thrust which inspired the yards of this period also compromised the integrity and organic arrangement of the urban texture irreversibly.

The town of Forlì covers a total area of 228,457 square kilometres. It is located at latitude 44°22' north and longitude 12°04' east, and is approximately 34 m above sea level.

Climate

The maximum temperature ranges from 6°C in January to 29°C in July and August. The average annual precipitation is 634 mm (Table 2.19).

Table 2.19 The climate of Forlì

	J	F	M	A	M	J	J	A	S	O	N	D
Precipitation mm	40	38	51	54	48	54	41	59	62	60	68	59
Max. temp.	6	9	13	17	22	27	29	29	25	19	11	7

The cities

Table 2.20 Population by age group in Forlì

Age	Total	Per cent
0–14	12,556	11.39
15–24	9,074	8.23
25–44	33,330	30.24
45–59	21,942	19.91
60–74	20,289	18.41
75+	13,018	11.81
Total	**110,209**	**100.00**

Population

In 2003, the population was just over 110,000 (Table 2.20).

Household structure

The household sizes were structured as shown in Table 2.21.

Housing stock

There are around 70,300 dwellings in the city, of which 19,620 are individual houses, 2,424 are condominiums and 48,253 are separate flats (apartments). The majority of dwellings (80%) are owner-occupied.

Table 2.21 Household size in Forlì

Household size (persons)	Number	Per cent
1	13,032	28.36
2	13,851	30.15
3	10,587	23.04
4	6,402	13.93
5	1,475	3.21
6	437	0.95
7	101	0.22
8 or more	61	0.13
Total	**45,946**	**100.00**

Geneva (Switzerland)

Geneva did not develop into an important centre until the end of the Middle Ages when its fairs, reaching their peak in the 15th century, first gave it an international reputation. Its independence was threatened, however, by Savoy, whose princes strove unsuccessfully from the 13th to the 17th century to force the town into

The cities

Table 2.22 The climate of Geneva

	J	F	M	A	M	J	J	A	S	O	N	D
Ave. temp.	1	3	6	8	14	17	19	19	14	11	5	2
Ave. max. temp.	4	7	12	14	20	22	25	25	20	15	8	5
Ave. min. temp.	−1	0	1	3	9	11	13	13	10	7	1	0
Ave. rain days	8	7	8	9	8	6	6	6	7	8	9	6
Ave. snow days	2	2	1	0	0	0	0	0	0	0	1	2

submission. At its time of gravest danger, during the first third of the 16th century, the city's autonomy was saved by the intervention of the Swiss cantons of Fribourg and Bern. When the Reformation triumphed in 1535, the city became a republic. Calvin made Geneva his home the following year, and it was through his genius that the city earned the name 'Protestant Rome'.

The International Committee of the Red Cross was founded in 1864, the first of many international organizations to settle there. Geneva's international role was confirmed after the First World War when it was chosen as the site for the headquarters of the League of Nations, the forerunner of the United Nations Organisation.

The city of Geneva, Onex and Versoix covers an area of approximately 29.22 square kilometers, is located at latitude 46°25' north and longitude 6°13' east and is approximately 416 m above sea level.

Climate

The average temperature ranges from 1°C in January to 19°C in July and August (Table 2.22).

Population

In 2001, the population was just under 420,000 (Table 2.23).

Housing stock

There are around 208,000 dwellings in the city (Table 2.24).

Table 2.23 Population by age group in Geneva

Age	Total	Per cent
0–19	91,600	21.83
20–64	267,573	63.76
65+	60,477	14.41
Total	**419,650**	**100.00**

The cities

Table 2.24 Age of the housing stock in Geneva

Age	Number	Per cent
Before 1900	13,456	6.47
1900–1920	19,319	9.29
1921–1946	23,016	11.07
1947–1960	29,808	14.34
1961–1970	47,686	22.94
1971–1980	33,927	16.32
1981–1985	9,696	4.66
1986–1990	9,393	4.52
1991–1995	9,490	4.57
1996–2000	10,509	5.06
After 2000	1,575	0.76
Total	**207,875**	**100.00**

Vilnius (Lithuania)

The Republic of Lithuania was formed in 1990, and Vilnius is the capital and the largest city in the country. The city covers an area of approximately 400 square kilometres and is located at latitude 54°41' north and longitude 25°19' east, and is approximately 156 m above sea level.

Climate

The climate of Vilnius is between continental and maritime. The average temperature ranges from −5°C in December to 17°C in July. The average annual precipitation is 661 mm (Table 2.25).

Household structure

The 2001 population of 542,000 formed 223,825 households, structured as shown in Table 2.26.

Table 2.25 The climate of Vilnius

	J	F	M	A	M	J	J	A	S	O	N	D
Ave. temp.	−3	−3	0	7	11	16	17	16	11	6	0	−5
Ave. max. temp.	−1	0	3	12	17	21	23	22	16	10	2	−2
Ave. min. temp.	−6	−6	−3	2	6	10	12	11	7	3	−2	−7
Ave. rain days	9	8	8	9	9	10	8	9	9	11	11	6
Ave. snow days	14	13	10	3	0	0	0	0	0	1	8	9

Table 2.26 Household size in Vilnius

Household size (persons)	Number	Per cent
1	73,993	33.06
2	52,747	23.57
3	47,001	21.00
4	37,195	16.62
5	9,362	4.18
6	2,534	1.13
7	670	0.30
8	191	0.09
9	75	0.03
10 or more	57	0.03
Total	**223,825**	**100.00**

Housing stock

There are around 201,200 dwellings in the city, of which 10,937 are individual houses, 4,654 are part of a house, and 179,648 are separate flats (apartments). The remaining 5,995 are hostels and other living quarters.

Table 2.27 Age of the housing stock in Vilnius

Age range	No. of residential buildings	Per cent
Pre 1919	1,750	7.37
1919–1945	3,577	15.07
1946–1960	2,794	11.77
1961–1980	3,966	16.71
Post 1980	11,436	48.18
Not known	212	0.89
	23,735	**100.00**

3 The surveys
Nathalie Röbbel

Lessons learned or how to deal with the real life of the survey

There is no doubt that theory and practice can differ very much. This is true of the LARES survey, the real life of which opened up many challenges. Dealing with these challenges has provided useful experience for the future.

Internationality

The study covered a range of geographical locations throughout Europe, which facilitated analysis of the relationships between housing and health under various national conditions. Housing stock variations, climate conditions and cultural differences were taken into account when designing the questionnaires and helped to ensure the building up of a comprehensive database. The internationality of the survey meant that the questionnaires had to be translated in seven languages. Translation 'biases' were mitigated by detailed definitions of all relevant technical and assessment terms and each set of questionnaires was tested in each country. However, a back-translation would have been an additional step for maximising the consistency of the survey tool.

This extensive international survey was only possible through the strenuous effort and commitment of the local municipalities and the WHO counterparts working at national level. The cities supported the implementation financially, practically and logistically. The cities covered the salary of the surveyors, provided free transport for the survey teams, covered the telephone costs and delegated a member of their staff for data cleaning. The samples, the promotion of the study through the media and the provision of the office with the equipment were also provided by the city municipalities. The commitment and hard work of each municipality was essential for the success of the surveys and the project.

The surveys

Sample

From the methodological point of view, the sampling process was shown to be sound and it represents good practice. Nevertheless, there were major problems in contacting the households during the survey because of the quality of the sources and practical problems – addresses changed, people moved, or a street no longer existed. In some cases, the samples contained double entries, so that the original sample size decreased, reducing the response rate. In other cases, secondary addresses, military barracks, etc., were still included in the sample; these were eliminated during the survey implementation.

In order to make the best use of the sample and to avoid losing information, the following aspects should be given priority:

- The sample should contain the following features: surname (family name), first name, gender, age, address, phone number, possibly the number of persons living in the same household, and family position of the selected person (e.g. father or daughter). This detailed information about the household structure can be used at a later stage for checking the completeness of the health questionnaires collected.
- It should be checked to ensure that there are no duplications (such as two individuals chosen from the same household).
- The sample should be provided in an electronic format so that the size of the sample given to each survey team can be adapted, depending on unexpected modifications in the team numbers and arrangements.
- In order to prepare the field work, the sample should be made available well in advance. Receiving the sample on the last day of the training sometimes reduced the available time for the training sessions as the sample had to be divided into different sections according to the number of survey teams.
- Nevertheless, the sample should be the most up-to-date version of all registered inhabitants in order to avoid mistakes in the attribution of streets, phone numbers, etc.

The burned house

Surveyor A and Surveyor T came into the office and took their schedule for the day. The first interview was in the outskirts of the city, so they decided not to lose time, took the necessary questionnaires for the day, checked the address again on the map and hurried to get the tram. It was a long way to the house, but they didn't bother too much as they were happy that they had got an additional interview. When, after a 50-minute ride they finally found the street, they started looking for the house. It was number 54, or at least it should

The surveys

> have been number 54. But even after turning around a few times they could not find it, only a wide open space. Fortunately, a neighbour came out of house number 50. The surveyors asked whether the lady knew where they could find number 54. Yes, indeed she could. The house burned down a few months before. Apparently, the change of residence of the family and the non-existence of this house were not mentioned in the sample received by the surveyors. They had lost more than 2 hours of their time.

Staff

There should be an adequate number of persons for carrying out the survey. This refers not only to the coordinating staff but also to the number of surveyors, the people responsible for the data entry and the people required to collect the Health Questionnaires. Guaranteeing sufficient staff is crucial not only for 'motivation' but also for the quality of the work.

The coordination and management of the survey in each city was carried out by two persons, one a representative of WHO and one a local person. A second WHO representative was present during the training and the first days of the field work. The WHO representative was responsible for the collection of the completed questionnaires and survey sheets every evening / morning, checking of the quality and completeness of the survey. The representative was the key person for any methodological questions arising during the field work and for coordinating the day-to-day activities. As well as providing assistance, the local person was in charge of all contacts and linkages between the town hall and the WHO representative.

It is clear that one coordinator is not sufficient. The presence of a second person looking after the performance of the survey teams and the other staff is essential. It also avoids the coordinator having to work very long hours each day. Ideally, the additional coordinator should be from the local authority and be able to provide local knowledge.

Similarly, there should be sufficient staff for carrying out the surveys and interviews. In one case, several members of the survey teams quit after a few days, which could have caused more serious problems if there had not been enough surveyors. It would appear that students with some interest in the background issues were very often more motivated and time flexible than professionals.

As with other staff, it is important to have an adequate number of persons for data entry. The experience from the first survey showed that one person was able to enter around eight sets of questionnaires into the computer per day. However, this was not enough to cope with the number of questionnaires completed each day. In the following surveys, the number of data entry personnel was increased. Clearly, the number of data entry staff will depend on the sample size.

The mystery of the boxes

The survey was complete, with no interviews left. Unfortunately, as only two people were entering data, the day the WHO representative left the city the data entry was not finished. It was agreed that the data entry process would go on, and as soon as it was finished the electronic data and all the paper questionnaires would be sent to the WHO office.

Six weeks later the boxes arrived at the WHO office. But could a big black round plastic bag contain the questionnaires that had so carefully been sorted by the coordinator? Yes, it could! All the questionnaires had been thrown together in one big plastic bag.

While sitting on the floor surrounded by thousands of questionnaires, the only thing that the coordinator could think of was, 'If we had had more data entry people, we would have been able to take the questionnaires with us directly and avoid having to re-sort them.'

Collecting the self-administered Housing and Health Questionnaires rather than relying on the households to send them back helped to increase the response rate. The collection was made by two support persons calling at the dwelling 2 or 3 days after the survey visit. Initially, only one person had been designated for this task, but this was not sufficient. These support staff also participated in the interviewer training; thus, they were able to answer questions from the households and could fill in if an interviewer became ill.

The rescuing taxi driver

The city was very big, and the distance between one interview and the next was huge. The temperature outside the survey headquarters was around −10°C. The questionnaire collector looked at the list for the day. It was a bad day! All the appointments were spread around the city. He counted how many buses he had to take in order to get to all the households – around 15. And, unfortunately, there was no car that could be used for picking up the questionnaires.

But the collector was lucky. It was the day that the survey teams received a visit from the head of the Department of Public Health of the national Ministry of Health. The collector is rescued – with the support of the representative of the Ministry of Health he was driven round the city to pick up the questionnaires.

The surveys

Local base set-up

In most cases, the life of the survey took place in one big room. This room, therefore, functioned as the data entry station, the coordination unit, the storage place for the completed and the blank questionnaires and survey sheets, the telephone centre, the training room, the social room, the dining room and much more. It was therefore necessary to have a room big enough to cope with all these functions.

It is also important that the room is accessible on evenings and weekends, and that there are enough telephone lines for all the survey teams and enough computers for all data entry persons. Also important is that the survey base should be located close to access to public transport.

The cut-off electricity

A new day and all the staff were slowly getting to the survey headquarters. There was a lot to do – interviews to be fixed, questionnaires to be checked and data to be entered. But the team could not get into the building. The electricity was cut off! The building was dark and not accessible! How long were they going to be shut out of the building? The prognosis was very bad – at least for the whole day the building would be shut. This meant a lost work day, dissatisfaction of those households who tried to contact the surveyors and a lot of lost interviews.

Training

An important element of the training was rehearsing and improving telephone call and personal visit techniques. First contact can be difficult, and only with some practice and experience were the surveyors able to explain the purpose of the survey efficiently and convince the households to participate. To deal with this, one part of the training was role-play sessions, in which each person had to make a few telephone calls while the training facilitators played the part of the householder. The various problems and challenges of this situation were then discussed, and advice and tips given to the surveyors.

On the second training day, the surveyors carried out a survey using the Housing Inspection Survey Sheet. The discussions triggered by this practical exercise were probably the most decisive and important discussions of the whole training and were thus a crucial element.

The surveyors' assessments made during training were kept until the end of the surveys to check for any variations or biases that should be taken into consideration for the analysis of the data.

The surveys

It would have been beneficial to extend the training and introduce special additional training for those making the initial telephone call; similarly, for those who would carry out the interviews, particularly giving some preparation for difficult situations. Finally, more practical exercises would have been useful.

Another option would be to use trained building professionals for the dwelling inspections (although some training would still be necessary to reduce variability), and to select others for the interviewing.

Implementation of survey

The pre-survey preparation time was very short in most cases. This short time created difficulties in making sure that everything was ready for the first day of the survey (telephone lines, computer, staff trained, etc.) ... and sometimes this tight timetable led to last minute copying of material.

Detention of an innocent dwelling

One major part of the training consisted in making an inspection of two dwellings as practical exercises. In this case, the visit to the dwellings was scheduled for the afternoon, but in the morning still no dwelling was available. By the afternoon there was still no dwelling available, so the head of the environmental unit of the public health centre offered her own flat for the inspection. Twenty-five people ran into the dwelling, looked in every room, asked questions and disappeared 2½ hours later.

Wrong questionnaire

It was the first day of the training. The surveyors arrived and the coordinator started the training. In the first break, after having given some information on the survey content and just begun with the introduction of the interview situation, the boxes with the questionnaires for the survey arrived. This was just in time, as during the afternoon session the surveyors were supposed to work with the Inhabitant Questionnaire.

During the afternoon the questionnaire was distributed and the trainer started to go through it question by question. But the surveyors started to get nervous. They were looking into their papers, then talking to each other. After a while one surveyor lifts his hand and cautiously explains that the questions that were being read out did not match exactly the questions in the distributed papers. An old version of the questionnaire had been copied. And there were only 2 days left before the survey was due to start.

The surveys

Only 2 weeks for a survey intended to achieve around 600 interviews is too short and in most cities the period was extended by a few days. Three weeks would have produced a higher response rate, better quality and a more relaxed atmosphere. Ideally, there should be sufficient time for revisits, allowing the survey teams to make up to five calls at an address before writing it off as a non-contact.

Time is also an important factor when planning the interviews. The estimated 60 minutes is only an approximation; some interviews were shorter and some longer. This needs to be taken into account when fixing appointments. Unfortunately, some interviewers often did not take into account the time needed for going from one interview to another.

During the training and the survey itself it was important to be very clear on the expected work standards and to make sure that each person involved fulfilled his/her duties. This included the surveyors keeping clear records of their addresses and their work progress, and reviewing and correcting every questionnaire before it was transferred to the data entry team. In this respect it was found that some additional effort had to be made in the collection of information about non-contacts and refusals to establish clearly the extent and nature of response bias. Records of survey outcomes need to distinguish clearly between addresses that are ineligible, non-contacts and refusals. A systematic approach in contacting houses with no telephone numbers needs to be developed to avoid losing them.

The pre-publicity was important; as was the press conference, and informing the local police about the survey. The letter signed by the municipality and WHO to inform the households about the interviews and survey helped, provided that it was sent out in good time. (It was noted that the highest amount of refusals came from those households where the letter didn't arrive.)

> ### The drunken man
>
> The two young ladies (S and C) were surveyors. They were going to the last interview of the day and were happy that afterwards they could go home and rest. When they finally arrived at the house, they started to feel uncomfortable. They didn't know why ... but as they had to do the interview, they plucked up their courage and rang the bell. When they entered the dwelling they realised that their initial feeling was right. The interviewee was completely drunk. S and C immediately tried to leave the house, but the drunken man wouldn't let them out. Fortunately, S managed to use her mobile and called the survey headquarters to ask for help. The coordinator immediately called the police, but was afraid that it would take time to explain the situation. But in his panic, the coordinator had forgotten that the police had been previously informed about the survey going on and that they should be prepared to intervene. Luckily everything went fine!

For any survey it is necessary to follow some basic steps for the security of the surveyors. All the LARES surveyors were provided with an identity card with their photograph. This identity card gave some authority and some official status to the surveyors, giving confidence to the interviewees. For the security of the surveyors it proved to be a good procedure to let them work in pairs (not only for methodological reasons but also for security reasons) and to provide them with insurance cover.

> **A broken shoulder**
>
> The atmosphere in the survey room was very tense. The study coordinators were pale. They had just received a telephone call from one of the surveyors. Her team partner had just had an accident. While trying to get on to the bus to go to an interview appointment, she had been hit and knocked down by a car. She had been immediately taken to the hospital, where she was to stay for a couple of days. She had suffered a broken shoulder, some abrasions and a bruised knee. Fortunately, the injuries were not severe and, fortunately, she had been insured by the town hall for all the time of the survey!

Conclusions

Overall, the survey methodology developed for the LARES study worked well. However, a number of improvements could be made to improve data quality and usefulness and to reduce bias. Unfortunately, most of these would increase the costs of such surveys.

Part II
The results of the analyses of the LARES data

4 Introduction

To make the most of the data gathered by the LARES project, WHO ECEH brought together a multidisciplinary and international team of experts. Working individually or in small groups, these experts analysed the data, concentrating on their own particular subject area. Coordinating meetings provided the opportunity for report backs and discussions on the progress of the analyses, and for cross-fertilisation, which sparked further ideas and insights. As a part of the coordination of the analyses, it was agreed that certain conventions or scores would be adopted (an explanation of these is given in Chapter 5).

The following chapters provide the main findings from the analyses. Each contribution has been provided by the expert(s) who carried out the analysis and therefore each has a personal approach, interpretation and opinion. What is clear is that the results and findings provide some new correlations between housing conditions and health that will make a significant contribution to the recognition of the public health importance of the housing environment.

Chapters 6–8 deal with aspects of indoor air quality, dampness and thermal comfort, respectively. In Chapter 6, Isabella Annesi-Maesano and David Moreau concentrated on the potential sources of indoor air pollution and the relationship with asthma and allergic diseases. A closely related area is that of dampness, mould growth and health, which is reported on in Chapter 7 by Peter Rudnai, Mihaly Varro, Tibor Malnasi, Anna Páldy, Simon Nicol and Alan O'Dell. Energy efficiency and thermal comfort are often linked to ventilation (and air quality) and dampness. The evidence provided by the study of the health effects of cold homes is reviewed by Ben Croxford in Chapter 8, followed by a report on the analysis of links between residential energy systems, socio-economic status and health given by Véronique Ezratty, Anne Duburcq, Corinne Emery and Jacques Lambrozo (see Chapter 9).

While the relationship between mental health and the housing environment is recognised, the evidence is often difficult to obtain. One of the less controversial aspects, that of feelings of safety and fear of crime in and around the home, and the findings from the LARES study, are discussed by Maggie Davidson in Chapter 10. This is followed by a review of the relationship between housing and mental

Introduction

health by Jérmone Fredouille, E. Laporte, and Mounir Mesbah (see Chapter 11). The approach adopted is based on that described by Mounir Mesbah in his contribution on building quality of life related housing scores (see Chapter 12).

Two different approaches to reviewing the relationship between the housing environment and the quality of life are then given. Chapter 13 features the contribution from Irene van Kamp, Annemarie Ruysbroek and Rebecca Stellato on the quality of the residential environment, and Chapter 14 features the contribution from Matthias Braubach on the relationship between health and the immediate housing environment.

The findings from analysis of the LARES data on noise and morbidity are reported in Chapter 15 from Hildegard Niemann and Christian Maschke. This is followed by a review of the findings on the relationship between housing factors and accidental injuries in the home by Richard Moore (see Chapter 16).

5 Scores and conventions

As the analysis of the data was to be carried out by a wide range of experts, standard 'scores' and conventions were adopted to allow for comparison of the results and findings. Below is an explanation of some of these.

Age bands

The database contained two sets of age groupings, breaking the sample down into 5 or 9 groups. For the general analyses these were amalgamated into three age bands (Table 5.1).

Where a specific group for adolescents was needed, it was suggested that this was taken to be the ages 12–16 years (inclusive).

Allergy scores

Two allergy scores were devised:

- ALLERAST, awhere there was at least one symptom of asthma or allergy in the previous 12 months[1]
- ALEST_DG, where there was at least one symptom of asthma or allergy diagnosed by a physician in the previous 12 months.[2]

It was decided that these variables were not only allergic status but also asthmatic status.

---

[1] See Appendix 1 Housing and Health Questionnaire, H_38_1_1, H_38_2_1, H_38_3_1, H_38_4_1, and H_38_5_1.
[2] See Appendix 1 Housing and Health Questionnaire H_38_1_2, H_38_2_2, H_38_3_2, H_38_4_2, and H_38_5_2.

Scores and conventions

Table 5.1 Age bands

Children	0–17 years	Infants	0–12 months
		Young children	1–4 years
		Children	5–9 years
		Teenagers	10–17 years
Adults	18–64 years	Younger adults	18–24 years
		Adults	25–29 years
		Older adults	30–64 years
Elderly	≥65 years	Young seniors	65–79 years
		Old seniors	≥80 years

Body mass index

A body mass index (BMI) was computed for residents of age 20–80 (inclusive). This BMI value and the categories 'underweight', 'normal', 'overweight', and 'obese' were then added to the database after the age groups.

Depression and psycho-social benefits

The responses to four questions in the Housing and Health Questionnaire (H_20 to H_23) were aggregated to give a depression screening tool (for adults) based on the SALSA approach.[3]

The seven responses to H_31 in the Housing and Health Questionnaire on the perception of the home were designed to measure the psycho-social benefits derived from the home.[4] Seven of the items were combined as an aggregate score to give three different dimensions, and a measurement of the psycho-social benefits derived from the home could be created by adding the seven variables.

Education level and occupational status

The education level question in the Housing and Health Questionnaire was categorised using ISCED 1997.[5] The question about the main profession of the father allowed for an open answer, but was recoded in the database according to ISCO 88.[6]

---

[3] Sleep disturbance, anhedonia, low self-esteem and appetite decreased. See Chapter 11 for an explanation and Brody *et al* (1998).
[4] See Kearns *et al* (2000).
[5] International Standard Classification for Education, 1997.
[6] The European Union variant of ISCO 88 (International Standard Classification of Occupations).

Scores and conventions

Health indices

Five scores were included in the database:

- Two related to respiratory conditions – one (RESP_IND) based on doctor-diagnosed, acute bronchitis and wheeze or whistling; and the other (RESP_ANY) based on self-reporting of either of the two respiratory symptoms.
- Two related to cardiovascular conditions – the first (CVD_IND) based on doctor-diagnosed hypertension, heart attacks and strokes; and the other (CVD_ANY) based on self-reporting of any of the three cardiovascular symptoms.
- Finally, an 'arthritis index' (ARTH_ANY) based on self-reported arthritis.

Housing Quality Score

The Housing Quality Score (HQS) was the sum of 10 variables from the dwelling inspection sheet to give the surveyor's evaluation of the quality of the dwelling. It included evaluation of the ceilings, floors, walls, doors, and windows in the kitchen, bathroom, corridor and room No. 1 (other rooms were not included as many homes had only one room).

Income

Income posed a problem, as the income question was based on the national currencies – euros for Angers, Bonn, Ferreira do Alentejo and Forlì; litas for Vilnius; crowns for Bratislava; forint for Budapest; and Swiss francs for Geneva.

While aware that any income categories would depend upon the city and country, and that the high- and low-income groups may represent very different percentages of the population, the approach suggested was that the lowest income groups for each country represent the 'less privileged' and the higher income groups the 'most privileged'.

Mould and dampness score

A mould and dampness score was created to be used when the analysis requires adjustment for 'mouldy home'. This score was based on one developed[7] using a continuous scale of exposure, taking into account both the data on mould and dampness in the dwelling, using data from the Household Questionnaire and the Housing Inspection Survey Sheet.

---

[7] By Alan O'Dell of the UK Building Research Establishment.

Scores and conventions

Noise variables

Scores were formed for 'general traffic noise' and for 'general neighbourhood noise'. For both, the original five scale variables were summed and then reduced to three scale variables – 'not at all' 'moderately' and 'strongly'.

For 'sleep disturbance' the variable used was H_27 from the Housing and Health Questionnaire.

Socio-economic status

A score to take account of socio-economic factors was created[8] combining the following variables:

- number in the household
- whether the household contains a couple/couples or single people
- highest education level of any adult in the household
- number of those in the household aged 18–59 and in full-time work
- number of full-time equivalent jobs held by people in the household
- number of people aged 60 or over in household
- size of dwelling in m^2 (banded)
- number of rooms in the dwelling.

The profession of the father was not included as, although it produced a slightly more reliable score, there were a significant number of cases with missing information on this variable. For this reason it was decided that it should be excluded so as to maximise the number of cases where the socio-economic status (SES) could be calculated. However, it could be included as a separate variable in the analysis.

The SES score did not use household income because, again, there was a substantial amount of missing data on this variable (however, it has a fairly high correlation, around 0.5, with household income).

The SES score, as devised, relates to the household. Consequently, for the data on individual health (where there is one set for each individual in the dwelling), the SES variables were taken to be the same for each person in that household.

References

Brody D.S. *et al* (1998) Identifying patients with depression in the primary care setting: a more efficient method. *Arch Intern Med* 158(22): 2469–75.

Kearns A., Hiscods R., Ellaway A., Macintyre S. (2000) 'Beyond four walls'. The psycho-social benefits of home: evidence from West Central Scotland. *Housing Studies* 15(3): 367–410.

---

[8]By Maggie Davidson of the UK Building Research Establishment.

6 Potential sources of indoor air pollution and asthma and allergic diseases

Isabella Annesi-Maesano and David Moreau

Introduction

Scientific interest in indoor air pollution started in earnest during the second half of the 1980s (Viegi *et al* 2004) mainly to investigate risk factors that may have been contributing to the rise in prevalence of diseases and conditions such as asthma, allergic rhinitis and eczema since the 1970s (Sly 1999). Nowadays, these diseases have become increasingly common in industrialised countries (up to one individual in 3) and are being found in developing countries, resulting in a huge socio-economic burden at world level (O'Connell 2004).

The development and phenotypic expression of asthma and allergies depend on a complex interaction between genetic factors, environmental exposure to allergens and non-specific adjuvant factors, such as infections, diet, tobacco smoke and indoor and outdoor air pollution. Only those factors that have significantly changed in the past decades are likely to have contributed to the increase in the prevalence of such diseases. One of these factors, indoor pollution, has increased through changes in the design and construction of dwellings, the introduction of new building and cleaning materials, of do-it-yourself products, and changes in human activities. Western lifestyles now mean that people generally spend more of their time indoors where the concentration of several pollutants can be many times higher than outdoors (Bardana 2001). Lastly, poverty, lack of investment in modern technology and weak environmental legislation have combined to cause high indoor pollution levels in some countries (Briggs 2003).

Combustion products, allergens and volatile organic compounds (VOCs) are the main indoor air pollutants found in dwellings (Table 6.1). Cooking, unvented gas and kerosene (paraffin) heaters, wood, oil, and coal burning, tobacco smoking, and penetration from outdoors are the main sources of indoor nitrogen dioxide (NO_2), and the concentration is often higher than outdoors. Using biomass

Table 6.1 Evidence of indoor pollutants (n = 3,373 dwellings)

Pollutant	Source	Prevalence
Combustion products		
Nitrogen dioxide (NO_2)	Gas ranges and pilot lights, unvented kerosene (paraffin) and gas heaters	Gas space & water heater: 17.0% connected to outside; 4.4% not connected. Gas stove: 6.8%
Respirable particles	Tobacco smoke, wood and coal combustion, fireplaces	Solid fuel (coal, wood): 2.1% Oil: 0.2%
Carbon monoxide (CO)	Gas ranges and pilot lights, unvented kerosene and gas heaters, wood and coal combustion, tobacco smoke	Kerosene: 0.1%
Environmental tobacco smoke (ETS)	Tobacco from cigarettes, cigars, pipes	1–15 cigarettes/day in the dwelling: 20.7% >15 cigarettes/day in the dwelling: 10%
VOCs and formaldehyde		
Aldehydes, aliphatic halogenated hydrocarbons, aromatic hydrocarbons, terpenes and formaldehyde	Furniture, solvents, paints, adhesives, cleaning products, combustion of gas, tobacco, and wood, insulation materials	Do-it-yourself activities and having brought new furniture: 64.9%
Allergens		
Acarids: house dust mites	Dust, bedding, carpeting Faeces (main source)	NA
Cats	Pets Saliva, dandruff	Cats: 14.8%
Dogs	Dandruff	Dogs: 20.95%
Rodents	Urine	Rodents: 3.1%
Birds	Feathers	Birds: 5.4%
Rats, mice	Pests Urine	Rats & mice: 3.9%,
Insects	Saliva and faeces	Mites: 4.4%. Cockroaches: 9.6%
Mites	Faeces	
Fungi (moulds)	Humidity, dampness	Dampness: 34.3% according to the inhabitants, 25.5% according to the surveyor Moulds: 23.5% according to the inhabitants, 39.9% according to the surveyor
Pollens	Plants	NA

Adapted from Viegi et al 2004. VOCs, volatile organic compounds; NA, not applicable.

Indoor air pollution, asthma and allergic diseases

(e.g. wood or coal for cooking and/or heating) can produce carbon monoxide (CO), nitrogen monoxide (NO) and particulate matter (PM). PM includes inorganic acids (e.g. sulphates or nitrates), smoke (containing polycyclic aromatic hydrocarbons), fine dust, residues of lead and asbestos, and can remain suspended for hours or days, especially in winter. Environmental tobacco smoke (ETS) is a main contributor to indoor PM.

VOCs include aromatic hydrocarbons, aldehydes, aliphatic halogenated hydrocarbons and terpenes, and sources include furniture, building materials, floor and wall coverings, paints, and urea formaldehyde foam insulation (UFFI). VOCs are also given off from cosmetics, adhesives, cleaning fluids, tobacco smoke and occupant activities. Indoor allergens, which may become airborne, are produced by mites, pets, pests, fungi (moulds) and other biological sources. Moulds can also be a source of other substances that have been shown to have an adverse impact on health, such as mycotoxins, microbial volatile organic compounds (MVOCs) and β glucans (O'Connell 2004; Viegi *et al* 2004).

There is consistent evidence that indoor air pollution increases the risk of asthma and allergic diseases as well as of intermediate phenotypes such as airways irritation, bronchial hyper-responsiveness and atopic sensitisation (Weiss 1994; Bernstein *et al* 2004; Viegi *et al* 2004). The presence of commonly known NO_2 sources (e.g. gas appliances) has been shown to be a risk factor for wheeze and asthma in children, adults, and the elderly, and some studies suggest a dose–response association. Greater effects on more susceptible subjects (i.e. patients with pre-existing mild or severe asthma) have been also observed.

CO has been scarcely studied in relation to allergic and respiratory health. However, an increased risk for wheezing attacks was found in Korean asthmatic children exposed to CO. Common indoor PM sources have been related to wheezing, cough and asthma attacks. Recently, an adverse effect of fine PM in classrooms on allergic sensitisation to indoor allergens was observed in children at the population level (Annesi-Maesano *et al* 2005), which confirmed previous experimental results. Involuntary second-hand smoking (passive smoking) is an important contributor to asthma in both children and adults. VOCs are associated with irritation symptoms of the upper respiratory tract and asthma, particularly in areas that are poorly ventilated. Formaldehyde exposure, even at relatively low levels, has been related to sensory irritation and asthma-like symptoms. Sources of allergens, including house dust mites, pets and cockroaches, can cause allergic sensitisation and give rise to allergic rhinitis, hay fever, asthma and atopic dermatitis. High levels of such allergens may increase bronchial hyper-responsiveness and asthma severity in asthmatic adults.

In this chapter we examine the relationships of indoor air pollution to asthma and allergic diseases using LARES data. We also discuss the combined role of indoor air pollutants, considering factors able to modulate both the exposure and the health outcome.

Indoor air pollution, asthma and allergic diseases

Methods

Measuring exposure

For all potential indoor air pollutants, except mould, the assessment of exposure was based on responses to the Inhabitant Questionnaire; for mould, the Housing Inspection Survey Sheet was used. The presence of a gas cooking stove, and solid fuel, gas, oil or kerosene as the major heating fuel was used as a proxy for exposure to combustion products – namely NO_2, PM and CO. Using the question – How many cigarettes (or other tobacco products) are smoked in the dwelling per day by all the residents – a three-class variable was generated to define exposure to ETS – no cigarettes; 1–15 cigarettes per day; and >15 cigarettes per day. Do-it-yourself activities and having brought new furniture into the dwelling in the past year were used to determine indoor exposure to VOCs. Potential sources of allergens covered by the study included dogs, cats, rodents, birds, cockroaches and mites. Lastly, a three-class variable was created for exposure to moulds according to whether the inhabitant answered 'never', 'seldom or sometimes', or 'often or permanently' to the question: 'Do you have problems with visible mould growth in your dwelling'.

Measuring allergic health outcomes

Only incidents of asthma and allergic diseases during the past 12 months were counted. To try to avoid underdiagnosis, allergic rhinitis was taken to include any nasal allergy (including hay fever), and problems with sneezing, or a runny or a blocked nose when the individual did not have a cold or influenza. Likewise, asthma was taken to include asthma attacks, and asthma-like symptoms, such as wheezing and whistling in the chest. Reports of eczema or any kind of skin allergy were also used. Information was available on whether the disease had been reported, whether a physician had diagnosed it and whether the individual had taken prescribed medicine for it, but for the analysis of the effects of indoor air pollutants, only those diseases confirmed by a doctor were considered.

Confounders

The following potential confounders were considered: sex; age; the interaction between age and sex; smoking habits; socio-economic status (SES) score[1]; and the city. Three age groups were defined for the purpose of the analysis – <18 years, 18–64 years, and >64 years. Those individuals smoking at least one cigarette a

---

[1] See Chapter 5.

Indoor air pollution, asthma and allergic diseases

day were considered to be active smokers. The city was included, as both health outcomes and air pollutants were likely to vary according to residential zones.

Epidemiological and statistical analysis

The odds ratio (OR) was used as a measure of the association between two qualitative variables. Two ORs were estimated to assess associations between indoor air pollution and asthma and allergies: first, the OR between the exposure to each indoor air pollutant and each health outcome after taking potential confounders into account; and, secondly the OR between each air pollutant and each health outcome after taking the other air pollutants and the confounders simultaneously into account. Logistic regression analysis was performed to estimate the adjusted odds ratio (aOR) after adjustment for potential confounders. To investigate any linear dependencies among variables, the collinearity was assessed. A marginal model (Liang and Zeger 1986) was applied in order to take account of the non-independence of data in individuals living in the same residential zone, and who share the same environment in terms of climate, pollens, social factors, food products and diet. The parameters of the marginal model were estimated by the generalized estimating equation (GEE) approach using SAS GENMOD with independent working correlation structure using the city as stratum. Version 8.2 of SAS System for AIX was used for statistical analyses. Statistical significance was provided by a p-value <0.05.

Results

Of the 3,382 dwellings in the LARES study, 3,373 provided useable information. Of these, a gas stove was present in 6.8% of the cases. The other fuels likely to produce combustion products were used more rarely for cooking (See Table 6.1). Gas space and water heaters were used in 21.4% of the dwellings, 17.0% being connected to the outdoors and 4.4% not connected. In 64.9% of the dwellings there were potential sources of VOCs; in 20.7% there was at least one smoker of 1–15 cigarettes per day and in 10% one smoker of at least 15 cigarettes. Pets were spread among the participants of the study, with one dwelling in five having a dog, 14.8% having a cat, 5.4% having a bird and 3.1% having a rodent. Cockroaches were present in 10% of the dwellings, mites in 4.4% and rats and mice in 3.9%.

Nasal allergies were the most frequent disease in the LARES study, followed by asthma and eczema (Figure 6.1). Of the 8,519 useable Inhabitant Questionnaires 27.8% reported nasal problems in the previous year and 12.9% reported suffering from nasal allergy (neither having a cold nor influenza). Nasal problems were reported as confirmed by a doctor for 10% of the respondents and nasal allergies for 8.4%. Wheezing and whistling in the chest in the previous year was reported by 10.4% of respondents and asthma actions by 2.2%. Asthma and

Indoor air pollution, asthma and allergic diseases

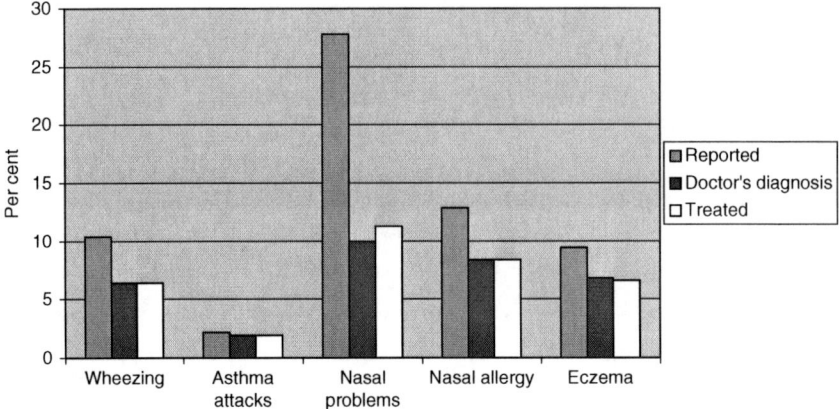

6.1 Prevalence of asthma and allergies in the past year (*n* = 8,519 individuals).

wheezing were confirmed by a doctor for 6.4% and 1.9% of the respondents, respectively. Lastly, eczema was reported by 9.4% of the individuals; 6.8% had a diagnosis of eczema and 6.6% had been treated for it.

Limiting the analysis to diagnosed diseases showed that women suffered more frequently than men from wheezing, nasal allergy and eczema (Table 6.2). Seniors had a higher risk for wheezing and a lower risk for nasal allergy and eczema. No differences in sex and age distribution were observed for the other diagnosed diseases. However, there were important significant variations in the geographical distribution of the allergic diseases (Table 6.3).

The more affluent individuals surveyed (an SES of >80) had more gas water heaters connected to the outside, more potential sources of VOCs, more pets and more infestations of mite (Table 6.4). Gas water heaters not connected to the outside and infestation of pests (but not mites) and cockroaches were related to a low SES. Neither ETS nor moulds depended on the SES in this study.

Table 6.2 Prevalence of doctor-diagnosed asthma and allergies in the past year by age and by sex (*n* = 8,519 individuals)

	Men	Women	Adolescents	Adults	Seniors
Wheezing or whistling in chest	5.1%	7.2%***	5.4%	4.8%	2.6%***
Asthma attacks	1.5%	1.9%	0.9%	1.6%	2.4%
Nasal problems	7.9%	10.7%	9.8%	9.2%	10.4%
Nasal allergy	7.3%	9.8%***	9.8%	9.2%	6.2%**
Eczema	5.0%	7.5%***	8.0%	6.3%	6.2%

Table 6.3 Percentage prevalence of doctor-diagnosed asthma and allergies in the past year by city (n = 8,519 individuals)

	Angers	Bonn	Bratislava	Budapest	Ferreira	Forli	Geneva	Vilnius	p
Wheezing	6.9	6.0	3.1	6.0	7.7	6.0	6.3	6.8	*
Asthma attack	2.6	2.0	0.7	1.2	2.0	1.4	3.3	1.4	**
Problem with nose	12.8	8.4	11.1	6.3	12.7	8.2	8.9	8.2	***
Nasal allergy	9.0	11.6	11.0	10.9	6.6	7.6	10.3	5.7	***
Eczema	7.9	8.8	8.3	5.7	4.6	7.2	7.9	3.8	***

Indoor air pollution, asthma and allergic diseases

Table 6.4 Percentage prevalence of indoor air pollutants according to percentiles of the socio-economic index

	<20	20–40	40–60	60–80	>80	p*
Combustion products						
ETS, number of cigarettes/day, %						
≤ 15	19.6	18.4	20.7	22.2	23.0	
> 15	8.1	10.1	11.6	10.5	9.0	NS
Gas water heater						
connected, %	12.0	16.5	15.2	18.3	21.5	
not connected, %	6.3	5.0	3.4	5.1	2.4	< 0.001
Gas stove, %	9.1	7.7	6.1	4.9	6.0	< 0.05
Solid fuel (coal, wood), %	3.2	2.5	2.0	0.9	1.4	< 0.05
VOCs						
New furniture, do-it-yourself works, %	54.2	61.9	66.7	69.4	73.6	< 0.001
Allergens						
Having a dog, %	10.3	17.9	24.9	24.6	29.1	< 0.001
Having a cat, %	8.7	14.4	16.2	16.3	19.2	< 0.001
Having a bird, %	2.50	4.93	4.98	7.04	8.19	< 0.001
Having a rodent, %	0.32	2.40	3.51	4.54	4.25	< 0.01
Presence of rats, mice, %	6.1	3.9	3.9	2.7	2.6	< 0.01
Presence of cockroaches, %	11.9	10.8	8.7	9.1	7.3	< 0.05
Presence of mites, %	2.3	3.6	3.5	6.9	6.2	< 0.001
Moulds						
Seldom, %	13.9	15.3	16.9	18.9	17.8	
Often, %	12.2	10.1	12.5	12.0	12.4	NS

ETS, environmental tobacco smoke; VOC, volatile organic compound.
* test.
χ^2 test.

Gas water heaters not connected to the outside were more likely to be in dwellings occupied by elderly people; individuals aged less than 65 years were exposed to more sources of VOCs than others; and exposure to ETS was found to be significantly related to age (0–17 and 18–64 years, respectively). Dwellings occupied by elderly people had fewer pets than the others, but had more infestations of rats and mice, whereas the presence of cockroaches and other pests was not found to be related to either sex or age.

After adjustment for confounders, various effects of indoor exposures were observed on diagnosed symptoms and diseases (Table 6.5). The odds of suffering from a wheezing were significantly increased in dwellings with rats, mice, cockroaches and moulds. Asthma attacks were significantly related to having a gas water heater not connected to the outside and also to the extent of moulds in the home.

Table 6.5 Prevalence of doctor-diagnosed asthma and allergies in the past year according to exposure to indoor air pollutants

	Wheezing		Asthma attacks		Nasal problems		Nasal allergy		Eczema	
	%	Adj OR	%	Adj OR	%	Adj OR	%	Adj OR	%	Adj OR
Combustion products										
ETS										
No	6.3		2.1	1.00	10.3		9.2	1.00	7.3	1.00
≤15 cig/d	6.5		1.3	0.63 [0.40, 0.99]	9.7		7.6	0.84 [0.69, 1.02]	5.8	0.83 [0.66, 1.05]
>15 cig/d	6.8		1.3*	0.60 [0.33, 1.10]	8.4		5.7**	0.58 [0.43, 0.78]	6.0*	0.87 [0.64, 1.16]
Gas water heater										
No	6.2		1.8	1.00	9.6		8.4		7.1	1.00
Connected	6.8		2.0	1.26 [0.77, 2.04]	11.0		8.3		6.4	0.92 [0.70, 1.20]
Not connected	8.7		3.8*	2.23 [1.12, 4.45]	11.3		8.7		2.9**	0.44 [0.23, 0.85]
Gas stove										
No	6.4		1.8		10.1		8.5		6.9	
Yes	7.0		2.7		8.6		8.1		6.3	
Solid fuel										
No	6.4		1.9		10.0		8.6	1.00	6.9	1.00
Yes	5.6		1.7		7.3		3.4*	0.43 [0.18, 1.07]	1.7**	0.35 [0.11, 1.11]
VOCs										
No	6.4		1.8		9.9		8.2		6.5	
Yes	6.5		1.9		10.0		8.5		7.0	
Allergens										
Having a dog										
No	6.5		2.0	1.00	9.9		8.7		7.1	1.00
Yes	6.2		1.3*	0.75 [0.47, 1.16]	10.1		7.6		5.8*	0.90 [0.72, 1.23]
Having a cat										
No	6.3		1.9		10.1		8.7		6.7	
Yes	6.8		1.8		9.5		7.3		7.2	

Adj OR: odds ratio adjusted for town, sex, age, interaction between age and sex, smoking habit and socio-economic score. ETS, environment tobacco smoke; cig/d,cigarettes per day.
*** $p < 10^{-3}$; **, $p < 0.01$; *, $p < 0.05$.

Table 6.5 (Cont'd)

	Wheezing		Asthma attacks		Nasal problems		Nasal allergy		Eczema	
	%	Adj OR	%	Adj OR	%	Adj OR	%	Adj OR	%	Adj OR
Rats, mice										
No	6.2	1.00	1.8		9.8	1.00	8.5		6.9	
Yes	10.5**	1.60 [1.09, 2.34]	1.5		13.7*	1.58 [1.14, 2.20]	8.7	5.1		
Cockroaches										
No	6.2	1.00	1.8		10.0		8.7	1.00	6.9	
Yes	8.1*	1.36 [1.02, 1.81]	2.1		10.2		6.3*	0.85 [0.63, 1.16]	6.6	
Mites										
No	6.9		2.2		9.8	1.00	8.1	1.00	6.5	1.00
Yes	6.4		1.8		13.7***	1.48 [1.09, 2.02]	13.7***	1.59 [1.17, 2.16]	12.0***	1.67 [1.20, 2.32]
Moulds										
No	5.4	1.00	1.5	1.00	8.6	1.00	8.5	1.00	6.8	1.00
Yes	8.1**	1.53 [1.16, 2.03]	3.5***	2.72 [1.74, 4.24]	14.8***	1.70 [1.37, 2.11]	10.5	1.46 [1.15, 1.87]	8.9**	1.55 [1.19, 2.02]

Adj OR: odds ratio adjusted for town, sex, age, interaction between age and sex, smoking habit and socio-economic score. ETS, environment tobacco smoke; cig/d, cigarettes per day.
*** $p < 10^{-3}$; **, $p < 0.01$; *, $p < 0.05$.

Table 6.6 Odds ratios between doctor-diagnosed asthma and allergies in the past year and indoor air pollutants – logistic regression models including all the air pollutants and the confounders at the same time

	Wheezing (Adj OR)	Asthma attacks (Adj OR)	Nasal problems (Adj OR)	Nasal allergy (Adj OR)	Eczema (Adj OR)
ETS					
No		1.00		1.00	
≤15 cig/d		0.60 [0.36, 1.01]		0.80 [0.64, 1.00]	
>15 cig/d		0.67 [0.34, 1.31]		0.59 [0.43, 0.82]	
Gas water heater					
None		1.00			1.00
Connected		1.43 [0.83, 2.45]			0.97 [0.71, 1.32]
Not connected		2.18 [1.01, 4.70]			0.52 [0.26, 1.01]
Rats and mice					
No	1.00		1.00		
Yes	1.50 [0.97, 2.32]		1.55 [1.08, 2.22]		
Cockroaches					
No	1.00				
Yes	1.00 [0.70, 1.43]				
Mites					
No			1.00	1.00	1.00
Yes			1.41 [1.00, 2.00]	1.58 [1.14, 2.20]	1.68 [1.21, 2.34]
Moulds					
No	1.00	1.00	1.00	1.00	1.00
Yes	1.45 [1.08, 1.95]	2.91 [1.84, 4.59]	1.64 [1.31, 2.06]	1.53 [1.20, 1.97]	1.55 [1.18, 2.04]

ETS, environmental, tobacco smoke; cig/d, cigarettes per day. Adj OR: odds ratio adjusted for town, sex, age, interaction between age and sex, smoking habit and socio-economic score.

Indoor air pollution, asthma and allergic diseases

Nasal problems, nasal allergy and eczema were associated with the presence of mites and moulds. Nasal problems were also more frequent in dwellings with infestations of rats and mice. There was a significant negative association of ETS in the home with asthma attacks, nasal allergy and eczema. The analysis of the joint effects of main indoor exposures adjusted for all other factors confirmed the results for moulds, rats and mice, gas appliances and ETS (Table 6.6), but the effect of mites and cockroaches disappeared. The results persisted when applying the marginal model.

Discussion

In the LARES study, asthma and allergic symptoms and diseases were significantly related to sources of potential NO_2 emissions, sources of potential allergens and the presence of moulds. This coincides with findings reported in the literature (Viegi and Annesi-Maesano 1999; Viegi et al 2004).

Although the cross-sectional nature of the LARES study did not provide evidence on causality, the data allowed for analyses of new dimensions of the relationship between exposure and health effects. First, sources of potential pollutants such as cockroaches, rats and mice, and VOCs, for which there is experimental evidence of health effects, were explored at population level. All but the VOCs were significantly related to asthma and allergies even after allowing for confounders. The analyses also confirmed the inverse relationship between ETS and asthma and allergies found in previous studies (Weiss 1994). This could be a result of under-reporting of active smoking when there is someone not well in the household. However, this could also be explained by a defence mechanism of individuals who have been diagnosed with allergies (Hjern et al 2001), which is recognised for nasal allergy and eczema but less for asthma (Annesi-Maesano et al 2004). Secondly, the concomitant role of various potential indoor air pollutants was also investigated. This affected the results only when the potential pollutants were highly correlated with one another (multicollinearity), as in the case of moulds and pests. Adjustment for confounders also contributed to a better understanding of the role of indoor air pollutants. The observed effects of possible indoor air pollutants did not depend on an individual's age, sex, and SES, or on whether the individual was an active smoker. Nor did it depend on the city of residence, even though a city effect was expected because of important variations in both the distribution of air pollutants and the health systems. In this respect, the data from the LARES study give a unique opportunity to dispose of data of heterogeneous cities on exposure and diseases.

A major limit of the present study results from the assessment of the exposure to possible indoor air pollution. Exposure is usually defined as the contact of the pollutant with the individual and is quantified according to two dimensions: intensity and duration (Viegi and Annesi-Maesano 1999). Such an exhaustive definition was not possible in the LARES study, as information on intensity and duration was not collected. However, epidemiological studies have shown that indirect methods for assessing indoor exposure through questionnaires can also be conclusive (Reijula and Sundman-Digert 2004). But this was not the case for VOCs, as the question was not sensitive enough on the duration of any exposure. Another limit derives from the self-reported assessment of health outcome. However, potential misclassification of asthma and other allergies was avoided by taking into account the doctor's diagnosis, which provided prevalences comparable to those of previous sparse studies.

The strategy chosen for the analysis did not clarify the issue of whether city and individual characteristics mediate (to some extent) asthma and allergies. However, it contributes to establishing the relationships between various indoor air pollutants and asthma and allergies after adjustment for these characteristics.

Conclusions

The analyses on the relationships between air pollution and allergic diseases suggest that reducing exposure to both allergens and adjuvant risk/protective factors may prevent manifestations of asthma and allergies. These measures may be applicable to the population generally, to children at risk of developing asthma and allergic disease (high-risk infants), to children with chronic disease and to the elderly (de Blay and Birba 2003).

References

Annesi-Maesano I., Oryszczyn M.P., Raherison C. *et al* (2004) Increased prevalence of asthma and allied diseases among active adolescent tobacco smokers after controlling for passive smoking exposure. A cause for concern? *Clin Exp Allergy* 34(7): 1017–23.

Annesi-Maesano I., Caillaud D., De Blay F. *et al* (2005) Adverse effects of particulate air pollution on allergic sensitisation and allergic and respiratory morbidity in a population-based sample of children. The French Six City Study. *Lancet* (submitted).

Bardana E.J. Jr (2001) Indoor pollution and its impact on respiratory health. *Ann Allergy Asthma Immunol* 87(6 Suppl 3): 33–40.

Bernstein J.A., Alexis N., Barnes C. *et al* (2004) Health effects of air pollution. *J Allergy Clin Immunol* 114(5): 1116–23.

Briggs D. (2003) Environmental pollution and the global burden of disease. *Br Med Bull* 68: 1–24.

de Blay F., Birba E. (2003) Controlling indoor allergens. *Curr Opin Allergy Clin Immunol* 3(3): 165–8.

Hjern A., Hedberg A., Haglund B., Rosén M. (2001) Does tobacco smoke prevent atopic disorders? A study of two generations of Swedish residents. *Clin Exp Allergy* 31(6): 908–14.

Liang K.Y., Zeger S.L. (1986) Longitudinal data analysis using generalized linear models. *Biometrika* 73: 13–86.

O'Connell E.J. (2004) The burden of atopy and asthma in children. *Allergy* 59 (Suppl 78): 7–11.

Reijula K., Sundman-Digert C. (2004) Assessment of indoor air problems at work with a questionnaire. *Occup Environ Med* 61(1): 33–8.

Sly R.M. (1999) Changing prevalence of allergic rhinitis and asthma. *Ann Allergy Asthma Immunol* 82(3): 233–48; quiz 248–52.

Viegi G., Annesi-Maesano I. (1999) Lung diseases induced by indoor and outdoor pollutants. In: Mapp CE (ed), Occupational Lung Disorders. *Eur Respir Mon* 4 (Monograph 11): 214–41.

Viegi G., Simoni M., Scognamiglio A. *et al* (2004) Indoor air pollution and airway disease. *Int J Tuberc Lung Dis* 8(12): 1401–15.

Weiss S.T. (1994) Smoking and asthma. *Compr Ther* 20(11): 606–10.

7 Damp, mould and health
Peter Rudnai, Mihaly J. Varro, Tibor Malnasi, Anna Páldy, Simon Nicol and Alan O'Dell

Introduction

Dampness in a dwelling can arise from four principal causes:

- capillary action of groundwater into the structure in contact with the ground, i.e. rising damp in the floor slab and walls
- penetration of the fabric or its joints by rainwater (or meltwater from standing snow)
- traumatic problems, such as burst pipes or overflowing tanks
- condensation – the deposition of moisture from the air onto surfaces.

Rising and penetrating dampness can generally be attributed to design, inadequate construction or disrepair. Traumatic problems may be a result of inadequate frost protection or disrepair.

Condensation can be caused by deficiencies in the design, construction and/or maintenance, or through unreasonable occupier behaviour. Moisture is produced by occupants through their normal biological and domestic activities. Relatively low levels of moisture are generated through breathing and are spread over 24 hours, but there are higher levels produced in peaks from cooking, clothes drying and bathing. A dwelling should be able to cope with a degree of moisture generation appropriate to its size, without resulting in problems of condensation.

Damp, mould and related illness

Moulds are present in all parts of the environment, both outdoors and indoors. They can grow and amplify indoors only when there is an adequate supply of moisture. House dust mites are present in all dwellings, but the numbers dramatically increase in damp conditions. As well as damp surfaces encouraging the formation of mould growth, high relative humidity can also encourage the proliferation of moulds and mites. Such problems can be minimised by not allowing relative humidity in a dwelling to rise above 70%, except for short periods, although reducing relative humidity below 40% is also undesirable in view of the possibility of increasing the incidence of respiratory discomfort and infection. Warm, dry well-ventilated homes are the ideal.

Mould spores and the detritus from dust mites are potent airborne allergens. Exposure to high concentrations of these allergens over a prolonged period can result in sensitisation of atopic individuals (those with a predetermined genetic tendency to sensitisation). Non-atopic individuals can become sensitised following exposure to very high levels of allergen over a prolonged period. Exposure can trigger allergic symptoms such as rhinitis, conjunctivitis, eczema, coughing and wheezing. When a sensitised individual is repeatedly exposed to an allergen, this can cause asthma. There appears to be a dose–response relationship associated with the exposure of sensitised asthmatic individuals to increasing humidity and house dust mite and mould levels (ODPM 2006).

Mould and fungal spores can also be carcinogenic, toxic and cause infections, the potential health effects varying with species. Toxins from some moulds (myotoxins) can cause nausea and diarrhoea, can suppress the immune system and have been implicated in cancers. These health effects are uncommon, but serious if they do occur.

As well as encouraging mould and mites, dampness in clothing and bedding may, by the process of cooling through evaporation, also prejudice the maintenance of body temperatures, particularly in young children and the elderly. Similarly, dampness can be prejudicial to health and safety through its action on the building fabric, lowering the ambient temperature, both by reducing the insulating capacity of external walls and by using up heat in the process of evaporation. Consequently, a marginal heating system can be rendered inadequate by persistent dampness. Persistent dampness will lead to the deterioration of the building fabric, with subsequent effects on the health and safety of the occupants.

Dampness is symptomatic of the quality and/or condition of a home, and it is known that living in a poor-quality home has a depressive effect on the mental health and well-being of the occupants (Douglas *et al* 2003).

Finally, the extent, location, frequency and persistence of any dampness of whatever cause will be particularly important in determining whether this is prejudicial to health.

Measuring the relationship between dampness and ill health

Many studies have found a consistent and significant relationship between respiratory symptoms and damp and mould in dwellings (e.g. Strachan 1993; Peat and Dickerson 1998). Whereas there is little dispute that the presence of dampness and mould growth will increase the likelihood of ill health, studies have found it very difficult to quantify the effect (Dedman *et al* 2001). Dampness is inextricably

Damp, mould and health

linked with other indicators of housing quality, the socio-economic factors of individuals, and location factors, all of which are also important determinants of health. It should also be recognised that people suffering from ill health are likely to spend more time in the home, resulting in higher levels of exposure.

Measuring the exposure is also problematic. Levels of mould spores, humidity and dampness may vary by room and day of assessment, and there are issues around the accuracy of the methods used to measure these specific aspects of housing conditions.

Even if independent associations are established, it may not be clear whether the poor health or the dampness came first. There is also the further complication of a possible time delay from exposure to effect, and it has been shown that poor health in adulthood may be the result of poor housing conditions in childhood (Marsh *et al* 1999; Dedman *et al* 1999).

A comprehensive, expert review of the risks and health hazards of domestic buildings identified mould and house dust mite allergens as some of the highest health risks (Raw *et al* 2001). Further work by Warwick University and the London School of Hygiene and Tropical Medicine to update the statistical base for the Housing Health and Safety Rating System (HHSRS) estimated that the overall likelihood of the most vulnerable individuals (children aged ≤14) showing symptoms of respiratory illness in England in all homes over a 1-year period was 1 in 464 (ODPM 2006). Some 89% of those who suffered through exposure to the risk had symptoms of coughing and wheezing only, whereas 10% had serious conditions and 1% had severe conditions.

Based on these reviews, it seems that an individual living in a damp/mouldy home is some 25 times more likely to suffer from respiratory illness than an individual who lives in a home free from dampness. Although there may be many reasons for this association, it is clear that there is a relationship between dampness and poor health.

Analysis of the WHO LARES dataset

The LARES database included information on conditions in 3,373 dwellings from eight European cities, and health data from 8,519 individuals. This database, with its composition from settlements of various sizes, with various climatic conditions, and various types of houses, provided a unique opportunity to study the housing conditions associated with mould growth and the health conditions of the people living in mouldy homes.

Methods

Data on dampness in the dwelling were derived from the Inhabitant Questionnaire, and also from the Housing Inspection Survey Sheet. Where possible both were used, since they offer complementary advantages; the Housing Inspection Survey Sheet provided a level of objectivity, but a snap-shot, and while the occupants' responses are likely to be more subjective, they have a more intimate knowledge of the dwelling and its problems throughout the year.

The data relate to 'mould growth', which is indicative of high humidity, and to 'dampness' per se, and again, both were used. It is recognised that some allergic conditions are possibly associated with mould spores, so there is a need for a specific 'mould' variable for some analyses. However, when 'damp' is being used in its own right, or as a background variable, it would be preferable to use all the indicators that are available. This suggests that it would be worthwhile to aim for separate measures of 'mould' and 'damp', and a combined measure.

Preliminary analysis showed that:

- From the household's perspective:
  - There is a strong association between the existence of mould within a room and the presence of other signs of damp.
  - There is a reasonably strong association between the presence of damp or mould in one room and its presence in other rooms.
- From the inspector's perspective:
  - There is an association between the presence of different symptoms of damp, but not as strong as those evident in the household data. It is weakest between 'condensation' and 'the smell of damp', and strongest between 'the smell of damp' and 'peeling wall-paper or paint' and also between 'mould' and 'peeling paper' (the strongest association with 'mould').
  - There is an association between symptoms in different rooms which is comparable with that found within the household data, and of quite a similar pattern.
- There is very good agreement between inspectors and households on the incidence of mould growth. For almost all rooms, the 'existence' of mould, as experienced by the household, lies somewhere between 'a few spots' and 'postcard-size patches', as reported by the inspectors.

We made use of additive scores obtained by counting the number of rooms affected, and by incorporating the information available on the relative seriousness of the problem (scale of mould; frequency and duration of mould and dampness). Separate indices of dampness, and mould growth, derived from households and inspectors, have been constructed, as well as various combination indices. For the initial analyses of the incidence of dampness, simple graphical methods and data mining techniques (CHAID) were used. For the relationship between dampness/mould and ill health, bivariate logistic regression has been used.

Results

Incidence of dampness/mould

The extent of mould growth reported in the LARES survey is summarised in Table 7.1. Data from surveyors and households agree on the most seriously affected rooms in the dwelling, and that mould growth occurs in around 1 dwelling in 10. In only about one-third of these cases are the areas of mould greater than about A3 size, and in only about one-half are they anything but temporary. Some 6.4% of households reported dampness that occurs often or permanently, compared with 5.6% who reported a similar frequency of mould growth.

The variation between the cities in the study is wide (Table 7.2). In Geneva and Bratislava only around 22% of households experience any problems of dampness, whereas in Forlì the percentage is 37% and in Ferreira over 70%.

Differences in construction methods, building materials and age of the building can change the propensity for problems associated with dampness and therefore might go some way to explaining inter-city variations. But other factors may be important. The internal environment of the dwelling will have an effect, and this will depend upon the heating and ventilation systems, the clothes-drying habits of the household and the intensity of use of the dwelling.

CHAID modelling was used to explore the relationship of some of these factors to dampness and mould problems. The results of modelling a range of the indices are summarised in Table 7.3. For each index, two values of the threshold (>0 and >2) were used. And in each case two models were produced, one allowing 'city' as an independent variable and one excluding it. In Figure 7.3, the shaded boxes indicate the extra variables which enter the model when 'city' is excluded.

Table 7.1 Summary of basic data on mould growth

Surveyor view	Percentage of dwellings affected by mould					Household view
	Any	>Postcard	>A3	>1 sq m	Some	
Kitchen	10.1	4.1	2.1	0.8	7.2	Kitchen
Bathroom	13.1	5.9	2.7	1.2	9.9	Bathroom
WC	2.5	1.1	0.5	0.2	0.9	WC
Corridor	4.7	2	0.9	0.4	2	Corridor
Room 1	7.6	3.4	2.3	1.1		
Room 2	9.7	4.8	2.7	0.9	6.3	Living room
Room 3	8.5	5.2	1.9	1.1	11.8	Bedroom
Room 4	3.2	1.2	0.7	0.3		

Damp, mould and health

Table 7.2 Per cent of dwellings with dampness and mould by city

	Per cent of dwellings with problems of dampness or condensation				
	Never/no	Seldom	Sometimes	Often	Permanent
Angers	63.5	7.3	12.0	7.3	9.9
Bonn	71.2	9.1	8.3	3.9	7.5
Bratislava	77.5	8.0	7.7	4.1	2.7
Budapest	68.2	10.4	5.9	9.7	5.9
Ferreira	27.6	13.2	23.4	23.9	11.8
Forlì	63.0	8.9	16.7	6.3	5.1
Geneva	78.9	5.5	8.6	4.0	3.1
Vilnius	71.6	6.2	9.9	7.1	5.2

	Per cent of dwellings with problems of visible mould				
	Never/no	Seldom	Sometimes	Often	Permanent
Angers	78.5	5.0	4.2	4.5	7.8
Bonn	81.3	5.7	4.4	1.8	6.7
Bratislava	87.6	5.0	2.1	1.5	3.8
Budapest	78.7	5.6	7.2	2.5	6.0
Ferreira	36.2	15.2	25.0	16.6	7.0
Forlì	75.6	9.7	8.1	3.8	2.8
Geneva	87.3	4.0	4.6	1.9	2.2
Vilnius	81.8	4.1	4.9	2.5	6.6

The different indicies produced different models, but there is something of a pattern:

- House type and building age do not seem to make a significant contribution, which indicates that it is not the superficial differences in the housing stock which cause the inter-city variations.
- However, the level of disrepair does appear important in virtually all the models. Disrepair is probably associated with rising or penetrating damp through the external envelope.
- The other significant variables are related to the heating in the dwelling – the existence of central heating and the perception of cold as reported by the household. These are likely to be associated with condensation.
- For several of the indices the 'city' variable appears in its own right, indicating that there is some variation which is not being explained by the more specific variables. In those cases where 'city' is important, when this variable is excluded from the analysis, its place tends to be taken by heating aspects linked to condensation.

Table 7.3 CHAID models of dampness and humidity indices

Dampness index	CHAID explanatory variables			
	First level	Second level	Third level	
Household mould >0 View	City	Disrepair	WinterCold	NumPeople
	Heating	Disrepair	Neighbourhood	WinterCold	NumPeople
Household mould >2 View	City	Disrepair	WinterCold	Disrepair	City
	Heating	WinterCold		BuildingAge	Disrepair
Household humidity >0 View	WinterCold	Disrepair	Heating	Climate	Heating	HouseType	NumPeople
	WinterCold	Disrepair	Heating	HouseType	Climate	Heating	HouseType	NumPeople
Household humidity >2 View	WinterCold	Disrepair	Heating	Neighbourhood Climate	Laundry
	WinterCold	Disrepair	Heating	Neighbourhood Climate	Laundry
Surveyor mould >0 View	Disrepair	City	Neighbourhood	WinterCold	Disrepair
	Disrepair	Heating	Neighbourhood Climate	WinterCold	Disrepair	Climate
Surveyor mould >2 View	Disrepair	City	Neighbourhood Heating	Heating
	Disrepair	Climate	Neighbourhood Heating	BuildingAge
Combined mould >0 View	City	Disrepair	WinterCold	NumPeople
	Heating	Disrepair	Neighbourhood	NumPeople	WinterCold
Combined mould >2 View	Heating	Disrepair	Disrepair	WinterCold
	Heating	Disrepair	Disrepair	WinterCold

HouseType – housing type, as specified in questionnaire.
BuildingAge – as specified, in questionnaire.
Neighbourhood – neighbourhood type, as specified in questionnaire.
Disrepair – 'none', 'minor', 'major' or 'severe', based upon a room by room assessment by surveyors.
WinterCold – winter temperature problems reported by households on a five-point scale from 'never' to 'permanent'.
Heating – existence and extent of central heating ('none', 'partial' and 'full').
Laundry – where laundry is dried ('outside', 'kitchen, etc.', 'living rooms, etc.').
Climate – three-point scale.
NumPeople – household size.

Damp, mould and health

- There does not seem to a particular link between the mould indices and the internal environment variables which are normally associated with condensation. Disrepair and heating seem to be equally associated with dampness and mould growth.

The predictions of the combined surveyor and household index are shown in Table 7.4. 'City' is not a significant independent variable in this model: the significant variables are disrepair and heating/coldness. The model gives reasonable predictions of the number of properties suffering mould for most cities, and reasonable predictions of the rank ordering of cities.

The relationship between illness and dampness/mould growth

For the majority of illnesses or conditions, the proportion of persons affected is relatively small. Since the proportion of dwellings with damp/mould problems is also small, it is unlikely that we shall be able to detect a relationship between the two factors unless the correlation is high.

The analysis of the relationship between the incidence of illness reported in the survey and dampness/mould has been standardised by using a common indicator. The indicator selected is a four-point scale based on the quantity of mould as observed by the inspector:

- no mould/dampness
- a little mould/dampness
- some mould/dampness
- much mould/dampness.

Figure 7.1 shows the distribution of all homes using this 'mould index' in the LARES study.

Bivariate logistic regression was undertaken for all chronic illnesses, acute illnesses and specific symptoms/conditions reported in the survey against this mould indicator. The formal identification of a relationship is complicated because there may be a particular threshold of 'mould' at which the relationship 'kicks in'. Even if a relationship could be detected this might not be a causal relationship, and it might not even be one which acts directly between the specific illness and mould without the intervention of other factors. For this exercise it was decided that, for a relationship between illness and mould to be considered significant, there must be:

- evidence of a dose effect
- a logistic regression significance of $p < 0.001$ at the highest dose (much mould dampness).

Table 7.4 Predictions of one of the CHAID models

City	Per cent of dwellings damp (index > 0)	Combined (surveyor/householder) mould index (index > 0)				Combined (surveyor/householder) module index (index > 2)			
		Explanatory variables	Actual number damp	Predicted number damp	Rank (actual: predicted)	Explanatory variables	Actual number damp	Predicted number damp	Rank (Actual: predicted)
Geneva	3%	Heating	7	13	1:1	Heating	0	1.8	1:2
Bratislava	6%		16	20	2:2		1	2.2	2:1
Bonn	8%	Disrepair	25	23	3:3	Disrepair	3	2.6	4:3
Vilnius	8%		42	59	4:7	Neighbourhood	8	8.9	6:6
Budapest	9%		32	35	5:6		8	7.2	7:7
Angers	11%	WinterCold	34	25	6:4	NumPeople	5	3.0	5:4
Forlì	13%		89	86	7:5	WinterCold	2	3.2	3:5
Ferreira	45%		89	86	8:8		16	14.1	8:8

HouseType – housing type, as specified in questionnaire.
BuildingAge – as specified, in questionnaire.
Neighborhood – neighbourhood type, as specified in questionnaire.
Disrepair – 'none', 'minor', 'major' or 'severe', based upon a room by room assessment by surveyors.
WinterCold – winter temperature problems reported by households on a five-point scale from 'never' to 'permanent'.
Heating – existence and extent of central heating ('none', 'partial' and 'full').
Laundry – where laundry is dried ('outside', 'kitchen, etc.', 'living rooms, etc.').
Climate – three-point scale.
NumPeople – household size.

Damp, mould and health

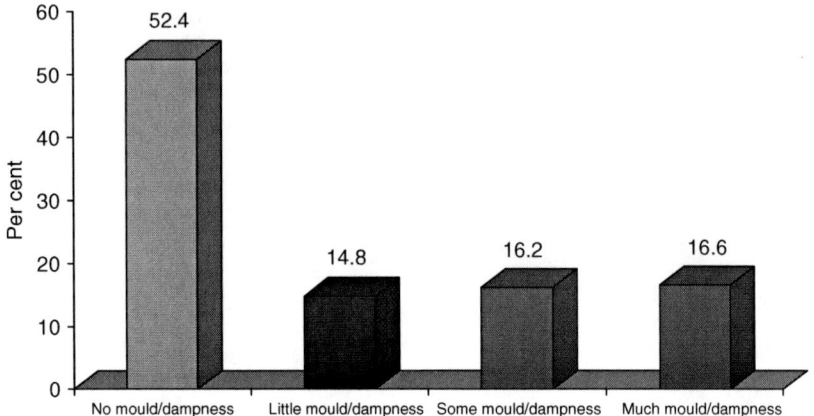

7.1 LARES – distribution of homes by mould indicator.

Analysis of Figures 7.2–7.5 shows that there seems to be definite relationships between mould and:

- anxiety/depression and migraine/frequent headaches, from the group of chronic illnesses
- diarrhoea and cold/throat illnesses, from the acute illnesses
- asthma, wheezing, eczema, watery eyes/eye inflammation and headaches, from the list of symptoms.

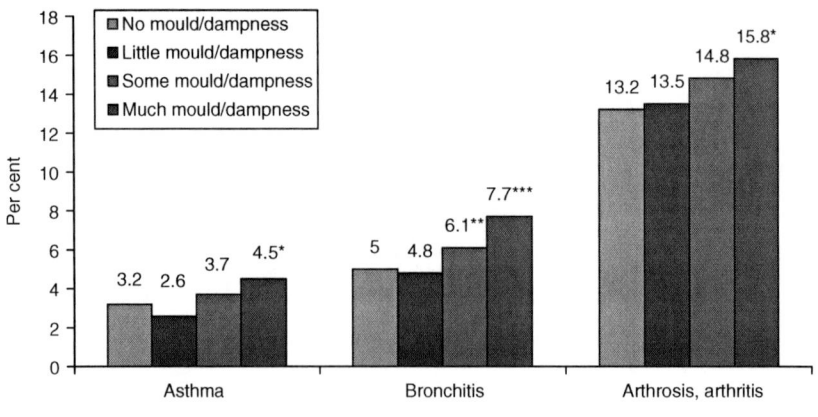

$^*p <0.05$ $^{**}p <0.01$ $^{***}p <0.001$

7.2 LARES – prevalence of some chronic diseases by mould indicator.

Damp, mould and health

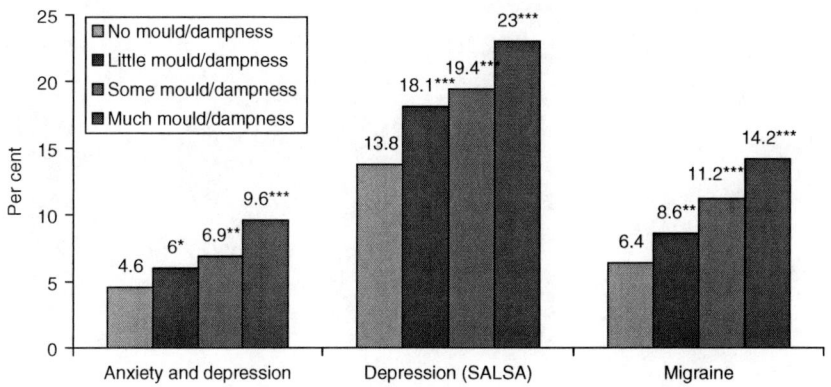

*p <0.05   **p <0.01   ***p <0.001

7.3 LARES – prevalence of some chronic diseases by mould indicator.

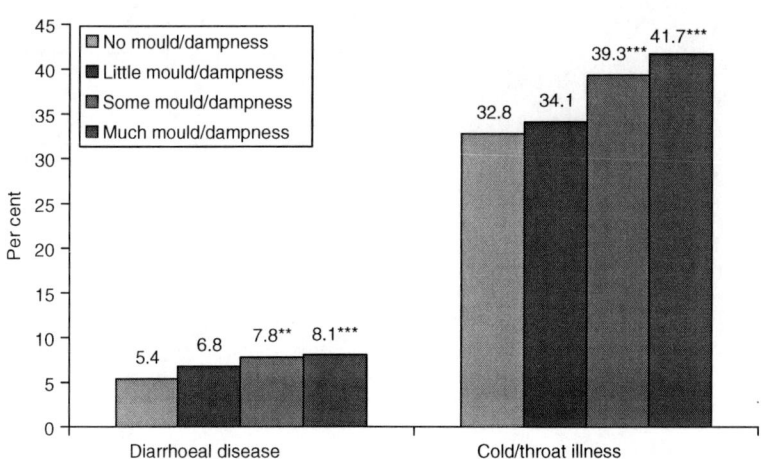

*p <0.05   **p <0.01   ***p <0.001

7.4 LARES – prevalence of people with some acute illnesses in the last 12 months by mould indicator.

Damp, mould and health

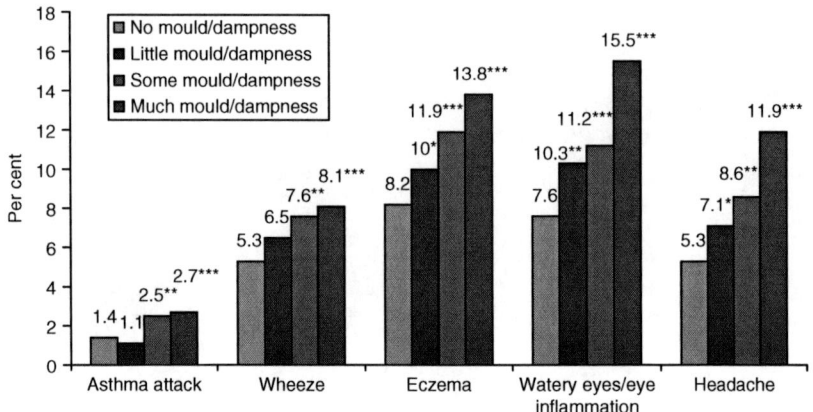

*p <0.05 **p <0.01 ***p <0.001

7.5 LARES – prevalence of some symptoms during the last 12 months by mould indicator.

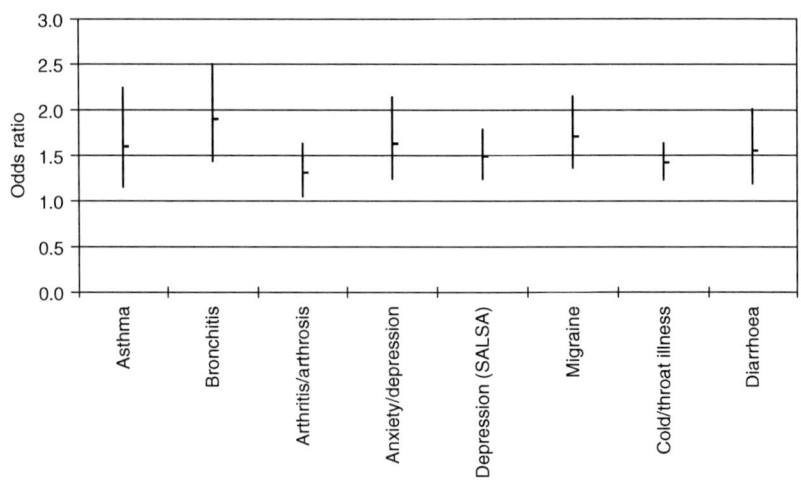

*Adjusted to age, sex, socio-economic status (SES), city, smoking and environmental tobacco smoke (ETS).

7.6 LARES – adjusted odds ratios* of some chronic and acute diseases among people living in homes with much mould/dampness (vs no mould/dampness).

Damp, mould and health

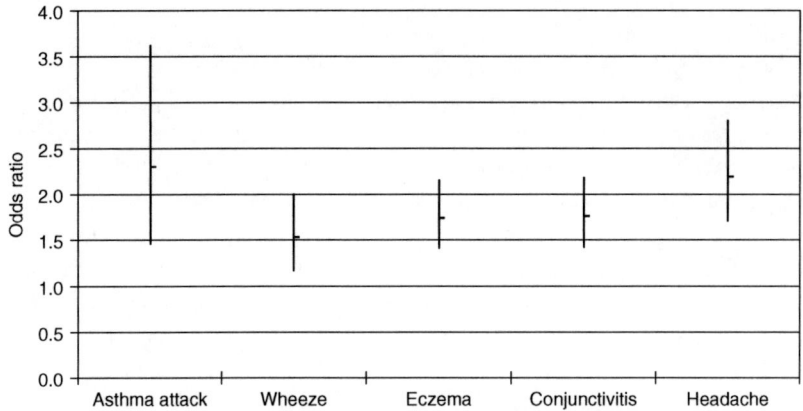

7.7 LARES-adjusted odds ratios* of the prevalence of some symptoms in the last 12 months among people living in homes with much mould/dampness.

Figures 7.6 and 7.7 show the association between those illnesses and symptoms: the logistic regression was shown to be significant, and remains significant even when adjusted for age, sex, socio-economic status, city, smoking and environmental tobacco smoke.

Discussion

Epidemiological studies have clearly demonstrated the link between dampness/growth of fungi in the indoor environment and health risk of the occupants, including irritations of the throat and eyes, allergies, asthma, depression and general symptoms such as tiredness, dizziness and headache (Jacob *et al* 2002; Zock *et al* 2002; Butler *et al* 2003; Moriske *et al* 2003). Some of these effects are related to allergy, whereas others are related to infection or toxicity (Terr 2004). Most of the studies could not derive a dose–response relationship between the measured concentration of fungi and the registered health problems.

The LARES survey was not designed to include any kind of measurements in the dwellings, but the detailed and well-documented inspection of the homes by the interviewers provided a good basis to create a four-graded mould variable that included not only the subjective statement of the occupants but also the judgment of the interviewers. In this way, for some chronic diseases, a clear-cut dose–response relationship was found between their prevalence and the degree of mould growth and dampness in the homes.

Questionnaire-based epidemiological studies often suffer from imprecision of the disease or symptom prevalence. We tried to avoid this trap by relying only on the diseases and symptoms diagnosed by a doctor, though reported by the occupants. Still, some recall bias cannot be excluded, as 31% of the occupants experienced an asthma attack during the last 12 months and considered that their health condition was related to the dwelling. In the case of other health problems, with the exception of frequent sneezing, runny or blocked nose and chronic bronchitis, most people did not consider the dwelling as a risk factor for their health status.

One-third of the sample population lived in homes with some or considerable mould and/or dampness, and suffered serious health problems. Asthma diagnosed by a doctor and attacks of asthma during the last 12 months were strongly associated with mouldy homes. There was also a significantly increased risk for doctor-diagnosed chronic bronchitis among people living in damp or mouldy houses. Nasal allergy, sneezing, runny nose, cold or throat illness, wheezing and eczema during the last year were also significantly associated with mould growth in the home. Other types of allergies and skin diseases, however, did not show significant relation to damp or mouldy houses.

Besides the respiratory symptoms, fatigue, headache, chronic anxiety and depression were also significantly associated with mouldy homes. The observed increased risk for arthritis may be the result of dampness rather than mould growth. The odds ratios (ORs) of cerebral stroke, heart attack and hypertension adjusted to age, sex, socio-economic status, city, smoking and environmental tobacco smoke indicated significantly increased risk associated with a high amount of moulds in the homes; however, in this case, there was no evidence of a dose–response relationship.

To test whether the given associations could be explained by the known role of anxiety in these cardiovascular conditions, we included doctor-diagnosed anxiety together with hypertension, or heart attack or cerebral stroke in the model. Although anxiety was very strongly associated with all the three conditions, mould still remained a significant independent determinant of these cardiovascular diseases. However, due to the cross-sectional nature of the survey, it is not possible to make any assumption on the temporal relationship of the exposure and these health outcomes.

It is recognised that the existence of a relationship does not imply anything about cause and effect or imply a direct connection between the illness and dampness/mould, since there could be other factors which mediate the relationship.

It might not actually be dampness and/or mould in the building that is the primary driving force in the relationship. It was shown earlier that one of the best predictors of dampness in a dwelling is the overall level of disrepair, and it could be that the relationship is between illness and general disrepair, or even between illness and the overall quality of the housing. Also, the physical symptoms are of a type that could be conceivably regarded as being brought on by the emotional response to circumstances.

These conclusions seem very reasonable; so it would be unwise to argue the case, from this data source, for direct cause-and-effect links between dampness/mould in a dwelling and the health of the occupants. Indeed, an analysis using multivariate procedures has indicated that the contribution of dwelling dampness/mould to anxiety and depression is very small compared to social and demographic factors. But, nevertheless, there is a residual 'damp/mould' effect that suggests its presence is a contributory factor to ill health.

Summary and conclusions

The LARES study adds to the knowledge base on disrepair and dampness and the relationship with the health of the occupiers. However, it is inevitably constrained by the small samples of significantly damp/mouldy homes and possibly related illnesses. The most significant associations between illness and the existence of dampness/mould seem to occur with mental or emotional conditions (such as anxiety or depression) and 'cold-like' symptoms.

More detailed analysis on the incidence of 'anxiety or depression' shows strong variation with age and gender of the person affected: older people are more prone to the condition than the young, and women more than men. However, there is a residual variation with dampness/mould; and as far as can be ascertained, given the small sample sizes, this relationship runs through most, if not all, of the age/gender categories. Further work shows that the role of dampness can be taken by other variables, notably age of building and city. This would suggest that something like 'housing quality' is the underlying factor, modifying the simple effects of age and gender of the person suffering the illness. But even 'housing quality' may be acting as a proxy for other social or economic factors that are the real causes.

The LARES study supports the view that poor-quality housing, of which dampness is a symptom, is more likely to contain occupants with poor health and negative well-being. It seems reasonable to conclude that design improvements and targeted action on affected homes could have a long-term benefit on the health of the occupants.

Recommendations

Although it appears difficult to pin down, there is strong evidence that a damp and mouldy home is not conducive to good health – particularly to vulnerable people who spend many more hours at home exposed to the risks.

To reduce the risks from dampness and mould, governments and agencies could:

- Carry out sample house condition surveys. These can show the extent of problems in the housing stock and the sort of situations in which dampness and mould growth can occur. They can also inform policies and actions at national and local level. Time series surveys can monitor the impact of housing and health policies.
- Produce guidance for homeowners/landlords to identify damp problems in their properties, point out the health risks and suggest solutions to rectify the situation.
- Make financial assistance (grants or subsidies) available towards the cost of improvement to the homes of those who cannot afford to fund the work themselves. This can be particularly effective if they are targeted on common problems that are simple to rectify.
- Produce building codes/regulations for new housing to ensure not only that homes are constructed to prevent the intrusion of dampness and problems of condensation but also that they are designed to prevent the proliferation of indoor allergens.
- Provide guidance for architects, builders and home owners who are undertaking repairs and improvements to help eradicate dampness and avoid the production of condensation.
- Provide guidance and advice to households on the health risks of living in damp and mouldy homes, and on how to avoid problems associated with high relative humidity levels and condensation.

References

Butler S., Williams M., Tukuitonga C., Paterson J. (2003) Problems with damp and cold housing among Pacific families in New Zealand. *N Z Med J* 116(1177): U494.

Dedman D., Gunnell D., Davey-Smith G., Frankel S. (2001) Childhood housing conditions and later mortality in the Boyd Orr cohort. *Journal of Epidemiology and Community Health* 55: 10–15.

Douglas M., Thomson H., Gaughan M. (2003) Health Impact Assessment of Housing Improvements: A Guide. *Public Health Institute of Scotland*, Glasgow.

Jacob B., Ritz B., Gehring U. *et al* (2002) Indoor exposure to molds and allergic sensitization. *Environ Health Perspect* 110(7): 647–53.

Moriske H.J., Szewzyk R., Leonidas M. (2003) Mould Guide – Guide for the Prevention, Investigation, Evaluation And Remediation of Indoor Mould Growth. Newsletter No. 32, WHO Collaborating Centre for Air Quality Management and Air Pollution Control, Berlin, December, pp 2–6.

Marsh A., Gordon D., Pantazis C., Heslop P. (1999) Home Sweet Home? The Impact of Poor Housing on Health. Bristol: The Policy Press.

Office of the Deputy Prime Minister (ODPM) (2006) Housing Health and Safety Rating System: Operating Guidance. London: ODPM.

Peat J., Dickerson J., Li J. (1998) Effects of damp and mould in the home on respiratory health: a review of the literature. *Allergy* 53: 120–8.

Raw G., Aizlewood C.E., Hamilton R.M. (eds) (2001) Building Regulation, Health and Safety. Watford: UK: Building Research Establishment.

Strachan D.P. (1993) Dampness, mould growth and respiratory disease in children. In: Burridge R., Ormandy D. (eds) Unhealthy Housing: Research, Remedies, and Reform. London: E and FN Spon.

Terr A.I. (2004) Are indoor molds causing a new disease? *J Allergy Clin Immunol* 113(2): 221–6.

Zock J.P., Jarvis D., Luczynska C., Sunyer J., Burney P. (2002) European Community Respiratory Health Survey: Housing characteristics, reported mold exposure, and asthma in the European Community Respiratory Health Survey. *J Allergy Clin Immunol* 110(2): 285–92.

8 The effect of cold homes on health: evidence from the LARES study
Ben Croxford

Introduction

Cold homes have been linked to poor health by many studies; the extreme example of this is the phenomenon of excess winter deaths (where more deaths are recorded between December and March than expected from the death rates in other months of the year). Some studies link particular health outcomes with temperature; one important study shows a minima in cardiovascular mortality at a daily mean temperature of about 20°C and an increase in mortality both as the temperature drops from this point and also as it rises (Wilkinson *et al* 2001). This relationship has been shown for many cities around the world with the minima consistently near 20°C, except for some tropical countries that have higher minima (Healy 2003).

Research also indicates that heart attacks and strokes in particular are more prevalent during winter as opposed to during the summer. These health outcomes are strongly associated with poverty (Asplund 2003) but Wilkinson *et al* (2001) found that cold-related mortality was greatest in the coldest homes. Healy found higher ratios of winter deaths to summer deaths in warmer climates than those of the coldest EU-14 countries (the highest was Portugal with 28% more deaths in winter months than summer; UK, 18%; mean, 16%). Other health outcomes linked with cold homes include the findings of Strusberg *et al* (2002), indicating that rheumatic pain is linked to climatic conditions, specifically humidity and temperature.

So, there is evidence linking cold homes with an increase in mortality. The underlying hypothesis of this chapter is that those living in cold homes also suffer more poor health. A plausible pathway for this is that those living in poverty are less able to heat and maintain their homes. This sets up a vicious circle where the occupiers can't afford to heat their home properly or to upgrade it sufficiently to reduce their fuel bills. The stress and worry of this situation, as well as the physical consequences, might be expected to have an effect on health long before the increased mortality outcome referred to in the literature. The work in this chapter presents evidence that could help decision makers act to help break this vicious circle, improving health as well as occupant comfort.

A home should be able to provide shelter from the elements, but poor insulation, a poor heating system and ill-fitting windows and doors can all contribute to a cold home. Wilkinson *et al* (2001) found five major determinants of cold, indoor temperatures for UK properties. Together with their consequences, these are:

- age of dwelling (the older, the colder)
- absence of, or dissatisfaction with, the heating system (more dissatisfied, more cold)
- cost of heating the dwelling (highest is colder)
- low household income (less is colder)
- household size (smaller is colder).

Even some relatively warm homes can 'feel cold' to some occupants. This reflects the fact that many factors affect an occupant's thermal sensation or 'thermal comfort'. Fanger (1970) states, 'Thermal comfort is that condition of mind that expresses satisfaction with the thermal environment'. However, he also found that thermal comfort is dependent on six main environmental variables: air temperature, relative humidity, radiant temperature, air speed, clothing level and metabolic rate (activity level).

If the home is both cold and has high moisture levels, a consequence can be mould and damp. The health effects of mould and damp are significant and important enough to be covered separately in another chapter.[1]

This chapter presents the findings from the LARES survey as follows: first, a description of the methodology used in the analysis is given; then the main health effects – respiratory health, cardiovascular health, arthritis and mental health – are analysed with respect to aspects of the home; there is a discussion of the consequences of the results of the analysis; and finally a consideration of improvements that could be applied to homes and the expected health benefit.

Methodology

Early in the design of the LARES survey a decision was taken that no physical measurements of the factors affecting thermal comfort would be made (temperature, humidity, ventilation rate).[2] Direct estimations of these factors are also not possible;

---

[1] See Chapter 7.
[2] See Chapter 1 on the survey design.

The effect of cold homes on health

however, information regarding occupant perception of thermal comfort is available through some questionnaire responses. Table 8.1 indicates possible ways to estimate the different variables from the LARES survey.

The effects of extreme heat weren't considered in this study, although this can be a significant health problem, particularly amongst vulnerable people in summer: see Valleron and Boumendil (2004) for information about the heatwave-related deaths in France 2003.

Some key variables remain unknown and will mean that most findings remain indicative. Most important amongst these variables is occupant behaviour: How do occupants 'use' the building? Factors include opening frequency of doors and windows, cooking habits, use of extract fans and bathing habits, all of which influence ventilation rate, heating gains and moisture production; these, in turn, affect both internal temperatures and humidities.

As indicated in the Introduction to this Chapter, several health outcomes have been associated with cold homes. The LARES dataset was used to test some of these associations in detail. Three main physiological outcomes were selected and also one more outcome that is attributable to mental health:

- any cardiovascular illness – doctor-diagnosed hypertension, heart attack and strokes
- any respiratory health problem – doctor-diagnosed acute bronchitis, wheezing and whistling
- any arthritis/rheumatic pain – self-reported
- belief that certain health problems affecting mental health are related to dwelling – this is related to the SALSA score.[3]

Each of these four outcomes is affected by many variables. In many cases the main cause of various illnesses is known (e.g. age and smoking status) but the

Table 8.1 Variables related to cold homes from the LARES survey

Required variable	Variables from LARES dataset
Indoor air temperature	Temperature complaints; heating system complaints
Indoor relative humidity	From mould and condensation questions
Air speed	From draughtiness and airtightness questions
Radiant temperature	Information on insulation
Clothing level	Can be adaptive, so more worn if cold; difficult to use this variable
Metabolic rate	Older people can be less active, so feel colder; age may be a factor

---

[3] See Chapter 11 for an explanation of SALSA.

The effect of cold homes on health

effect of minor variables is not known. The analysis techniques used here allow for investigation of these minor variables, excluding the influence of known variables such as gender or age. The size and range of this dataset allows analysis of the effect of these minor variables while compensating for the effect of these 'confounding variables'.

The variables used in the analysis are split into five separate blocks:

- personal
- household status
- perceived housing characteristics
- climate
- city.

The analysis aims to answer the question, 'Given a case where all other variables remain equal, are certain aspects of the home implicated or associated with a particular health outcome?'

Personal, household and perceived variables

The individual confounding variables used in the model are listed in Table 8.2.

Climate

Climatic data is used as a variable to explain possible city-to-city differences. The climatic data were generated using the program Meteonorm 4 (Meteotest 1999). Air temperature, relative humidity and absolute humidity were used in the model.[4] The more water present in the air, the higher the home temperature has to be to reduce the relative humidity to below 70%, which is considered important to prevent mould growth (Oreszczyn and Pretlove 1999).[5]

The climate variables selected were those considered as being most important in determining the effect on indoor hygrothermal conditions during winter.

City

'City' is used in the analysis as a variable to compensate for cultural and population differences that may exist between populations of different cities. It is known, for example, that diet changes between cities. By using City within the

---

[4] Absolute humidity is a measure of the total amount of water in the air at a given time. Relative humidity is the ratio of the amount of water in the air at a given temperature compared with the maximum the air can possibly hold at that temperature expressed as a percentage.
[5] See also Chapter 7.

The effect of cold homes on health

Table 8.2 Variables used in the logistic regression model

Variable type	Variable	Notes
Personal	Age	
	Gender	Some cases with no valid gender are excluded
	Height	
	Weight	
	BMI adult	Not valid for child age group
	Smoking status	
	Alcohol consumption	
	Exercise status	
Household status	Socio-economic status (SES)	See Chapter 9
	Number of inhabitants	
	Mental health indicator (SALSA)	Not valid for child age group
	Fuel poor?	if >10% income spent on heating (definition of fuel poverty from Boardman 1991)
Perceived household characteristics	Problems with cold in winter or transient season?	
	Dissatisfaction with heating system	
	Dissatisfaction with thermal Insulation	
	Dissatisfaction with draughtiness	
	Mouldy or damp home (MOULD_SCORE)	(see Chapter 7 for details)

analysis the effect of unknown city-to-city differences can be compensated for, making the analysis more robust.

General analysis comments

Certain variables have been transformed from a five point scale to a binary variable. For example where respondents were asked to rate their dissatisfaction with their heating system, 'often' or 'permanent' were aggregated and compared with 'never' or 'seldom'; the neutral cases were discarded. This allows the difference between occupants who were generally dissatisfied with their heating (for example), to be compared with the set who were generally satisfied. It also reflects how people answer questionnaires. It is sometimes difficult to separate people who responded 5 compared to those who responded 4 on a five-point scale, but the assumption here is that they were clearly different to those who responded 2 or 1.

The effect of cold homes on health

Detailed analyses using the full health dataset with each health outcome as the dependent variable and the set of possible environmental variables were selected as the independent variables. The technique used was logistic regression. The program Statview (1998) was preferred over SPSS for ease of use. The model was tested with and without the blocks of variables mentioned in the previous sections and the effects of these blocks of variables on the dependent variables investigated and the overall model fit are considered and commented on.

For the health outcomes, no city had a particularly high prevalence of any one outcome, so it was not considered necessary to exclude a particular city from the analysis or to test the validity of the findings for each city in turn. However, Ferreira do Alentejo had an extreme incidence of mould, in part due to climate and to the high prevalence of homes with no heating system, so this city was excluded from some analyses to ensure that any relationship found was true with and without this city.

Age is an important factor for each health outcome; some of the health outcomes have a very different aetiology depending on age, so the overall model was split into three age groups.[6] Age was kept in the model, as there can be a variation, dependent on age, within each of these three age groups.

For each block of variables tested, the odds ratios and the 95% confidence intervals were calculated for each of four housing characteristic variables selected as most likely to be indicators of poor hygrothermal conditions:

- Problems with cold in winter or transient season?
- Dissatisfaction with thermal insulation.
- Dissatisfaction with heating system.
- Dissatisfaction with draughtiness

The hypothesis tested is 'that people who find their homes to be cold are more likely to report having certain health symptoms'.

Results

From the distribution of variables in the LARES dataset there are several points that are apparent. First, the distribution of health symptom prevalence by city was different for each health symptom. Bonn and Vilnius had the highest prevalence of respiratory health problems, Bratislava and Vilnius had the lowest prevalence of arthritic problems, whereas Vilnius, Ferreira do Alentejo and Budapest had the highest prevalence of cardiovascular problems. The distribution of cardiovascular problems for occupants over 60 years old indicated some similarities between the

---

[6] Age is split into three rather than any more groups to keep the numbers in each group high for each city. Adults are between 19 and 60, children are younger and seniors are older than adults. See also Chapter 5 on Scores and Conventions.

Table 8.3 Summary of all statistical analyses

Factor	Age group	Housing factor, direction of effect (OR 95% CI)	Comments
Respiratory problems reported	Child	2.1 times *more* prevalent if dissatisfied with heating system (OR = 2.1, 95% CI 1.0–4.38) 4 times *less* prevalent if dissatisfied with draughts (OR = 0.25, 95% CI 0.13–0.49)	No changes when tested with and without Ferreira do Alentejo
	Adult	None	No changes when tested with and without (city 3) Ferreira do Alentejo and (city 4) Bonn*
	Senior	1.97 times *more* prevalent if house cold in winter (OR = 1.97, 95% CI 1.03–3.76) 2.39 times *more* prevalent if dissatisfied with insulation (OR = 2.39, 95% CI 1.07–5.36)	Relationship seen is slightly strengthened by excluding Ferreira do Alentejo from the the analysis
Cardiovascular problems reported	Child	N/A	Too few cases for analysis
	Adult	None	
	Senior	None	Positive association found with MOULD_SCORE*
Arthritis problems reported	Child	N/A	Too few cases for analysis
	Adult	None	
	Senior	1.92 times *more* prevalent if house cold in winter (OR = 1.92, 95% CI 1.16–3.16)	
Belief that mental health problems are related to dwelling	Child	7.7 times *less* prevalent if dissatisfied with insulation (OR = 0.13, 95% CI 0.02–0.99)	Positive association found with MOULD_SCORE†

OR, odds ratio; CI, confidence interval.
*Bonn had a high prevalence of respiratory illness reported, Ferreira do Alentejo had the highest prevalence of mould.
†See Chapter 5 and Chapter 7.

The effect of cold homes on health

Table 8.3 (Cont'd)

Adult	1.79 times *more* prevalent if house cold in winter (OR = 1.79, 95% CI 1.07–2.98) 1.67 times More prevalent if dissatisfied with insulation (OR = 1.67, 95% CI 1–2.81) 1.82 times more prevalent if dissatisfied with heating system (OR = 1.82, 95% CI 1.14–2.91)	
Senior	None	Positive association found with MOULD_SCORE Almost significant association found with poorly rated insulation.

two groups. The distribution of smokers across the eight cities was very similar, with an average of about 25%.

The distribution of 'problems with cold in winter or transient season' showed Ferreira do Alentejo and Vilnius as having the highest prevalence. However, considering the mean temperature in winter, Ferreira do Alentejo was the warmest city and Vilnius the coldest. (Ferreira do Alentejo is only cold for a short period of the year and many homes do not have heating, and some have rooms with no windows.)

A factor discussed in the Chapter 7 is that the prevalence of mould is far higher in Ferreira do Alentejo than in any of the other seven cities, which can be explained in part by the high absolute humidity for the city. In winter the air is relatively warm and can hold a higher level of moisture than in the other cities and, as most homes have no heating, if the indoor temperature drops, condensation forms on the cold surfaces and provides ideal conditions for mould growth.

The results of all the analyses are presented in summary form in Table 8.3. Individual analysis results are commented on in the following sections and conclusions are drawn from these analyses in the Discussion section. The results cover each of the three age groups. All analyses with the Child age group exclude the body mass index (BMI) and the mental health variable SALSA, as these variables are not valid for this age group.

Specific findings

Climate variables seem to produce similar effects to the City variable, indicating that a large part of the difference seen between cities may be explained by climatic differences. All the analyses for Child age group do not include BMIADULT or SALSA as variables as these are not valid for this age group.

A more detailed discussion of each of these analyses is presented in the next paragraphs.

Respiratory problems reported

Of the entire dataset, the prevalence of reported respiratory conditions is shown in Table 8.4 by age group.

Child

In all cases there was a strong negative relationship with draughts, interpreted as the draughtier a home is perceived the less likely children will suffer from respiratory symptoms. There was a slight positive relationship between poor heating system and respiratory symptoms. Further analysis shows that MOULD_SCORE[7] was a significant variable. An explanation could be that when the home is cold and there is insufficient ventilation, mould can be a problem. The analysis was tested with and without Ferreira do Alentejo, and in no case were the results changed from 'significant' to 'not significant' or vice versa. However, climate variables seemed to produce similar effects to the City variable, indicating that a large part of the difference seen between cities may be explained by climate differences.

Adult

None of the four housing factors chosen were found to be statistically significant in any of the combinations of variables. This was also tested without Ferreira do Alentejo and Bonn.

Table 8.4 Prevalence of respiratory symptoms

	No symptoms	Some symptoms	Total
Child	1399	201	1600
Adult	5147	458	5605
Senior	1104	210	1314
Total	7650	869	8519

---

[7]Developed by by Alan O'Dell of the UK Building Research Establishment, see Chapter 5.

The effect of cold homes on health

Senior

'Temperature cold in winter?' and 'Dissatisfied with insulation?' were both significant in explaining respiratory symptoms amongst the senior section of the population surveyed. The relationship seen was slightly strengthened by excluding Ferreira do Alentejo from the analysis.

Cardiovascular problems reported

The prevalence of reported cardiovascular problems is shown in Table 8.5 by age group.

Child

As there were only 13 cases for the Child category with cardiovascular disease (CVD) problems, the analysis was only carried out for Adults and Senior age groups.

Adult

None of the four housing factors chosen was found to be statistically significant in any of the combinations of variables.

Senior

None of the four housing factors chosen was found to be statistically significant in any of the combinations of variables. Mould was found to be a statistically significant factor and is dependent on cold damp conditions (see Chapter 7).

Arthritis problems reported

The prevalence of reported arthritis problems by age group is shown in Table 8.6.

Table 8.5 Prevalence of CVD symptoms

	No symptoms	Some symptoms	Total
Child	1587	13	1600
Adult	4755	850	5605
Senior	690	624	1314
Total	7032	1487	8519

CVD, cardiovascular disease.

The effect of cold homes on health

Table 8.6 Prevalence of arthritis symptoms

	No symptoms	Some symptoms	Total
Child	1580	20	1600
Adult	4851	754	5605
Senior	684	630	1314
Total	7115	1404	8519

Child

Again, as there were so few reported symptoms for the Child category, this analysis is not reported.

Adult

None of the four housing factors chosen were found to be statistically significant in any of the combinations of variables.

Senior

'Do you have problems with cold in winter or transient season?' was the only factor found to be statistically significant in any of the combinations of variables.

Discussion

Four main areas of health symptoms were considered in this analysis:

- a respiratory index (including acute bronchitis and wheezing and whistling)
- cardiovascular problems (hypertension, heart attacks and strokes)
- arthritic pain
- an indication of mental health problems

From the literature we expect colder homes to have a higher prevalence of these health complaints. Some clear findings from this investigation appear to back up this hypothesis. It should be noted that the factors within the home that are used in this analysis are responses to questions asked by the surveyor to the head of the household and these responses are used as an indicator of possible causes of cold homes. Consequently, 'Dissatisfied with insulation' is an opinion on the thermal qualities of the insulation and not necessarily an accurate assessment.

Respiratory symptoms were found to be linked in different ways to different housing factors for children and for seniors. Draughty homes were linked to

The effect of cold homes on health

fewer symptoms, whereas poor heating systems were related with increased prevalence of respiratory problems for children. For seniors, having problems with cold temperatures in winter and being dissatisfied with the home's insulation were both associated with increased prevalence of respiratory symptoms.

Cardiovascular problems were strongly linked to age, weight and gender, but, after compensating for these, only MOULD_SCORE was found to be a factor from all the housing factors considered.[8]

Arthritic problems were very strongly linked to age; however, within the senior age grouping, 'problems with cold temperatures in winter' were also significantly associated with arthritic problems. It is important to note that arthrosis, degeneration essentially due to age, was classified in the same category as arthritis, so this may have led to a confusing picture resulting from the analysis.

It is likely that those with ill health show indications of depression, but investigating the prevalence of 'those that believe that their mental health symptoms are related to their home' showed some interesting findings. This variable was associated with problems with cold in winter, dissatisfaction with heating system, poor insulation and MOULD_SCORE; all can be considered variables symptomatic of a cold home. Given that there exists a link between depression and health, it seems plausible to hypothesise that cold homes may increase depression and therefore possibly affect health further.[9]

Recommendations for possible improvements

In this report the main hypothesis was that cold homes and also homes that are perceived as being cold are detrimental to human health. The data presented from the LARES study tend to back up this hypothesis.

This dataset allowed us to look in detail for particular factors that may be related to certain health outcomes. The dataset is important as it combines factors from different subject areas for a large number of respondents. There are questions of reliability about the dataset,[10] which is inevitable for one covering such a wide geographical range and population range. Despite these limitations and after compensating for age, gender, smoking status, socio-economic status, city effects and climate effects, significant associations were found between health symptoms and housing factors.

Cold, damp homes are relatively simple to improve but require resources; the improvements may well improve the quality of living and also the health of the

---

[8]See also Chapter 7.
[9]See Chapter 11.
[10]See Chapter 1.

occupants. The weight of evidence presented in this chapter and others suggests that money spent on improving poor housing is likely to reduce money spent on dealing with health problems.

A recent study backing this finding shows that respiratory symptoms improve in new energy-efficient homes (Leech *et al* 2004), the indication being that it is the improved living conditions that are responsible for improved respiratory health.

Actions taken to improve housing will be strongly specific to each city; this must be taken into account in implementing any improvements.

References

Asplund K. (2003) Down with the class society! *Stroke* 34: 2628–9.

Boardman B. (1991) Fuel Poverty: From Cold Homes to Affordable Warmth. London: Belhaven Press.

Fanger P.O. (1970) Thermal Comfort. Analysis and Applications in Environmental Engineering. Copenhagen: Danish Technical Press.

Healy J.D. (2003) Excess winter mortality in Europe: a cross country analysis identifying key risk factors. *Journal of Epidemiology and Community Health*, Vol 57(10).

Leech J.A., Raizenne M., Gusdorf J. (2004) Health in occupants of energy efficient new homes. *Indoor Air* 14: 169–73.

Meteotest (1999) www.meteotest.ch.

Oreszczyn T., Pretlove S. (1999) Condensation Targeter II: modelling surface relative humidity to predict mould growth in dwellings. *Building Serv Res Technol* 20/3: 143–53.

Statview (1998) SAS Institute.

Strusberg I., Mendelberg R.C., Serra H.A., Strusberg A.M. (2002) Influence of weather conditions on rheumatic pain. *Journal of Rheumatolology* 29(2): 335–8.

Valleron A.J., Boumendil A. (2004) Epidemiology and heat waves: analysis of the 2003 episode in France. *C R Biol* 327(12): 1125–41.

Wilkinson P., Armstrong B., Landon M. (2001) Cold Comfort: The Social and Environmental Determinants of Excess Winter Deaths in England, 1986–1996. Foundation by The Policy Press (ISBN 1 86134 355 8). Summary available at http://www.jrf.org.uk/knowledge/findings/housing/n11.asp.

9 Residential energy systems: links with socio-economic status and health in the LARES study

Véronique Ezratty, Anne Duburcq, Corinne Emery and Jacques Lambrozo

Introduction

As well as being critical aspects of housing quality and affordability, energy fuel sources, energy efficiency and domestic heating and cooking systems have a direct impact on the resident's health and comfort.

There is nothing new about health hazards from indoor air pollution caused by poor-quality energy supplies and equipment. Modern archaeological pathologists have revealed the disease burden from this pollution in ancient cultures. The study of ancient Egyptian mummies with preserved internal organs (such as lungs) has shown cases of anthracosis that may have resulted from breathing indoor air polluted by open fires for cooking and heating.

Nowadays, the problem of access to, and cost of, different energy sources, which primarily affects developing countries, leads to the use of biomass fuels for indoor cooking and heating and thus to high levels of indoor air pollution. According to the World Health Report 2003, 'Shaping the Future', indoor air pollution is responsible for 36% of the total number of lower respiratory infections worldwide and 22% of the cases of chronic obstructive pulmonary disease. In 2002, lower respiratory tract infections constituted the second leading cause of mortality in children, accounting for 1.8 million deaths throughout the world. In the 51 countries of the WHO European region, it is estimated that in the age group 0–4 years, 4.6% of all deaths are attributable to indoor air pollution from the use of solid fuels (Valent *et al* 2004).

In developed countries, cooking and heating can also affect respiratory illnesses, albeit to a lesser degree, but especially in children (Burr *et al* 1999; Triche *et al* 2002). Achieving levels of indoor air pollutants that are acceptable from a health point of view requires eliminating or controlling the sources of these compounds (Raw *et al* 2004) and maintaining adequate ventilation in homes (Engvall *et al* 2003).

At the same time, inadequate heating, which is also linked to the cost of fuel, particularly in energy-inefficient housing, also leads to poor health (Gemmell 2001).

We must also be aware that building energy use accounts for nearly 50% of energy consumption in some European countries. Consequently, by choosing appropriate energy sources and making homes more energy efficient, we can reduce harmful pollution and save residents money too, while ensuring that homes, nonetheless, maintain a temperature range adequate for human health. This calls for balanced decision making.

The LARES survey provides substantial data from household reports about their energy systems (household appliances and use) and possible energy savings.

The aim of the analyses discussed in this chapter was to assess the links between the quality of residential energy systems,[1] socio-economic status (SES) and common diseases.

Methods

As described elsewhere,[2] the LARES project provided three sources of data:

- the Housing Inspection Survey Sheet (one per household, $n = 3,373$)
- the Inhabitant Questionnaire (one per household, $n = 3,373$)
- the Housing and Health Questionnaire (one per person in each household, $n = 8,519$).

The statistical analysis was performed with SAS® V8.2 software after importing the two principal databases, which were furnished in SPSS format, and the database appendix, which covered SES.

---

[1] In this chapter, the term **'residential energy systems'** is used to cover, in a simple and global way, different aspects related to energy in the dwelling. The aim was to take into account, in a relevant way, all the data collected in the survey that were related directly or indirectly to the energy issue. These data were classified according to their relationship with the building, the indoor air quality, the energy efficiency and the home equipment for heating and cooking so that it was possible to build indicators that covered all the aspects related to energy in the dwellings.

[2] See Chapter 1.

Residential energy systems, SES and health

The statistical analysis covered the following four main topics:

1. Description of the residential energy systems and the potential energy savings estimated by respondents. This was analysed by general description of the housing, weather-tightness, ventilation system and home equipment for cooking and heating city by city, overall and as a function of the household SES. A specific analysis by residents' age group was also performed to compare energy equipment and satisfaction levels for the elderly (≥65 years old) with those of the younger population.
2. Construction of indicators characterising the quality of each household's energy systems according to specific aspects (weather-tightness, ventilation, mould/dampness and thermal comfort). The aim of this step was to allow the identification of the systems that are inefficient or not optimal in given domains.

For both of these first two analyses, standard statistical tests were used to compare different groups of households or people in the descriptive statistical analyses: χ^2 test or Fisher's exact test, as appropriate, for the qualitative variables, and Student's t test for the quantitative parameters.

3. Characterisation of households with a 'home energy problem': first, in terms of socio-economic characteristics; secondly, in terms of housing characteristics (including age of building, housing type and location of the dwelling). Multivariate analyses with logistic regression models were performed to identify the factors explaining the quality of household energy systems. In particular, to study the association between these indicators and SES, and between these indicators and different components of the SES. For Geneva, these indicators were also crossed with the heating cost index (HCI) developed by the canton's energy department (ScanE[3]).
4. Analysis of the relationship between the indicators assessing the quality of home energy systems and the health status of residents (for the 12 months preceding the survey), for some common diseases and symptoms. Multivariate analyses with logistic regression models were conducted to study the statistical relationships between household energy system indicators and selected health features. Depending on the parameters studied, the analyses therefore involved either:

- the household (axes 1, 2 and 3, based on the 3,373 housing units, except for the analysis by age group), or

---

[3] http://www.geneve.ch/scane. This was provided by Cédric Lambert, Centre universitaire d'écologie humaine de Genève, CH-1211 Genève 4.

- the inhabitants of the household, assigning the same housing characteristics to all the inhabitants of a given household (axis 4, based on 8,519 persons).

City effect

To take into account any possible city effect, we chose an approach that was both feasible and relevant in view of our topic.[4] We analysed the pooled data, adjusting it by including two city indicators: mean temperature in July and mean temperature in January for each city.

Definition of indicators

The SES score developed for the LARES project was applied to all members of the same household.[5]

For allergies, we used the following three variables: responses to the question 'Allergy without asthma'; and the two scores constructed for the LARES project, ALLERAST and ALEST_DG.[6]

Four indicators were constructed to characterise the weather-tightness of the roof and windows, the ventilation, mould/dampness problems and temperature problems in the dwelling, respectively.

1. **Quality indicator for weather-tightness**
   A problem associated with weather-tightness was identified when it was reported that the roof was not waterproof, that the windows were not airtight or that the windows were only single-glazed.
2. **Quality indicator for ventilation**
   Reports about the ventilation systems by the inhabitants and the surveyors were inconsistent, and in some cases, contradictory. However, as the inconsistencies and contradictions go in both directions, there appeared to be no clear over- or underestimation by the surveyors. These discordances are probably associated with a problem of definition and understanding of the different types of ventilation systems. To overcome this problem, we used a global variable derived in five or in two categories. We defined 'a ventilation problem' in the dwelling where there was no or free ventilation with windows but without air vents (i.e. no behaviour-independent ventilation system). Based on the variables in the Housing Inspection Survey Sheet concerning

---

[4]Based on recommendations made by Paul Wilkinson, London School of Hygiene and Tropical Medicine, London.
[5]This SES score was devised by Maggie Davidson *et al*, Building Research Establishment, Garston, UK.
[6]See Chapter 5.

Residential energy systems, SES and health

the existence of ventilation and windows in three rooms of the home (kitchen, bathroom and toilet), we created three new variables with five categories for each:

- forced ventilation
- natural ventilation without windows (air vents only)
- natural ventilation with windows (windows ± air vents)
- window ventilation without air vents ('no ventilation' reported but window in the room)
- no ventilation.

From the three variables defined above, we created an overall indicator for the home, considering the room for which the response was most favourable.

3. **Mould or dampness problem**
   An indicator was created for the LARES project[7] that uses a continuous scale of exposure and takes into consideration data on both mould and dampness, based on perception of the household and the surveyors' assessment. The score was defined in four groups with the tertile cut-off points. It was grouped in two categories for our analysis – no or little mould/dampness versus some or much mould/dampness.
4. **Problem with temperature (thermal comfort)**
   We identified such a problem when a household reported a problem 'often or permanently' during the winter or the spring/autumn season versus never, seldom or sometimes.

Methods for multivariate analyses

First, Axis 3 – the characterisation of households with a home energy problem. Each dichotomous indicator was analysed with a logistic regression model based on households ($n = 3,373$ housing units). We tested several models (Table 9.1):

- Model 1 presents the association between each indicator and SES (bivariate analysis).
- Model 2 adjusts model 1 by taking into account the 'city effect' (average temperatures in July and in January per city).
- Model 3 further includes the housing type, classified in three categories:
  o (prefabricated) panel block buildings
  o multifamily apartment blocks (up to six units and more than six units)
  o one-family houses (detached, semi-detached and terraced).

---

[7]Created by Alan O'Dell, Building Research Establishment, Garston, UK, and David Moreau.

Table 9.1 Variables used in the analyses models

For all the models	Supplementary variables for the thermal comfort and 'cold home' models	Supplementary variables for the 'mould' model
SES	Connection to central heating	Problem with temperature
Climate zone	Additional heating devices	Cold home
Housing type	Heating system in all inhabitable rooms	No ventilation
At least part of the unit located directly below the roof	Waterproof roof	Laundry dried in the dwelling most of the time
Floor (first or ground floor/ or not)	Single-glazed windows	
Age of building	Windows not tight	

SES, socio-economic status.

- The final model (model 4) takes into account all of the following explanatory variables.

Model 4 is derived from a stepwise procedure with SAS® that began by testing all of the variables and then successively eliminating, one by one, those not significant at 5%. The model obtained considers only the variables significantly associated ($p < 0.05$) with the indicator studied.

Secondly, Axis 4 – the analysis of the relationship between the home energy systems indicators (as described above) and the health status of household members (for the 12 months preceding the survey) for some common diseases and symptoms.

We selected diseases or symptoms that occur frequently and appeared relevant to housing-related public health issues. The health survey specifically asked if these diseases had been diagnosed by a physician or treated with prescription drugs.

Multivariate analyses with logistic regression models were performed, bivariate first, and then multivariate, both adjusted for relevant parameters (Table 9.2).

Results – by city

Socio-economic characteristics of households and characteristics of homes

On average, 1.8 family members per household have an income. A majority of inhabitants are homeowners in Vilnius (94%), Bratislava (90%), Budapest (86%), Ferreira do Alentejo (89%) and Forlì (84%) and renters in Geneva (92%).

Of the total 3,373 dwellings, 60% (2,024) had been renovated (not including minor work performed by the occupants). In Budapest it was 87%. This rate is lower in Geneva (37%) and Forlì (42%).

Residential energy systems, SES and health

Table 9.2 Health variables and adjustments

Health variables studied	Adjustment for					
	Sex	Age*	SES†	Smoking‡	BMI*	Alcohol‡
Hypertension (high blood pressure)	x	x	x	x	x	
Asthma	x	x	x	x	x	
ALLERGY, ALLERAST, ALEST_DG	x	x	x	x	x	
Gastric or duodenal ulcer	x	x	x	x		x
Migraine and frequent headache	x	x	x	x		
Cold or throat illness	x	x	x	x		
Diarrhoeal diseases	x	x	x	x		
Health in general	x	x	x	x		

*Used as a quantitative parameter.
†Used in five categories.
‡Grouped into three categories: never/in the past/now.

The habitable space averages 80 m², with substantial variations by city (58 m² in Vilnius and 157 m² in Ferreira do Alentejo), with an average of four habitable rooms (roughly three in Vilnius and six in Forlì).

Weather-tightness and insulation: these characteristics vary greatly by city

There are wide variations between the eight cities in the weather-tightness and insulation characteristics. For example there is at least one non-airtight window with draughts in 40% of the housing units, especially in Vilnius (64%) and Bratislava (48%). In Bratislava 96% of windows are double-glazed (83% in Bonn and 81% in Vilnius), whereas Ferreira do Alentejo has essentially only single-glazed windows. Forty-one per cent of the homes are located on the ground floor (houses included), and 11% of the units in multi-family apartment houses are on the top floor (this information is an estimate since specific information about the location of the top floor is not available).

Ventilation: many housing units lack appropriate ventilation

We found that many housing units lacked appropriate means of ventilation.

Whereas very few dwellings have no ventilation system at all, even windows (except in Ferreira do Alentejo, with 12%), the percentage of households with no behaviour-independent ventilation system (no ventilation or window without air vents) is rather high, especially in Forlì (80%), Ferreira do Alentejo (28%), Bonn (52%) and Budapest (44%). However, residents' perceptions of their systems are not consistent with these observations: satisfaction is highest at Forlì (3.9 on a scale of 1–5).

Residential energy systems, SES and health

Heating system: particularity of Ferreira do Alentejo

Most homes have heating in every room, except in Ferreira do Alentejo where the opposite is true.

On average, 77% of households have central heating, but only 1% in Ferreira do Alentejo. (There was no information given on the fuels used for central heating.) In the absence of central heating, the fuels used are specific to each city: gas in Forlì (88%), Budapest (84%) and Bratislava (79%); electricity in Angers (83%); and solid fuel in Vilnius (64%). Additional supplementary heating devices are used by 31% of the households, on average (although by only 23% according to the investigators), a figure that reaches 94% in Ferreira do Alentejo. The energy source for these supplementary heating devices is electricity in 61% of cases.

The percentage of income spent on heating appears to differ substantially by city. In Vilnius 77% of the households spent more than 10% of their income on heating, 58% in Budapest and 47% in Bratislava. However, as 28% of the respondents did not give any answer to this question, this result is not particularly reliable.

Results – by age

The elderly are less well equipped but more satisfied. Globally, those aged 65 years or older live in homes that present different energy problems (more units on the ground floor, old, small, etc.) than the homes of younger residents. However, although the housing units occupied by the elderly seem somewhat less well equipped (fewer with double-glazing and with central heating), they appear more satisfied with their heating system, their home insulation, and their ventilation.

The homes of the isolated elderly (≥65 years old and living alone) differ somewhat from those of elderly people not living alone: they more often live in multifamily apartment blocks, less often on the ground floor, and have smaller dwellings. They also own their units less often. There are few differences in terms of equipment but their heating expenses are proportionally greater. They report the same levels of satisfaction for the quality of their heating, ventilation, and insulation. Thermal comfort is similar in winter and during the spring and autumn, but they report fewer temperature problems in summer than the non-isolated elderly.

Results – multivariate analysis: evaluation of associations between SES and home energy indicators

The results of the multivariate analysis are similar whether we take the SES score or its components into account. However, for mould and dampness problems we found no relation with SES for the overall score, although we did find

Residential energy systems, SES and health

correlations between the probability of this problem and some score variables (such as number of occupants, size of unit, etc.).

We found that the 'weather-tightness' indicator is significantly associated with SES after adjustment for city effect and other variables. We found that the wealthier classes have a lower risk of weather-tightness problems. This indicator is also associated with housing type: the probability of having a weather-tightness problem is higher in panel blocks and in one-family houses. It is closely related to the age of the building: the older the building, the greater the risk of this problem. Dwellings without any part under the roof are also more likely to have a weather-tightness problem (roof or windows). These results appear paradoxical but may be explained by the fact that households will invest less to improve the tightness of their windows when there is no part under the roof. On the contrary, households living in an apartment located under the roof or in a house will try to have the best weather-tightness and insulation they can so that the heating does not cost them too much.

The bivariate analysis of the 'ventilation problem' indicator shows that, paradoxically, the highest social classes have the greatest risk of not having a behaviour-independent, that is, forced ventilation or air vents. But when we take housing type into account the relationship is reversed, and the poorest have the greatest risk of no ventilation equipment. After taking the city effect into account, the final multivariate model shows the importance of the age and type of building (in particular, one-family houses have a higher risk than multi-family apartments). SES is no longer significant in this model. These results ('ventilation problem' indicator related to type of housing, independent of SES) may be explained by the fact that the newest apartment buildings meet regulatory requirements of each country. These requirements are more demanding in terms of air changes, and new buildings are therefore generally equipped with forced ventilation or free ventilation through air vents, unlike older houses and/or buildings (that predate the 1970s oil shock).

The 'mould/dampness' indicator is not linked with the SES when we use the SES score. After taking the SES components into account, the probability of mould problems is significantly greater for larger households, smaller housing units, one-family houses, in areas with higher January mean temperatures, in ground-floor dwellings and in units with temperature problems. The result of the multivariate analysis of the relationship between the unit floor space and mould or humidity is difficult to interpret. In particular, there is no linear relation in the bivariate analysis.

The 'perceived temperature problem' indicator is significantly associated with SES in the bivariate analysis and remains associated (at the same order of magnitude) after adjustment for city effect and type of housing but not in the final model. This type of problem is explained most especially by the housing unit's heating and insulation characteristics. When we take the SES components into account, only the size of the dwelling is associated with perceived temperature problems: the household's social, demographic and cultural characteristics are not.

The results of our evaluation of the associations between Home Energy Indicators and diseases and symptoms are summarized below:

- Reporting **bad or very bad health** is significantly associated with perceived temperature problems odds ratio [OR] = 2.6), weather-tightness problems (OR = 2.4), and mould or dampness (OR = 1.7).
- After adjustment for relevant parameters, **hypertension** is significantly associated with temperature problems (OR = 1.8), weather-tightness problems (OR = 1.2), and mould or dampness (OR = 1.2).
- **Asthma** is significantly linked with ventilation (OR = 1.5), mould or dampness (OR = 1.7) and perceived temperature problems (OR = 1.5).
- None of our four indicators is significantly associated with the global variable that assesses **allergy** prevalence (**excluding allergic asthma**):
  - **Allergy assessed by the ALLERAST** score (corresponding to self-reported symptoms) is significantly associated with mould or dampness (OR = 1.1) and perceived temperature problems (OR = 1.2)
  - **Allergy assessed by the ALEST_DG score** (symptoms diagnosed by a physician) is significantly associated with weather-tightness problems (OR = 1.1), mould or dampness in the dwelling (OR = 1.3) and perceived temperature problems (OR = 1.5).
- **Gastric and duodenal ulcers** are significantly associated with perceived temperature (OR = 1.9) and weather-tightness problems in the dwelling (OR = 1.6).
- **Migraine and frequent headaches, cold and throat illness, and diarrhoeal diseases** are significantly associated with problems in the quality of household energy systems.

Discussion

The results we observed for common diseases like asthma and hypertension are consistent with the literature. Indeed, there is increasing evidence that mould in homes constitutes a risk factor for respiratory illness (Dharmage et al 2002). A low ventilation rate may enhance the risk but there are fewer data available, especially in residential (compared with office) buildings (Bornehag et al 2004). There is also extensive literature on the influence of temperature changes on hypertension (Rosenthal 2004).

Some of the results reinforce hypotheses already proposed. In particular, numerous studies of sick building syndrome (SBS) have assessed the affect of some building characteristics (water-tightness, moulds and humidity, ventilation) on the non-specific symptoms found in this syndrome (such as headaches, respiratory symptoms, and nasal and eye mucus irritation).

Other results are original, such as those observed for the common digestive diseases we selected (diarrhoeal diseases and gastric/duodenal ulcers). However, these findings, which constitute new paths for research, must be confirmed by further studies because of limitations in both the collection and analysis of the data.

Self-administered questionnaires were used to collect the occupant health data. The questions asked and conditions of data collection were optimised but there is no guarantee about the type of response, even though residents were asked if the diagnosis was made by a physician and/or if medication was taken for the condition. In particular, some diseases are defined by specific criteria (e.g. diarrhoea by number of stools per day) that could not be ascertained. The value of self-reported data depends on many factors and may lead to either an overestimate or an underestimate of health problems. Thus, despite the quality and volume of the data collected from a very large sample for diseases or symptoms with high prevalences, it is appropriate to be prudent and to verify the 'trends' observed by studies of smaller samples but with stricter criteria.

This is a large sample, and significant results are not difficult to obtain. The corollary is that it is important to pay attention to their real pertinence.

The construction and validation of new indicators enabled us to conduct analyses that would otherwise have been impossible and to take into account parameters that involve many complex elements, often understudied, such as residential ventilation. The indicators were constructed principally from data reported by the residents or investigators and are not based on measurements. It would be interesting to cross these indicators with objective indicators available in this domain.

This was possible for Geneva, for which an HCI is available. Crossing the HCI with our indicators shows correlations that tend to indicate that the residents' perceptions of the quality of their energy system is fairly reliable.

The approach of decomposing the SES score in the analysis enabled us to refine and detail the interpretation of some results. The SES score mixes together several types of information – in particular, the household composition, highest educational level, employment situation and size of unit. The advantage of this type of indicator is that it takes several interesting dimensions into account and summarises them; the disadvantage is that it is not necessarily very specific, which can lead to a loss of power compared with a specific variable and that we do not know exactly what it actually characterizes.

This led us to use several simultaneous approaches: models with SES, then models including the different components taken into account, to specify which specific factor might be involved with this or that energy indicator (e.g. to know which parameter mattered most: sometimes the number of persons in the apartment, sometimes the floor space of the apartment, sometimes the household social status).

This breakdown of the SES adds something to the level of explanation, especially for mould and dampness. It would have been interesting to complete this analysis by considering the occupation of the head of the household. But the variable explored in the study was 'father's occupation'; we cannot know what people really understood by this title and what they replied (occupation of the head of the household or occupation of the father of the person who completed the questionnaire?). The ambiguous formulation of this question makes it difficult to interpret the answers.

Recommendations for possible improvements

Citizens' energy choices cannot be easily influenced, but interventions at other levels can be promoted to improve energy efficiency and thermal comfort while not compromising health.

The problems raised and the areas for improvement proposed by inhabitants are strongly specific to each city; this should be taken into account in the recommendations that follow.

Problems of insulation and tightness affect thermal comfort, especially in winter and in summer. These problems are associated with SES, with the local climate and with the type of housing.

In our study, we found significant associations between the weather-tightness problem in the dwelling and common diseases such as asthma, allergies and hypertension. Consequently, improving the quality of weather-tightness could lead not only to better thermal comfort, better energy efficiency and energy savings but also to better health for the residents.

However, recommendations for improving buildings (fixing window and roof weather-tightness, installing double-glazed windows and better thermal insulation envelopes) must be accompanied by verification of the ventilation systems in the units so that homes that are uncomfortable in the winter or energy inefficient are not synonymous with homes with poor indoor air quality and condensation problems.

Therefore, the following actions should be considered:

- Improve the information that users receive about ventilation: in this large survey conducted in eight different European countries, the definition of the different ventilation systems was poorly understood by many subjects and was also difficult to understand for the investigators, despite their training. According to one survey,[8] half of French residents do not know how their home is ventilated.
- Promote improving quality of ventilation, in particular by better use of natural ventilation in the dwelling to reach a balance between indoor air quality, energy

---

[8]CSTB and CETE Study of 'the sociological aspects of indoor air management', a paper given during the ADEME 1987 'ventilation days' meeting.

economy, thermal comfort, urban lifestyle (5–10 minutes of open windows can suffice), outside noise (acoustic comfort) and protection against break-ins.
- Revise the regulations concerning adequate air change rates.

Conclusion

For this study on the possible associations between 'home energy systems, SES and health', we used indicators constructed by other teams and developed three new indicators to assess the problems of air- and water-tightness, ventilation and temperature in homes.

These findings, which confirm some known data, as well as the new and original results, should help us choose the directions for research in this emerging domain so that more specific studies assessing the relationship between energy systems in the home and health can be performed.

References

Bornehag C.G., Sundell J., Sigsgaard T. (2004) Dampness in buildings and health (DBH): Report from an ongoing epidemiological investigation on the association between indoor environmental factors and health effects among children in Sweden. *Indoor Air* 14 (Suppl 7): 59–66.

Burr M.L., Anderson H.R., Austin J.B. *et al* (1999) Respiratory symptoms and home environment in children: a national survey. *Thorax* 54: 27–32.

Dharmage S., Bailey M., Raven J. *et al* (2002) Mouldy houses influence symptoms of asthma among atopic individuals. *Clin Exp Allergy* 32: 714–20.

Engvall K., Norrby C., Norback D. (2003) Ocular, nasal, dermal and respiratory symptoms in relation to heating, ventilation, energy conservation, and reconstruction of older multi-family houses. *Indoor Air* 13: 206–11.

Gemmell I. (2001) Indoor heating, house conditions and health. *Epidemiol Community Health* 55: 928–9.

Raw G.J., Coward K.D., Brown V.M., Crump D.R. (2004) Exposure to air pollutants in English homes. *J Expo Anal Environ Epidemiol* 14 (Suppl 1): S85–S94.

Rosenthal T. (2004) Seasonal variations in blood pressure. *Am J Geriatr Cardiol* 13: 267–72.

Triche E.W., Belanger K., Beckett W. *et al* (2002) Infant respiratory symptoms associated with indoor heating sources. *Am J Respir Crit Care Med* 166: 1105–11.

Valent F., Little D'A., Bertollini R. *et al* (2004) Burden of disease attributable to selected environmental factors and injury among children and adolescents in Europe. *Lancet* 363: 2032–9.

10 Perception of safety and fear of crime
Maggie Davidson

Introduction

Definitions and incidence

This chapter focuses on people's perceptions of safety when returning home in the dark, which has strong overlaps with their fear of crime. Fear of crime and for personal safety in general are serious problems throughout Europe, and indeed most of the world, although the International Crime Victim Survey (ICVS) carried out through the UN indicates that this varies markedly by country. Results from the 2000 survey showed that in Finland and Sweden just 3% of those questioned said that they felt very unsafe walking alone after dark, compared with 10% in Poland and Switzerland and 14% in Australia (Van Kesteren *et al* 2000).

The British Crime Survey (BCS) is a large-scale survey run by the British Government that includes questions on fear of crime and feelings of personal safety. In 2002/2003, 13% of all adults said they felt very unsafe walking alone after dark (Simmons and Dodd 2003). Community surveys in Britain have also shown that fear of crime and disorder are important issues for local communities, often coming top of the concerns.

How is fear of crime linked to health?

The BCS has also shown strong links between the fear of crime and general health. Just 10% of those in good or very good health say that they feel very unsafe walking alone after dark, compared with 33% of those who say that their general health is bad or very bad. Logistic regression analysis of data from the British Household Panel Survey shows links between fears for personal safety and both general health and mental health, taking account of confounding factors such as age, sex and socio-economic status (Penvalin and Rose 2003).

However, it may be that people in poor general health may have heightened awareness about physical safety, and may also see themselves as more likely to be the victims of crime. Feelings of fear, especially if extreme or prolonged, may manifest themselves in a number of other mental and physical symptoms.

Safety and fear of crime

Concern about crime may seriously curtail activities outside the home, and the independence and initiative that parents allow their children. Fear of crime can also be associated with social isolation and disintegration and can reinforce these negative characteristics; the fewer the number of people who go out at night, the more unsafe the streets are perceived to be. The impact of these fears on quality of life issues is difficult to quantify. The 2002 BCS reported that 7% of households felt that fear of crime had a major impact on their quality of life, and a further 33% felt that it had some impact, although the nature and severity of this impact was not assessed.

Crime itself may also represent a threat to health in the form of injuries caused, or in extreme cases death. Vandalism to common areas and facilities can make these more dangerous to use: for example, where handrails to stairs are damaged or broken glass is present. The dumping of rubbish can block entrances or stairs and may also attract vermin. Fear of crime, especially if this involves fear of being outside, is also likely to result in people spending more time inside their home and increase their exposure to potential problems such as exposure to mould and other allergens, noise, pests, etc. In this way, fear of crime may exacerbate health problems caused by other factors.

In addition, there are the financial implications. Pascoe and Bartlett (2000) estimate that introducing effective crime prevention measures to social housing in England would save around £250 per dwelling per year on general management costs and responsive maintenance.

What are the main determinants of fear of crime and how does housing fit in?

The two main surveys of crime, the ICVS and BCS, both stress that while the fear of crime is largely a rational response to actual levels of crime, it is often inconsistent with the incidence of crime. For example, the BCS in 2001/2002 found that 41% of respondents were worried about being a victim of mugging, but only 0.8% of them were actually mugged in that year. The BCS also indicates that fear of crime is closely linked with the age, sex and socio-economic group, type of area, social cohesion and visible signs of anti-social behaviour. Women, older people, those in poorer areas or areas lacking social cohesion and those where there are problems like vandalism and graffiti are more likely to feel unsafe.

The incidence of crime (and therefore fear of crime) is linked to the design and maintenance of housing and its immediate environment. Studies with convicted burglars suggest various factors as important in reducing the risk of crime in social rented housing estates (Pascoe 1993, 1999), including good lighting to streets and common areas, dwellings overlooking streets and good-quality doors and windows.

Other studies have suggested a link between dwelling type and stressful living conditions, such as increased fear of crime, social isolation, reduced privacy and lack of play areas for children (Gabe and Williams 1993). A reduced fear of crime and increased feelings of safety were reported by residents following housing improvement schemes (Halpern 1995; Woodin *et al* 1996; Ambrose 2000; Blackman *et al* 2001).

Taking design too far, however, and so creating fortress-like dwellings may have negative effects; in particular, making access for emergency services difficult (DETR 1999), increasing social exclusion and reducing a wider sense of community.

It seems that the relationship between fear of crime and the built environment are complex for two main reasons:

- The factors to be considered are not just physical or technical but also relate to how the buildings and space are managed and the involvement of the occupants in that process.
- Although there may be guidelines for the design of estates and dwellings (Pascoe 1993, 1999) the solutions are not solely or mainly technical. Like many housing-related issues, there is no single simple answer. What is clear, however, is the importance of involving the occupants fully in the process of deciding on physical and management improvements. This process of working with the residents is probably as important, or possibly more important, than the physical solutions that are put in place. The consultation process itself can be used to build communities, communication, trust and confidence (sometimes referred to as 'social capital') that are central to combating fear of crime (see AIC 2003).

Whereas crime, fear of crime and anti-social behaviour are caused by social factors, the design, maintenance and management of buildings and their immediate environment can have a deterrent effect on the occurrence of crime. The question is: How much of an effect is this and can it be demonstrated that fear of crime is linked to some of these aspects if we control for other factors? This is where the LARES study and analysis comes in.

Methods

The main analysis was concerned with investigating how far fear of crime could be linked to design, condition and management of buildings and their immediate environment. This involved three stages:

- deciding on a dependent variable to represent fear of crime
- initial analysis of raw data
- building and testing a model using logistic regression.

Additional simple analysis was also carried out to establish how the fear of crime was related to other problems in the home (principally moulds, damp, cold and noise) to see whether it might act as an aggravating factor in connection with any of these problems. No attempt has been made to demonstrate conclusive linkages

Safety and fear of crime

between health problems and fear of crime; in fact, the analysis has treated both general health and signs of depression as confounding variables for the reasons outlined in the Introduction.

Main analysis – deriving a measure for fear of crime

The LARES study included four questions related to this fear of crime:

1. 'Do you feel safe when returning to your home when it is dark?'
2. 'Would you encourage your children to play on the local playgrounds?'
3. 'What are the major reasons for your dissatisfaction with the area?'
4. 'Does your home feel safe?'

We decided not to combine these into single individual scores for the following reasons:

- One question (No. 4 above) was asked of all people, the other three of just one person in the household.
- Initial analysis had suggested that different confounding factors may operate for the different aspects – e.g. age and sex are much more strongly related to feeling safe returning home after dark than to feeling safe in the home.
- Common sense suggests that the independent variables one might use would be different: for example, feeling safe in the home may be related to a history of accidents, design of stairs within the home, etc., which should have no causal link with feeling safe outside after dark.
- Perceived safety of play areas is only relevant to, and can only be reliably answered by, people with children of appropriate ages.

The analysis focused on 'Do you feel safe when returning to your home when it is dark?' (No.1 above). This question was felt to relate most directly to fear of crime. This question had three response categories ('yes', 'to some extent' and 'no, not at all'). Standard multiple regression was therefore not an option. We decided to combine the 'yes' and 'to some extent' categories. The dependent variables used were only those where there appeared to be some evidence of a relationship within the LARES data.

Initial analysis

The first stage was to examine the raw data to establish:

- The extent of missing data on key variables.
- Whether the overall incidence of fears for safety reported in LARES was broadly in line with other studies.

Safety and fear of crime

- What simple relationships existed between fears for safety and factors relating to the occupants, neighbourhood characteristics and the dwelling and immediate environment and whether these were similar to those found in other work.

The results indicate that the overall levels of fear of crime were higher than those reported in the ICVS or BCS, with 19.5% of households in the LARES sample saying that they did not feel at all safe returning home when it is dark. Part of the reason for the difference is because the question wording is slightly different to that used in these other surveys which ask how safe people felt 'walking in the area after dark'. The LARES study also shows huge variations by city and the three cities with particularly high levels of fear (Vilnius, Bratislava and Budapest) make up about half of all cases in the data set (see Figure 10.1).

The same respondent characteristics are linked to fear of crime as in the BCS. Women, older people, those in poor health and those from lower socio-economic groups are more likely to express fear than those from other groups (see Table 10.1).

The analysis also indicated that a number of variables related to building design and condition were related to feelings of safety after dark, in particular dwelling type, lighting to common areas and condition of shared spaces (Table 10.2).

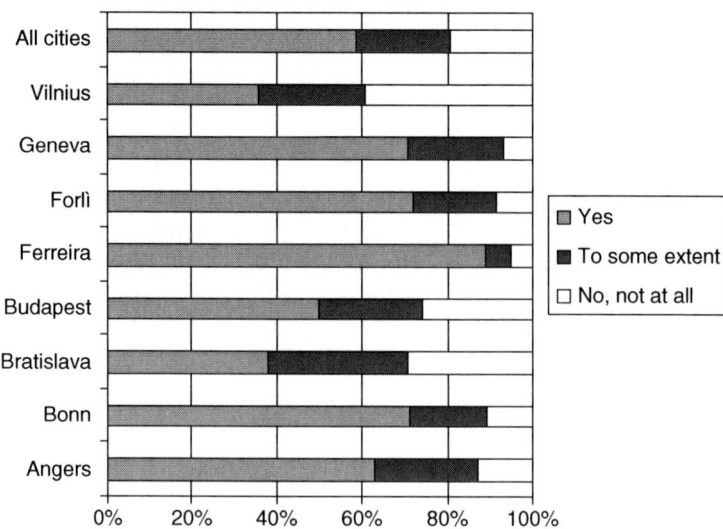

10.1 Percentage of respondents indicating whether they feel safe returning home when it is dark by city.

Table 10.1 Simple analysis of LARES data on per cent of households feeling unsafe returning home after dark – respondent characteristics

Personal characteristics		Feel safe returning home when it is dark			Total
		Yes	To some extent	No, not at all	
Age	20–39 years	63.2	21.6	15.2	100.0
	40–59 years	60.2	22.1	17.7	100.0
	60–79 years	53.2	20.6	26.2	100.0
	≥ 80 years	48.4	25.8	25.8	100.0
Gender	Female	53.4	22.9	23.7	100.0
	Male	69.3	19.4	11.3	100.0
SES score	Bottom 20%	51.3	19.9	28.8	100.0
	20th–40th percentile	57.7	21.5	20.8	100.0
	40th–60th percentile	55.2	25.2	19.6	100.0
	60th–80th percentile	59.7	22.3	17.9	100.0
	Top 20%	70.4	20.4	9.2	100.0
Health status	Very good	74.1	17.4	8.4	100.0
	Good	63.4	22.1	14.5	100.0
	Fair	50.9	23.3	25.8	100.0
	Bad	48.8	21.8	29.4	100.0
	Very bad	46.5	15.5	38.0	100.0
Signs of depression	Depressed	49.0	21.7	29.3	100.0
	Not depressed	61.0	21.8	17.1	100.0
All households		**58.8**	**21.7**	**19.5**	**100.0**

Another group of variables measured whether matters relating to the overall management of blocks and common areas, the presence of vandalism and the proportion of vacant dwellings was linked to fear of returning home after dark (Table 10.3).

One rather surprising finding was that there were higher levels of fear of crime in buildings with housekeepers than in those without. This raises the question of whether the presence of a housekeeper could be a response to residents' fears rather than a factor that could be associated with increased or reduced levels of fear. For this reason, it was omitted from the later regression analysis.

Looking at variables related to the overall design of the immediate environment and facilities present, play areas for children and having a place to sit and relax appear to be strongly related to fear of crime (Table 10.4). As expected, there are also clear links with problems like graffiti, litter and dog excrement.

Safety and fear of crime

Table 10.2 Simple analysis of LARES data on per cent of households feeling unsafe returning home after dark – building design and condition aspects

Building design and condition variable		Feel safe returning home when it is dark			
		Yes	To some extent	No, not at all	Total
Dwelling type	House	73.2	15.7	11.2	100.0
	Small apartment block	66.9	21.1	12.1	100.0
	Larger apartment block	54.0	23.1	22.9	100.0
	Panel block	39.0	29.3	31.8	100.0
Lighting of common areas	Working and sufficient	60.6	21.6	17.8	100.0
	Working but inadequate	39.9	25.2	34.9	100.0
	Present but not working	34.2	13.2	52.6	100.0
	Not present	59.1	9.1	31.8	100.0
Fire detection equipment	Yes	60.7	22.5	16.7	100.0
	No	58.9	21.5	19.5	100.0
In case of fire, easy escape from building	Yes	62.6	21.0	16.4	100.0
	No	51.4	23.3	25.3	100.0
Streets and pathways can be overlooked	Yes	60.8	21.5	17.7	100.0
	No	52.0	23.2	24.8	100.0
Most spaces and play areas can be overlooked	Yes	56.6	23.9	19.6	100.0
	No	57.0	19.8	23.2	100.0
	Not relevant	57.0	19.8	23.2	100.0
Lowest floor level of dwelling	Base, ground or first	68.5	17.6	13.9	100.0
	Second floor or above	57.0	19.8	23.2	100.0
Number of windows with gap and draughts?	None	59.1	21.7	19.2	100.0
	1 or more	51.1	22.2	26.7	100.0
Condition of shared spaces	Well maintained	63.4	21.9	14.7	100.0
	Not well maintained	49.3	25.5	25.3	100.0
	Run down	46.8	19.4	33.9	100.0
	Mix of conditions	66.7	9.1	24.2	100.0
All households		**58.8**	**21.7**	**19.5**	**100.0**

Safety and fear of crime

Table 10.3 Simple analysis of LARES data on per cent of households feeling unsafe returning home after dark – management of blocks and common areas

Management of blocks and common areas		Feel safe returning home when it is dark			Total
		Yes	To some extent	No, not at all	
Inhabited dwellings in building	All dwellings inhabited	59.7	21.6	18.7	100.0
	Under 10% empty	52.3	23.9	23.9	100.0
	11–20% empty	62.1	13.8	24.1	100.0
	21–30% empty	53.3	20.0	26.7	100.0
Signs of decoration	Yes	52.9	22.6	24.5	100.0
	No	51.7	25.2	23.1	100.0
Signs of vandalism	Yes	36.0	25.0	39.0	100.0
	No	56.2	24.5	19.3	100.0
Presence of housekeeper	Yes	49.5	25.2	25.3	100.0
	No	65.2	19.2	15.6	100.0
All households		**58.8**	**21.7**	**19.5**	**100.0**

Finally, there also appeared to be relationships between feeling safe and characteristics of the area, as shown in Table 10.5.

Logistic regression

In the initial model, all of the above variables, with the exception of presence of housekeeper, were entered to establish which were the key ones to use in a reduced model.

It is surprising that condition of shared/common spaces did not appear to be significant. When adjusted for all other variables, the odds ratios (ORs) for both minor and major problems were less than 1.2. Some association was expected, especially as the other three variables relating to condition of the immediate environment (graffiti, litter and dog excrement) showed a reasonably strong association.

The regression with the reduced set of variables was conducted in six stages so that the effect of adjusting for different types of variables could be gauged (Table 10.6).

Findings

Dwelling type

Initially this appeared to have a strong relationship with fear of returning home after dark, with apartment blocks showing an OR of around 1.4 and panel

Safety and fear of crime

Table 10.4 Simple analysis of LARES data on per cent of households feeling unsafe returning home after dark – immediate environment facilities, design and problems in the area

Immediate environment		Feel safe returning home when it is dark			Total
		Yes	To some extent	No, not at all	
Enough recreational areas for children	Yes	61.7	23.0	15.3	100.0
	To some extent	50.5	26.9	22.6	100.0
	Not really	57.3	17.2	25.4	100.0
Enough recreational areas for teenagers	Yes	61.7	22.7	15.6	100.0
	To some extent	53.6	25.2	21.2	100.0
	Not really	57.5	19.7	22.7	100.0
Place where to sit and relax	Yes	61.7	22.5	15.8	100.0
	No	52.1	20.3	27.6	100.0
Open or green space that belongs to building	Yes – private garden	70.5	18.0	11.4	100.0
	Yes – commonly shared area	48.6	25.9	25.5	100.0
	No open space	62.0	19.2	18.8	100.0
Parking sites close to buildings	Yes	57.3	22.3	20.4	100.0
	No	65.3	19.2	15.5	100.0
Graffiti	No graffiti at all	65.1	20.8	14.1	100.0
	One or two	48.9	23.1	28.0	100.0
	Three to five	44.7	21.6	33.7	100.0
	Six or more	35.3	28.0	36.7	100.0
Amount of litter	1 Very dirty / littered area	40.0	24.0	36.0	100.0
	2	42.6	23.3	34.1	100.0
	3	55.2	21.7	23.1	100.0
	4	60.9	21.8	17.3	100.0
	5 Not at all dirty / littered	66.1	21.0	12.9	100.0
Dog droppings	1 Extreme amount	42.7	24.0	33.3	100.0
	2	40.1	23.0	36.9	100.0
	3	56.4	22.0	21.6	100.0
	4	63.1	20.6	16.3	100.0
	5 No excrements at all	62.2	23.0	14.8	100.0
All households		**58.8**	**21.7**	**19.5**	**100.0**

Safety and fear of crime

Table 10.5 Simple analysis of LARES data on per cent of households feeling unsafe returning home after dark – area characteristics

Area characteristics		Feel safe returning home when it is dark			
		Yes	To some extent	No, not at all	Total
Surveyor's classification of neighbourhood type	Houses	76.5	13.8	9.7	100.0
	Apartment blocks	58.8	21.9	19.3	100.0
	Mixed	55.9	23.4	20.7	100.0
	Panel blocks	38.4	29.9	31.7	100.0
Housing circumstances	Urban centre close to busy street	59.9	22.2	17.9	100.0
	Urban centre at less busy street	62.8	19.8	17.3	100.0
	(Sub)urban neighbourhood close to busy street	53.1	21.7	25.2	100.0
	(Sub)urban neighbourhood at less busy street	56.0	24.0	20.0	100.0
	Rural area close to busy street	76.9	14.3	08.8	100.0
	Rural area at less busy street	73.9	15.8	10.3	100.0
All households		**58.7**	**21.7**	**19.5**	**100.0**

blocks an OR of 2.1 compared with houses. However, when city was added at the final stage, the OR reduced to close to 1.0, indicating no real association with dwelling type.

Lighting to common areas

This variable showed a strong relationship with fear of returning home after dark at all stages for situations where the lighting was not working or not present. When we added City, the OR shifted but there was still an increased likelihood of fear of crime of at least 1.6.

Overlooking open space

Being unable to overlook open space does appear to be linked to fear of returning home after dark. The OR actually increased slightly when we controlled for

Safety and fear of crime

Table 10.6 Results of stages of regression analyses

	Odds ratios at each stage					
	1	2	3	4	5	6
Apartment block	1.433	1.493	1.669	1.571	1.507	1.093
Panel block	2.078	2.178	2.313	2.208	1.877	0.974
Common areas, lighting not working	2.225	2.546	2.203	2.134	2.108	1.624
Common areas, lighting not present	1.926	2.05	2.199	2.122	2.182	2.734
Cannot overlook open space	1.301	1.389	1.396	1.329	1.359	1.292
Dwelling above ground level	1.281	1.413	1.426	1.425	1.406	1.292
Vandalism in common areas	1.517	1.622	1.496	1.476	1.415	1.177
Limited recreation facilities for children	1.242	1.269	1.254	1.209	1.207	1.150
No recreation facilities for children	1.567	1.619	1.627	1.659	1.695	1.764
No place to sit outside and relax or talk	1.635	1.572	1.485	1.500	1.496	1.599
Small amount of graffiti	1.523	1.456	1.482	1.463	1.510	1.167
Larger amount of graffiti	1.697	1.768	1.848	1.910	1.999	1.546
Major amount of graffiti	1.590	1.648	1.734	1.692	1.779	1.484
Immediate environment very dirty/littered	1.270	1.471	1.273	1.100	1.091	0.997
Large amount of dog excrement	1.484	1.424	1.355	1.457	1.472	1.456
Excessive amount of dog excrement	1.007	1.053	0.863	0.885	0.865	0.840

demographics and health but reduced to around 1.3 when we controlled for the main confounders and other dwelling design and condition variables.

Floor level of dwelling

The final ORs when we controlled for the main variables were very similar to that for overlooking open space, and there may be some association but not particularly strong.

Vandalism in common areas

Problems with vandalism initially appeared to have some association with fear of crime; however, the relationship virtually disappeared when we controlled for City. While a stronger relationship was expected, it may be that if the respondents had been asked about vandalism in the general area, rather than just common areas of flats, this may have been found.

Safety and fear of crime

Recreational areas for children

Lack of recreational facilities for children showed some relationship with fear of crime when adjustments were made for key confounding variables including City. Where respondents said there were not enough facilities, the OR was about 1.8.

Place to sit outside and relax or talk

Having nowhere to sit outside to relax or talk appeared to be related to fear of crime. When we controlled for the other key variables the OR was still about 1.6.

Graffiti to surrounding buildings

There appeared to be some relationship as higher levels of graffiti showed ORs of around 1.5 when adjusted for the other key variables. However, there was no linear relationship between the amount of graffiti and fear of crime. This may be because of a 'threshold' effect rather than a gradual effect. However, it is more likely to be a result of problems in assessing this aspect. Work on the English House Condition Survey has shown that assessments of problems in the local area are highly subjective and variable even after thorough training using real examples with feedback and discussion about assessments. Also, assessment will be influenced by the route taken through the area.

Litter in the immediate environment

Litter in the immediate environment showed a fairly weak relationship when adjustments were made for the other dependent variables. Once we controlled for all confounders, any effect disappeared. Although it is likely that there is some relationship between litter and fear of crime, it did not show in this analysis. Again, this may be because of the subjectivity of assessment. Questioning occupants about how serious a problem it was for them may have shown a stronger association.

Dog excrement in the immediate environment

Dog excrement in the immediate environment shows some relationship with fear of crime, although the highest ORs are associated with the second highest rather than the highest category, with an adjusted OR of just under 1.5. A lack of a linear relationship probably arises for similar reasons as for graffiti and may possibly indicate a 'threshold' effect.

Safety and fear of crime

Different patterns in different cities

The City variable had a very large impact on the associations between the dependent variables and fear of crime. We therefore carried out logistic regression using all of the key variables for five of the cities in turn to assess how far different factors might be operating in different situations.

The results for some of the key variables showed some interesting differences and similarities. Lighting to common areas, recreational areas for children and graffiti were associated with an increased likelihood of feeling not at all safe in all of the five cities. Being unable to overlook open space and having nowhere to sit and relax in the immediate environment were linked to increased fear of crime in all cities except Bonn.

Discussion

Overall, the results from the logistic regression across all cities adjusting for City and the individual regression analyses within City suggest that certain aspects of the buildings and the immediate physical environment were associated in their own right with fear of crime. These were:

- dwellings with common stairs where the lighting does not work or is not present
- inadequate recreational areas for children
- having nowhere to sit and relax in the immediate environment
- graffiti to surrounding buildings
- dog excrement in the immediate environment
- dwellings where the windows do not overlook open space
- flats located above ground floor level.

These are all the sorts of factors that one would expect to show associations based on previous work, although as far as we are aware, this is the only survey and analysis that has been able to demonstrate these linkages statistically.

Obviously, the results need to be interpreted with caution because there are a number of additional factors that could be important but for which no information was collected in the survey. These include prior victimisation, actual recorded crime in the city and level/type of press coverage before the survey.

Relationship between fear of crime and other problems

Some simple initial analysis was carried out to see how far fear of crime was related to other problems in the dwelling that may be linked to health (Table 10.7).

Safety and fear of crime

Table 10.7 Percentage of households in each 'feeling safe returning home after dark' category having other problems

	Yes – safe	To some extent	Not at all safe	Simple ratio of not at all safe: yes, safe
Current problem with mice	3.2	4.2	4.5	1.406
Current problem with cockroaches	6.6	10.3	17.0	2.576
Have permanent problems with temperature at least 1 season	15.7	13.8	27.4	1.745
Dissatisfied with heating (code 1)	3.3	3.2	7.0	2.121
Draughts described as permanent	6.0	8.2	13.8	2.226
Dissatisfied with air quality (code 1 or 2)	7.2	10.2	16.3	2.264
Damp score over 1.0	12.8	12.2	18.7	1.461
Strongly annoyed by general neighbourhood noise	3.8	6.5	13.2	3.474
Strongly annoyed by general traffic noise	5.6	10.7	17.5	3.125
Strongly annoyed by neighbour flat noise	5.8	9.2	14.8	2.552
Strongly annoyed by road traffic noise	8.8	13.5	18.2	2.068

This was to assess whether fear of crime might increase exposure to these conditions and therefore increase the risk or severity of the health outcomes. If we compared households who said they did not feel at all safe after dark with those who felt safe, then there may be much higher proportions of the former group experiencing problems with their heating, air quality, noise, pests and dampness. It is therefore very likely that fear of crime will act in combination with these problems to increase risks to health.

Conclusions

There is ample evidence that fear of crime is linked to general and mental health problems and reduced quality of life, although no causal linkage has been proved. LARES and other surveys have demonstrated that fear of crime is a common problem in Europe and that the residents of certain cities are particularly badly affected. The logistic regression has also indicated that there are aspects related to the design, maintenance and management of buildings and the immediate environment that are strongly associated with fear of crime (as represented by returning home when it is dark). This occurs even when we take into account the key confounding variables related to occupants and location.

There are also indications that those who are afraid when returning home after dark are more likely to live in homes with other problems that are likely to be detrimental to their health, including problems with heating, certain types of pests, dampness, noise and air quality. If the fear of going out forces people to spend more time at home, it may act to exacerbate and amplify the negative effects of these factors on occupants' health. Analysis of English House Condition data over several years supports the view that dwellings with multiple problems are the rule rather than the exception.

Recommendations for policy

The analysis of individual cities has indicated that a 'one size fits all' approach is inappropriate. More attention needs to be focused on the management of dwellings and on how residents can be involved in that process. Research carried out in the UK has demonstrated that even some of the worst social housing estates in terms of crime can be turned around by the application of intensive local management and increased tenant participation (DETR 1999; Cole *et al* 2001). The results of these exercises and methods used to involve residents and build communities need to be brought to a wider audience, including practitioners and those in charge of finances for housing.

However, some of the worst problems are amongst owners living in large apartment blocks or panel blocks that are suffering from poor design combined with years of neglect. Further research and development is needed to devise ways of bringing together these groups of owners to collectively improve the design, condition and management of their housing environments. It needs to be emphasised that the costs of investing in their housing and immediate environments may be rather less than the costs of simply picking up the pieces in terms of increased spending on the criminal justice and health systems.

References

AIC (2003) Working with communities to prevent and reduce crime. Australian Institute of Criminology, AIC Crime Reduction Matters, July 2003, No. 5.

Ambrose P. (2000) A drop in the ocean; the health gain from the Central Stepney SRB in the context of national health inequalities. London: The Health and Social Policy Research Centre, University of Brighton.

Blackman T., Harvey J., Lawrence M., Simon A. (2001) Neighbourhood renewal and health: evidence from a local case study. *Health and Place* 7(2): 93–104.

Cole I., Hickman P., Whittle S. (2001) On-the-Spot Housing Management. A Development Guide for Policy Makers and Practitioners. London: DTLR, October.

DETR (1999) National Strategy for Neighbourhood Renewal Report of Policy Action Team 5 – Housing management: effective housing management in the most deprived areas. Department of the Environment, Transport and the Regions, August.

Gabe J., Williams P. (1993) Women, crowding and mental health. In Burridge R., Ormandy D. (eds), Unhealthy Housing: Research, Remedies and Reform. London: E & FN Spon.

Halpern D. (1995) Improving mental health through the environment: a case study. In Halpern D. (ed.), Mental Health and the Built Environment: More than Bricks and Mortar? London: Taylor & Francis.

Pascoe T. (1993) Domestic burglaries: the burglar's view. BRE Information paper IP19/19.

Pascoe T. (1999) Crime prevention through environmental design: a view of current and future burglary research. Paper presented at the International Forum on Crime Prevention, 6–7 April 1999, Tokyo.

Pascoe T., Bartlett P. (2000) Making crime our business: a crime audit for Registered Social Landlords. CRC.

Penvalin D.J., Rose D. (2003) Social Capital for Health: Investigating the Links between Social Capital and Health Using the British Household Panel Survey. Health Development Agency, University of Essex.

Simmons J., Dodd T. (eds) (2003) Crime in England and Wales 2002/3 Home Office Statistical Bulletin, July.

Van Kesteren J.N., Mayhew P., Nieuwbeerta P. (2000) Criminal Victimisation in Seventeen Industrialised Countries: Key-findings from the 2000 International Crime Victims Survey. The Hague: Ministry of Justice, WODC.

Woodin S., Delves C., Wadhams C. (1996) Just what the doctor ordered: a study of housing, health and community safety in Holly Street, Hackney. London Comprehensive Estates Initiative, Hackney Housing Department.

11 Housing and mental health

Jérmone Fredouille, E. Laporte and Mounir Mesbah

Introduction

While causal effect of housing on mental health does not seem to be considered as controversial (Freeman 1984), we found only few epidemiological studies in the literature. Moreover, if these studies reveal psychic disorders related to typologies of housing, they do not establish a pathogenic hierarchy of factors.

In Table 11.1, Evans (2003) lists some known direct and indirect links between mental health and housing factors.

On the whole, the psychic disorders usually linked with housing are anxious disorders (anxiety, psychological distress), thymic disorders (depression, sadness, tiredness) and psychosomatic disorders (Dalle 1969; Lefebvre 1984; Evans 2003). There is also the exacerbation of psychiatric conditions or of Alzheimer's disease.

These identified psychic disorders are important in European countries, although their prevalence varies across countries. Reported results depend on the measurement techniques used and on the geographic (rural or urban) and demographic (age, gender, marital status, employment) characteristics of the study sample. Two recent studies give some insights (see Table 11.2): the 2001 Outcome of Depression International Network (ODIN) study (Ayuso-Mateos *et al* 2001) gives estimates of the prevalence of depressive disorders in Europe; and the more recent European Study of the Epidemiology of Mental Disorders project (ESEMeD/MHEDEA, 2004a).

The ESEMeD project (2004b) also examined the impact of mental health on work days lost and on quality of life. It shows a similar impact of anxiety and of depression on work loss days, but a greater impact of depression than anxiety on quality of life.

These two studies show high prevalence of both depression and anxiety in Europe. The results justify the interest given to environmental factors as potentially high risks, and housing conditions in particular appear to be significant.

Table 11.1 Direct mental health effects of housing factors

Housing factors	Direct mental health effects
High rise, multiple dwelling units	Psychological distress (anxiety and depression)
Higher floors	More mental health problems
Housing quality (structural quality, maintenance, upkeep, amenities like private bath or central heating, physical hazards)	Psychological distress
Insecurity	Psychological distress
Residential crowding	Negative effects, physiological stress
Loud exterior noise sources	Psychological distress
Malodorous air pollutants	Negative effects and behavioural reaction
Behavioural toxins	Anxiety, depression, irritability and concentration difficulties
Insufficient daylight	Sadness, fatigue and depression

Housing and mental health

A primary function of housing is to provide shelter and refuge from the outside world. It is from the reality of this shelter that stems a feeling that something stable and permanent can be achieved (Winnicot 1971). Hence, a dwelling is defined as a holding space, a physical and psychological envelope within which intimacy will develop and where each individual will find an opportunity to be himself or herself. What was just a house will become a home, and integrity of body and mind are dependent upon this possibility.

A roof under which there is shelter, together with its various conveniences and spaces, does not completely explain what is involved in living somewhere. The prime consequence of homelessness is a lack of stable social relations. Owning or having a home is a symbol of social belonging, and losing it will be felt as falling out of society. Housing induces taking roots and allows the development of supportive and mutually helpful social bonds (Paquot 1996). Security and quality of life depend very much on the establishment of good relations with neighbours, which in turn depends on various circumstances, including how the building is spatially organized, the quality of the building and its upkeep. These factors influence how people look at each other, and whether they perceive others as a nuisance, as potentially dangerous, or even as outright foes.

Those parts of a building which are shared between households function as a border zone between self and others, and tensions may arise when they fail to act as buffer zones or when neighbours try to use them as private spaces.

Table 11.2 Recent mental health studies in Europe

Study	Sample size	Countries	Results
ODIN	8764 adults (18–64 years)	UK, Ireland, Norway, Finland, Spain	Prevalence of depressive disorders: 8.56% (95%CI: 7.05–10.37) Women: 10.05% (7.80–12.85) Men: 6.61% (4.92–8.83)
ESEMeD	21425 adults (18 or older)	Belgium, France, Germany, Italy, The Netherlands, Spain	Any mood disorder, lifetime prevalence: 14% (13.4–14.6) Women: 18.2% (17.3–19.1) Men: 9.5% (8.7–10.3) Any anxiety disorder, lifetime prevalence: 13.6% (13.0–14.2) Women: 17.5% (16.6–18.4) Men: 9.5% (8.7–10.3)	Any mood disorder, 12-month prevalence: 4.2% (3.8–4.6) Women: 5.6% (5.1–6.1) Men: 2.8% (2.3–3.3) Any anxiety disorder, 12-month prevalence: 6.4% (6.0–6.8) Women: 8.7% (8.0–9.4) Men: 3.8% (3.3–4.3)

Housing and mental health

A number of the psychological processes contributing to the development of individual personality are based upon housing characteristics, and the personalisation of a space of intimacy in a home allows for feelings of being separate and an individual (Lugassy 1989).

Of course, housing conditions cannot be the only potential factors of psychiatric decompensations and nor are they the most important. Psychiatric decompensations certainly have a multifactorial aetiology, where housing conditions act to reveal psychic vulnerability or as a trigger to the appearance of psychic disorders.

Material and methods

In this work, using data from the LARES study, we analysed the associations between mental health and housing conditions. The data used was from the Housing Inspection Survey Sheet, giving relatively objective information on the housing conditions, and the Housing and Health Questionnaire, providing self-reported health status from all residents in the selected dwellings. For reasons that we explain later, we did not use data from the Inhabitant Questionnaire, and only individuals >18 years old were considered.

Mental health measurement instrument

The Housing and Health Questionnaire contains a lot of items about quality of life or, more generally, about the mental health status of the inhabitants. This was a self-completed questionnaire, and, as no physician was involved, mental health could be evaluated only through this questionnaire. For this, measurement instruments of Depression, Anxiety or Mental Quality of Life were used, and psychometrically validated scores were derived.

1. **Depression scale**
   The Housing and Health Questionnaire includes four items about depression-related symptoms which provides a SALSA[1] index. If two or more symptoms of four are present, the SALSA index (Brody *et al* 1998) indicates a high probability of major depression (APA 1994). We performed a confirmatory analysis by analysing those items of the SALSA using the Stepwise Cronbach Alpha Curve (SCAC). An increasing SCAC allows a unidimensional psychometrically validated simple score of depression to be built based on the number of symptoms present.[2]
2. **Anxiety scale**
   Questions about symptoms of anxiety (as defined in Diagnostic and Statistical Manual-IV, 300.02 (APA 1994) or in International Classification

---
[1]See Chapter 12.
[2]The SALSA final measure, as originally defined, can be obtained by dichotomising this validated score.

of Diseases-10, F41.1 (WHO 1993) were selected and analysed using the SCAC to build a unidimensional psychometrically validated score of anxiety.
3. **Quality of Life scale**
    Questions in the Housing and Health Questionnaire about Mental Quality of Life were identified and analysed, again using the SCAC, to build a unidimensional psychometrically validated score of Quality of Life. During this step, we take into account that most of the Quality of Life items included in the Housing and Health Questionnaire were extracted from the MOS 36-Item Short-Form Health Survey (SF-36), a proven multi-purpose health survey (Ware and Sherbourne 1992).

The relationships between these three mental health scales and housing conditions from the Housing Inspection Survey Sheet were investigated by logistic regression models, including individual 'prognostic' factors from the Housing and Health Questionnaire, using an ad hoc preliminary logistic regression study.

Population analysed

The three different mental health scales only fit well with information on adult symptoms. This is because the SALSA index has been validated for those aged ≥18 years old (Brody *et al* 1998), and the MOS SF-36 includes some items validated only for those aged ≥14 years old (Ware and Sherbourne 1992). For Anxiety, some of the items examined can describe anxiety in children, but we know that anxious disorders are less easy verbalized by children than adults, and more often expressed as physical symptoms (Messerschmitt 1994). For these reasons, our study is limited to the subpopulation of adults >18 years, providing 6920 valid questionnaires.

Risk factors investigated

1. **Individual factors**
    Demographic and sociological characteristics are likely to alter well-being or mental disorder levels. For each mental health aspect investigated, we tested our three scales against all General Information items of the Housing and Health Questionnaire, except the only single open question. The City variable and the SES score[3] were also considered.
2. **Housing factors**
    Housing conditions in the LARES survey were investigated by two questionnaires – the Inhabitant Questionnaire and the Housing Inspection

---

[3] Developed by Maggie Davidson of the UK Building Research Establishment.

Housing and mental health

Survey Sheet. We analysed only the more objective housing variables from the Housing Inspection Survey Sheet. Even if results from this source are also influenced by the subjectivity of the surveyors, it is, of course, independent of the subjectivity of the inhabitant.

The Housing Inspection Survey Sheet contains 248 closed questions, all of which were used. Open questions were not analysed. For each categorical non-ordinal variable (individual or housing factors) we generated and analysed new dichotomous variables (dummy variables), each corresponding to a specific level of the original variable.

Statistical analysis strategy

The statistical problem is to analyse the effect of housing conditions on mental health. Housing conditions are defined by the set of housing factors, and mental health is defined by the set of three validated scales for Depression, Anxiety and Quality of Life. It is well known that mental health is mainly affected by individual factors, so that examination of the effect of the housing factors must be adjusted on an individual basis. The choice of a statistical strategy is dependent on the nature and the number of the response variables (quantitative or categorical) and on the explanatory variables involved in the analysis. Our choice was to focus on the three response variables summarising mental health already described.

It is difficult to prove causality of the effect of a factor and a response variable in an observational transversal study. Nevertheless, one can at least avoid many pitfalls and bias, and recover useful and reliable information about causality.

For each response variable (Depression, Anxiety or Quality of Life), we applied the following analysis strategy.

Step 1: analysis of individual factors

i   Identification of individual factors marginally associated with the response using marginal analysis.
ii   Building a multiple logistic regression model with explanatory variable set, including all previously identified individual factors.
iii   Then removing those individual factors not significantly associated with the response in this multiple logistic model. So, for each mental health variable, we identified a set of individual significant factors.

Step 2: analysis of housing factors adjusted on individual factors

i   Identification of housing factors marginally associated with the response using marginal analysis, removing non-significant factors.

ii For each of those housing factors marginally associated, examining its effect in a multiple logistic regression model with as explanatory variable the set of individual significant factors identified in Step 1, stage iii, and the considered housing factor. At this step, we obtained, for each housing factor, an odds ratio (OR) measuring this effect adjusted on the set of individual factors. If this OR is non-significant, the housing factor is removed.

Step 3: Multiple analysis of housing factors adjusted on individual factors

i For each housing domain, we built a multiple logistic regression model with explanatory variable set, including the set of individual significant factors (Step 1, stage iii) and all previously significant housing factors identified in Step 2, stage ii. This gave, for each housing factor, an OR measuring this effect adjusted on the set of individual factors and the set of housing factors of the same domain. Again, if this OR is non-significant, the housing factor is removed.

ii Then, we built a multiple logistic regression model with explanatory variable set including the set of individual significant factors (Step 1, stage iii) and all previously significant housing factors identified in stage i of Step 1. This gave, for each housing factor, an OR measuring this effect adjusted on the set of individual factors and the set of all other significant housing factors. Once again, if this OR is non-significant, the housing factor is removed.

Results

Validation and scores construction

SCAC was used to validate the four items defining Depression in the SALSA index and the items in the questionnaire relating to SF-36 and Quality of Life.

Four items were used to build a score for Anxiety, varying from 0 to 100. The reliability was high (more than 0.73) but the SCAC was not an increasing one. This suggested removing one item – Need time to get to sleep – but after validating it with another item in the questionnaire on previously observed anxiety and depression, it was decided not to remove it.

Statistical investigation of housing factors associated with mental health

Results of the statistical analysis are summarized in Tables 11.3A and 11.3B (Quality of Life), Tables 11.4A and 11.4B (Anxiety) and Tables 11.5A and 11.5B (Depression). Following the chosen strategy, we first analysed individual factors.

Housing and mental health

Table 11.3A Individual risk factors of a good Quality of Life

Label	Odds ratio
Sex (male)	1.212 (1.191; 1.233)
Married, living with spouse	1.060 (1.022; 1.099)
Married, separated from spouse	0.899 (0.838; 0.964)
Single	1.057 (1.016; 1.099)
Divorced	0.944 (0.898; 0.992)
Widowed	0.867 (0.825; 0.911)
Level of education (0 no, 4 high)	1.059 (1.051; 1.068)
Full-time work	1.042 (1.021; 1.063)
Student/pupil	1.068 (1.031; 1.108)
Unemployed	0.914 (0.884; 0.945)
Taking care of household	1.124 (1.081; 1.170)
Smoke daily more than 15 cigarettes	0.799 (0.778; 0.821)
Problem with drinking	0.881 (0.864; 0.898)
Amount of sport (1 low, 5 high)	1.115 (1.106; 1.124)
Socio-economic score	1.027 (1.019; 1.034)
Angers	1.233 (1.191; 1.277)
Vilnius	0.866 (0.840; 0.892)
Bonn	1.207 (1.166; 1.250)
Budapest	0.876 (0.849; 0.904)
Ferreira	1.183 (1.141; 1.225)
Forlì	1.104 (1.069; 1.141)
Geneva	1.285 (1.238; 1.334)

Only those individual factors significantly associated (at the 5% level) with mental health responses marginally and globally (in the multiple final model) are presented. Similarly, housing factors were analysed in multiple models, and only significantly associated factors (at the 5% level) with mental health responses marginally and globally (in the multiple final model) are presented.

The ORs with 95% confidence interval are shown. The number of significant factors seems to be high, but it is low considering the high number of factors investigated. More individual than housing factors remain in the final model. This is the direct consequence of the statistical strategy chosen: the set of individual factors built into first step of the analysis, and no individual factors can be removed in Steps 2 or 3. Nevertheless, most of the time, these individual factors remain strongly associated with the responses in Steps 2 or 3. This is a confirmation that in relation to mental health, the individual human profile is more important than environmental factors. The number of significant factors is higher when Quality of Life is the response, and lower when the response is Depression.

The OR between Anxiety and Depression (Risk of Anxiety when Depressed) was 2.684 (2.611; 2.759). The OR between Quality of Life and Depression (Risk of Good Quality of Life when Depressed) was 0.383 (0.376; 0.390).

Table 11.3B Housing risk factors of a good Quality of Life

Labels	Multifamily No	Multifamily Yes
Housing information		
Neighbourhood: mainly semi-detached houses	1.169 (1.060; 1.288)	
House type: multifamily apartment block – up to 6 units	1.438 (1.331, 1.554)	1.113 (1.065; 1.163)
Location: in a (sub)urban neighbourhood close to a busy street	1.115 (1.050; 1.185)	
Location: in a rural area close to a busy street	1.699 (1.519; 1.901)	
General aspects		
Window quality in the flat: single-glazed windows	1.123 (1.062; 1.188)	
No mould growth visible		1.050 (1.027; 1.073)
Smell of dampness/mould	0.725 (0.659; 0.799)	
Condensation signs at windows	0.747 (0.689; 0.809)	0.858 (0.801; 0.920)
Faults, disrepair		
Faults at several places of the same element	0.845 (0.743; 0.962)	
Number of faults		0.858 (0.801; 0.920)
Kitchen		
Gas water heater connected to the outside, in the kitchen	0.809 (0.760; 0.860)	1.103 (1.049; 1.159)
Deep freezer	0.906 (0.835; 0.982)	0.870 (0.821; 0.923)
Kitchen sink, one or two		0.835 (0.725; 0.961)
Kitchen workspace next to the sink	1.108 (1.037; 1.184)	
Extract above the cooking place connected to the outside		1.073 (1.022; 1.126)
Extract above the cooking place not connected to the outside	1.097 (1.025; 1.173)	1.139 (1.089; 1.192)
Bathroom		
Hot water is available in the bathroom	1.561 (1.258; 1.937)	1.287 (1.048; 1.581)
Type of floor to the bathroom is tiles	1.135 (1.005; 1.283)	
Type of floor to the bathroom is PVC/plastic	1.406 (1.200; 1.646)	0.844 (0.753; 0.945)
No toilet inside or exclusive	1.220 (1.072; 1.388)	1.160 (1.026; 1.312)
Wash-hand basin in the toilet with cold and warm water	1.100 (1.026; 1.179)	
Total number of showers and/or bath tubs (max. 3)	0.898 (0.866; 0.931)	

(continued)

Table 11.3B (Cont'd)

Label	Multifamily	
	No	Yes
Safety, accessibility		
Doorsteps in the door frames to the entrance door	0.886 (0.840; 0.935)	0.872 (0.828; 0.918)
Doorsteps in the door frames between the rooms		1.057 (1.000; 1.118)
Most streets or pathways can be overlooked from the dwelling	1.166 (1.096; 1.241)	1.073 (1.026; 1.123)
There are no open spaces and play areas		0.928 (0.886; 0.971)
Steps and staircase		
Stairs are heavily damaged and unsafe	0.217 (0.137; 0.344)	
Stairs have adequate, light equipment operational and sufficient		1.102 (1.042; 1.164)
Stairs are slightly damaged or loose/heavily damaged and unsafe		1.251 (1.164; 1.344)
There are many height differences where people can stumble		0.911 (0.869; 0.956)
There are any signs of decoration or appropriation in the staircase		1.089 (1.050; 1.130)
There are signs of vandalism in the staircase		1.118 (1.050; 1.191)
Housing environment		
No open garden or shared space	1.673 (1.408; 1.987)	1.362 (1.209; 1.535)
These space are well maintained/taken care of	1.491 (1.295; 1.716)	1.322 (1.175; 1.488)
These space are not well maintained but also not run-down	1.365 (1.180; 1.579)	1.335 (1.183; 1.506)
These space are not maintained and run-down	1.593 (1.323; 1.918)	
No graffiti at all		0.922 (0.868; 0.980)
Amount of litter: 1, very dirty; 5, not at all	1.031 (1.000; 1.063)	
Amount of dog droppings: 1, extreme; 5, no excrements		0.974 (0.953; 0.995)
Vegetation/greenery visible, on public grounds	0.881 (0.835; 0.929)	0.916 (0.880; 0.954)
Vegetation/greenery visible, on facades/windows/balconies	1.105 (1.052; 1.162)	1.071 (1.032; 1.111)
There is a park or green open space close to the dwelling	1.100 (1.044; 1.159)	0.950 (0.912; 0.990)

Discussion

For several reasons, these results must be taken with caution. Missing data can invalidate the results and many marginal associations can disappear after multivariate adjustment. This is not for confounding reasons or spurious associations, but because the sample population analysed, in practice, will be different. The great number of the examined variables did not allow us to propose an easy-to-make solution for this problem. Nevertheless, assuming that missing data were missing at random, it can be reasonably expected that the associations found are true, albeit conservative. However, it could mean that some associations found to be non-significant could be significant.

Mental health and housing conditions

Our analysis of the LARES database makes it possible to propose a typology of the dwelling driven by a high significant level of probability of anxiety or depression (Tables 11.4A, 11.4B, 11.5A and 11.5B):

1. *Dwellings not correctly fulfilling their functions of protection from the outside:* windows that cannot be closed; single-glazed windows; visible mould growth; condensation signs at windows; heavily damaged stairs; etc.
2. *Dwellings lacking a pleasant environment:* located in a rural area near a busy street; multifamily apartment block up to 6 residential units; without streets or pathways overlooked from the dwelling through windows; and without open spaces and play areas overlooked from the dwelling through windows.

Table 11.4A Individual risk factors of Anxiety

Label	Odds ratios
Sex (male)	0.794 (0.774; 0.814)
Married, living with spouse	0.899 (0.870; 0.929)
Single	0.909 (0.873; 0.945)
Level of education (0 low, 4 high)	0.928 (0.916; 0.939)
Unemployed	1.120 (1.066; 1.176)
Smoke daily more than 15 cigarettes	1.291 (1.239; 1.346)
Problem with drinking	1.118 (1.086; 1.151)
Amount of sport (from low to high)	0.916 (0.905; 0.928)
Socio-economic score	0.974 (0.964; 0.984)
Angers	1.090 (1.040; 1.142)
Vilnius	1.261 (1.215; 1.309)
Budapest	1.227 (1.175; 1.280)
Ferreira	1.122 (1.070; 1.177)

Table 11.4B Housing risk factors of Anxiety

Label	Multifamily No	Multifamily Yes
Housing information		
Multifamily apartment block – up to 6 residential units	0.745 (0.680; 0.817)	0.877 (0.840; 0.915)
Location: in the rural area close to a busy street	0.797 (0.721; 0.880)	0.799 (0.740; 0.863)
General aspects		
Window can be closed in the flat		1.044 (1.019; 1.070)
Window quality in the flat: double-glazed windows	0.922 (0.863; 0.986)	0.960 (0.928; 0.993)
Amount of mould growth visible	1.039 (1.011; 1.068)	1.021 (1.006; 1.036)
Condensation signs at windows	1.223 (1.125; 1.331)	1.080 (1.032; 1.131)
Faults, disrepair		
Faults at several places of the same element		1.052 (1.004; 1.102)
Kitchen		
Kitchen workspace next to the sink		0.942 (0.912; 0.972)
Bathroom		
Hot water is available in the bathroom	0.665 (0.540; 0.821)	0.736 (0.571; 0.948)
Safety, accessibility		
No spaces available to be overlooked through windows		1.074 (1.038; 1.111)
Steps and staircase		
Stairs are heavily damaged and unsafe	2.190 (1.482; 3.237)	
Housing environment		
One or two graffiti	1.140 (1.029; 1.262)	1.070 (1.033; 1.108)
Vegetation/greenery visible, on public grounds	1.105 (1.042; 1.171)	1.055 (1.022; 1.089)
Vegetation/greenery visible, on facades/windows/balconies	0.904 (0.851; 0.960)	0.951 (0.923; 0.981)
Parking site close to building	1.094 (1.030; 1.161)	1.056 (1.018; 1.095)

3. *Dwellings with degraded or not very attractive common parts:* with visible faults, disrepair or evidence of deterioration at several places; without signs of decoration or adequate management in the staircase; without adequate working lighting in staircase; with visible graffiti; and without vegetation/greenery visible in the immediate housing environment.
4. *Dwellings lacking certain elements of comfort:* without kitchen workspace next to the sink, hot water in the bathroom or lift in the building.

Table 11.5A Individual risk factors of Depression

Label	Odds ratios
Sex (male)	0.695 (0.605; 0.799)
Married, separated from spouse	1.980 (1.259; 3.106)
High level of education	0.869 (0.814; 0.927)
Full-time work	0.689 (0.589; 0.805)
Student/pupil	0.694 (0.528; 0.914))
Smoke daily more than 15 cigarettes	1.511 (1.224; 1.866)
Problem with drinking	1.504 (1.299; 1.742)
High amount of sport	0.816 (0.762; 0.873)
Socio-economic score	0.913 (0.866; 0.963)
Bonn	0.493 (0.372; 0.654)
Ferreira	1.572 (1.287; 1.923)
Forlì	0.578 (0.462; 0.723)
Geneva	0.675 (0.512; 0.888)

Similarly, it is possible to propose dwelling typology driven by highly significant decrease in quality of life (Tables 11.3A and 11.3B). This includes the factors previously described and also:

1. *Dwellings lacking other elements of comfort:* no gas water heater in the kitchen, no fridge, no kitchen sink, no exhaust system above the cooking place, no toilet, or no wash-hand basin in the toilet, a small number of showers, floor in the bathroom without tile, etc.
2. *An unpleasant or badly maintained environment:* absence of garden or open or green space that belongs to the building, badly maintained gardens or spaces, accumulation of waste in these spaces, absence of park or open space accessible to the public near the dwelling, presence of dog droppings in the neighbourhoods.

About causality between mental health and housing conditions

It is well known in clinical psychiatry that individuals with psychiatric problems can neglect the maintenance of their housing so much so that it becomes unhealthy. The classical Diogenes syndrome (Kocher and Chabert 1993) is an illustration and, in these very exceptional situations, alterations of housing and psychic disorders are combined and mutually worsened.

In the very large majority of cases, the pathogenesis of housing does come into question. It will be obvious when the individual does not have any or only few possibilities of action on their housing: e.g. absence of parks, difficult district, external degradations and defects of architectural design. So, it is not easy to establish evidence about the causal relationship.

Table 11.5B Housing risk factors of Depression

Label	Multifamily	
	No	Yes
Housing information		
Location: in the rural area close to a busy street	1.812 (1.058; 3.103)	
Faults, disrepair		
At least one fault at several places of the same element	0.485 (0.343; 0.686)	
Safety, accessibility		
Most streets or pathways can be overlooked from the dwelling		1.286 (1.009; 1.638)
Steps and staircase		
The steps or the staircase have handrails	0.627 (0.422; 0.931)	
The lift serves all floors in the building		1.377 (1.025; 1.849)

Conclusion

The LARES study, by the diversity and the extent of its sample, makes it possible to confirm the psycho-social concepts often deduced from more restricted studies or individual assumptions of responsibility.

From our analyses, we have shown that the housing factors that can affect the quality of mental life of their inhabitants are numerous – the 42 items in Table 11.3B. Among these, the 15 items in Table 11.4B are in addition significantly related to anxious disorders, and the 5 items in Table 11.5B are significantly related to depressive disorders.

This graduation of the pathogenesis of housing (which goes from housing causing deterioration of the Quality of Life, to housing giving true anxious or depressive disorders) seems to be one of the great findings in the LARES study. It supports the concept of a 'dose effect' of housing factors. Indeed, it makes it possible to establish a hierarchy of the technical, architectural or urbanistic interventions to improve the global housing quality by elimination or reduction of deteriorations of housing related to a high level of anxiety or depression.

Thus, by establishing a very solid statistical association between housing conditions and the presence of statistically higher anxious or depressive disorders among inhabitants, the LARES project makes it possible to reaffirm the fundamental functions of housing:

- It must be able to function as a refuge (shelter), providing adequate protection from the outside (windows, damp-proof, protection from noise and cold, etc).

- It must provide, in a flexible and pleasant way, a bridge between the interior and the external world (this includes the importance of the opportunities to observe the outside, since housing and a pleasant and peaceful local environment are not isolated).
- Lastly, each dwelling is a kind of social representative of the inhabitants. Its degradation (graffiti, staircases), its lack of decoration or light, constitute an equivalent of a degradation of the individual and influence depressive or anxious states.

The taking into account of these important functions of housing should guide those responsible for creating new residences and those responsible for the rehabilitation of old or decayed housing. This is not to ignore certain elements of domestic comfort, such as well-equipped kitchens, or that certain characteristics of the immediate environment, such as gardens and open spaces, are significant, and that their absence will deteriorate the quality of life of the inhabitants.

References

American Psychiatric Association (APA) (1994) Diagnostic and Statistical Manual-IV. Washington, DC: American Psychiatric Association.

Ayuso-Mateos J.L., Vázquez-Barquero J.R., Dowrick C. et al (2001) Depressive disorders in Europe: prevalence figures from the Outcome of Depression International Network (ODIN) study. *Br J Psychiatry* 179: 308–16.

Brody D.S., Hahn S.R., Spitzer R.L. et al (1998) Identifying patients with depression in the primary care setting: a more efficient method. *Arch Intern Med* 158: 2469–75.

Dalle B. (1969) Existe-t-il une psychopathologie de l'habitat? *Confrontations Psychiatriques* 4: 109–19.

ESEMeD/MHEDEA 2000 Investigators (2004a) Prevalence of mental disorders in Europe: results from the European Study of the Epidemiology of Mental Disorders (ESEMeD) project. *Acta Psychiatr Scand* 109 (Suppl. 420): 21–7.

ESEMeD/MHEDEA 2000 Investigators (2004b) Disability and quality of life impact of mental disorders in Europe: results from the European Study of the Epidemiology of Mental Disorders (ESEMeD) project. *Acta Psychiatr Scand* 109 (Suppl. 420): 38–46.

Evans G.W. (2003) The built environment and mental health. *J Urban Health* 80: 536–55.

Freeman H.L. (1984) Housing. In: Freeman H.L. (ed), Mental Health and the Environment. London: Churchill Livingstone, 197–225.

Kocher Y., Chabert M.J. (1993). Le syndrome de Diogène. *Gérontologie et Société e*. 64: 132–44.

Lefebvre P. (1984) Hygiène mentale et grands ensembles en Europe occidentale. *Annales Médico-Psychologiques* 4: 527–32.

Lugassy F. (1989) Logement, corps, identité, coll. Emergences, ed Universitaires.

Messerschmitt P. (1994) Les troubles anxieux et le concept de névroses de l'enfant. In: Canoui P., Messerschmitt P., Ramos O. (eds), Psychiatrie de l'Enfant et de l'Adolescent. Paris: Maloine.

Paquot T. (1996) Architecture et exclusion. In: L'Exclusion l'État des Savoirs, edition la Découverte. Paris.

Ware J.E., Sherbourne C.D. (1992) The MOS 36-Item Short-Form Health Survey (SF-36):I. Conceptual framework and item selection. *Med Care* 30: 473–83.

Winnicot Q.W. (1971) The place where we live. In: Playing and Reality.

World Health Organization (WHO) (1993). The International Classification of Diseases, 10th edn. Classification of Mental and Behavioral Disorders: Diagnostic Criteria for Research. Geneva: World Health Organization.

12 Building Quality of Life-related Housing scores using the LARES study – a methodical approach to avoid pitfalls and bias

Mounir Mesbah

Introduction

The main goal of this work is to use established scientific knowledge, modern statistical techniques and the large database provided by the LARES study (Bonnefoy *et al* 2003, Bonnefoy *et al* 2004; WHO 2005) to develop and validate simple scores and indicators measuring Health. These Quality of Housing scores are based on responses to variables (questions) included in two of the LARES instruments: from the Housing and Health Questionnaire (HH) completed by inhabitants and from the Housing Inspection Survey Sheet (HI) completed by the surveyors. In a second step, again using the same database, and using the health scores and indicators created, a prognostic model was developed with Housing Conditions as explanatory and Health scores as response variables.

This model will help to predict various Health domains: Mental (Depression, Anxiety), Quality of Life, Accidents, Noise, Allergy, by the intermediate of these Housing scores. This model and these scores will help inform policymakers in the joint fields of housing and health.

The large database provided by the LARES survey provided the opportunity to build and validate these scores statistically. Figure 12.1 shows an overview of the global model, explaining inhabitant health in terms of Housing Conditions

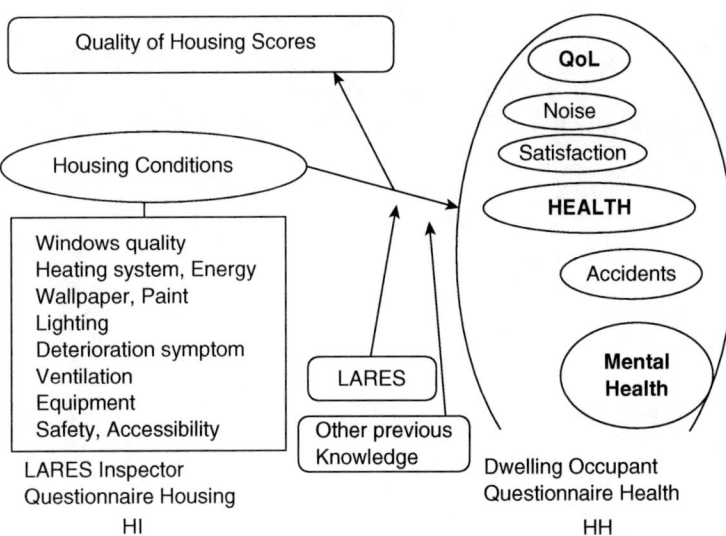

12.1 Overview.

(including various fields) using the LARES survey and previous knowledge. This model will allow us to produce Quality of Housing Scores.

At this stage, two different (but similar and complementary) questions can be investigated:

- **Question A** – analysis of causal effect of Housing Conditions (HI) on Health (HH).
- **Question B** – Creating scores based on (computed with) Housing Conditions (HI) that predict accurately Health Conditions (HH).

In a first step, both Questions A and B can be interpreted by Figures 12.2 and 12.3, but:

- Question A means that we are interested in individual (human) risk factors related to their Housing Condition, and we are looking for a scientific explanation.
- Question B is more related to an operational decision; we are focussing on the dwelling risk factor, whatever the profile of the individual.

Question A – analysis of causal effect of Housing Conditions (HI) on Health (HH)

To be able to state that a specific Housing Condition is a risk factor we must show that there is a strong relation between that Housing Condition and Health,

Quality of Life-related Housing scores

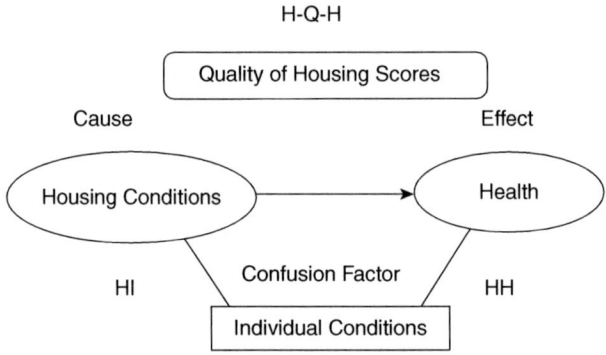

12.2 Health explained by Housing Conditions, after adjustment on individual profile.

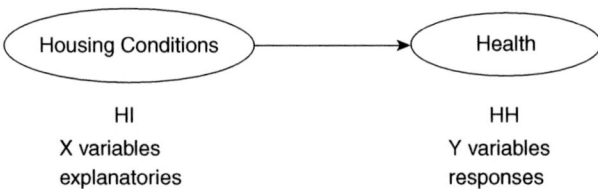

12.3 Health explained by Housing Conditions, without adjustment on individual profile.

whoever is living in that house. So, we must analyse the relation between HI (as an explanatory variable X) and HH (as a response variable Y) after taking into account the effect of individual factors (see Figure 12.4). The effect of the specific Housing Condition on Health must be significant, whatever the individual factor.

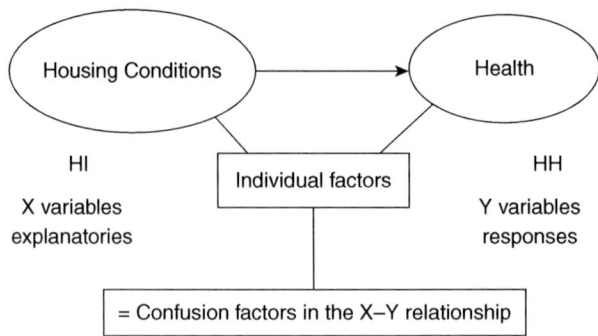

12.4 Causal relationship between Housing Conditions and Health.

Quality of Life-related Housing scores

Question B – Creating Quality of Housing Scores (H-Q-H) driven by Health Conditions, i.e. building scores computed with Housing Conditions (HI) that predict Health Conditions (HH) (see Figure 12.5)

Of course, it is not realistic to build an operational H-Q-H score for the possible profiles of every individual. We are more interested in the 'dwelling profile', for some individual profiles. For instance, we can focus on:

- the 'worst healthy people' – those individuals most vulnerable in terms of their health or
- the 'mean healthy people' – the mean health profile of individuals' profile (i.e. the intermediate health condition level).

But we have to be aware that these 'worst healthy people' or 'mean healthy people' profiles are different from one country to another. Even if one treats Europe as a homogeneous continent, at least in terms of health (more than in terms of socio-economic status), local policymakers must optimise their decision by applying our methodology to their local data.

Defining the 'worst healthy' is difficult, so we avoid this political question (i.e. choosing between 'worst' and 'mean' healthy) by choosing the easiest (in term of technical work) strategy, which is fortunately a conservative approach. When we select factors marginally associated to health housing factors and then include individual factors, we can expect to lose some associations, but we cannot discover new associations – hidden factors.

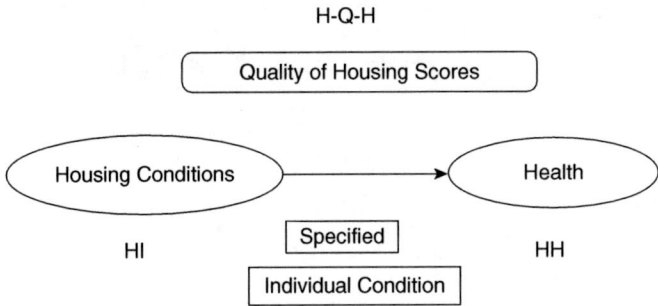

12.5 Quality of Housing scores.

Material and methods

This work is based on the LARES data from the Housing and Health Questionnaire (HH) completed by all inhabitants in the selected dwellings, and the Housing Inspection Survey Sheet (HI) completed by the inspectors.

Quality of Life-related Housing scores

For reasons explained in Chapter 11, data from the Inhabitant Questionnaire is not used, and only data from the Housing and Health Questionnaire completed by people >18 years old is considered in this work.

Measurement theory: statistical background.

The parallel model describing the unidimensionality of a set of variables

Let $X_1, X_2, \ldots, X_k$, be a set of observed variables measuring the same underlying unidimensional latent (unobserved) variable. We define X_{ij} as the measurement of subject i, $i = 1, \ldots, n$, given by a variable j, where $j = 1, \ldots, k$. The model underlying Cronbach's Alpha is just a mixed one-way ANOVA model:

$$X_{ij} = m_j + a_i + e_{ij}$$

where m_j is a varying fixed (non-random) effect and a_i is a random effect with zero mean and standard error s_a corresponding to subject variability. It produces the variance of the true latent measure ($t_{ij} = m_j + a_i$). The error e_{ij} is a random effect with zero mean and standard error s corresponding to the additional measurement error. The true measure and the error are uncorrelated:

$$\text{cov}(a_i, e_{ij}) = 0$$

These assumptions are classical in experimental design. This model defines relationships between different kinds of variables: the observed score X_{ij}, the true score t_{ij} and the error e_{ij}. It is interesting to make some remarks about assumptions underlying this model. The random part of the true measure of individual i is the same whatever might be variable j. The quantity a_i does not depend on j. The model is unidimensional. One can assume that in their structural part all variables measure the same thing (a).

Reliability of an instrument

A measurement instrument gives us values that we call observed measures. The reliability r of an instrument is defined as the ratio of the true over the observed measure. Under the parallel model, one can show that the reliability of any variable X_j (as an instrument to measure the true value) is given by:

$$\rho = \frac{\sigma_\alpha^2}{\sigma_\alpha^2 + \sigma^2}$$

which is also the constant correlation between any two variables. This coefficient is also known as the intra-class coefficient. The reliability coefficient r can be easily interpreted as a correlation coefficient between the true and the observed measure.

When the parallel model is assumed, the reliability of the sum of k variables equals:

$$\tilde{\rho} = \frac{k\rho}{k\rho+(1-\rho)}$$

This formula is known as the Spearman–Brown formula. Its maximum likelihood estimator, under the assumption of a normal distribution of the error and the parallel model, is known as Cronbach's alpha coefficient (CAC) (Cronbach 1951; Kristof 1963):

$$\alpha = \frac{k}{k-1}\left(1-\frac{\sum_{j=1}^{k}S_j^2}{S_{tot}^2}\right)$$

where

$$S_j^2 = \frac{1}{n-1}\sum_{i=1}^{n}(X_{ij}-\bar{X}_j)^2$$

and

$$S_{tot}^2 = \frac{1}{nk-1}\sum_{i=1}^{n}\sum_{j=1}^{k}(X_{ij}-\bar{X})^2$$

It is easy to show a direct connection between CAC and the percentage of variance of the first component in principal component analysis (PCA) that is often used to assess unidimensionality (Moret *et al* 1993). The PCA is usually based on an analysis of the latent roots of the correlation matrix of k variables R, which, under the parallel model, looks as follows:

$$\mathbf{R} = \begin{bmatrix} 1 & \rho. & .. & ..\rho \\ \rho. & 1 & \rho. & ..\rho \\ .. & \rho & 1 & \rho.. \\ \rho. & .. & .\rho & 1 \end{bmatrix}$$

This matrix has only two different latent roots: the greater root is

$$\lambda_1 = (k-1)\rho+1$$

and the other multiple roots are

$$\lambda_2 = \lambda_3 = \lambda_4 = \ldots = 1-\rho = \frac{k-\lambda_1}{k-1}$$

So, using the Spearman–Brown formula, we can express the reliability of the sum of the k variables as

$$\tilde{\rho} = \frac{k}{k-1}\left(1 - \frac{1}{\lambda_1}\right)$$

This clearly indicates a monotonic relationship, which is estimated by a (CAC) and the first latent root λ_1, which in practice is estimated by the corresponding value of the observed correlation matrix and thus the percentage of variance of the first principal component in a PCA. So, CAC is also considered as a measure of unidimensionality.

The Spearman–Brown formula indicates a simple relationship between CAC and the number of variables. It is easy to show that the CAC is an increasing function of the number of variables. This formula is obtained under the parallel model.

Stepwise Cronbach alpha curve

A step-by-step curve of CAC can be built to assess the unidimensionality of a set of variables (Moret et al 1993; Curt et al 1997). The first step uses all variables to compute CAC. Then, at every successive step, one variable is removed from the scale. The removed variable is one which leaves the scale with its maximum CAC value. This procedure is repeated until only two variables remain. If the parallel model is true, increasing the number of variables increases the reliability of the total score, which is estimated by Cronbach's alpha. Thus, a decrease of such a curve after adding a variable would cause us to suspect strongly that the added variable did not constitute a unidimensional set with the other variables.

Factorial analysis

Factorial analysis models generalise the previous simple parallel model ($X_j = \mu_j + \alpha + \varepsilon_j$, the subject subscript i is forgotten without risk of confusion) from one true component α to p true components θ_1 ($k << p$, and with $\theta_1 = \mu_j + \alpha_j$):

$$X_j = a_{11}\theta_1 + a_{12}\theta_2 + \ldots + a_{1p}\theta_p + E_j$$

In the factor analysis setting, this is usually written as:

$$X = AU + E$$

where A is the factor loading matrix and U and E are independent.

PCA can be considered as a particular factorial analysis model with $p = k$, and without error terms (E is not in the model). In PCA, components (θ_1) are chosen orthogonal ($\theta_1 \perp \theta_m$) and with decreasing variance (amount of information).

Quality of Life-related Housing scores

In practice, a varimax rotation is often performed after a PCA to allow a better interpretation of the latent variable in terms of the original variables. It allows a clear clustering of the original variables in subsets (unidimensionals). In each subset, one expects unidimensional variables.

Modern measurement models and graphical modelling

Modern ideas about measurement models are more general. Instead of arbitrarily defining the relationship between observed and truth as an additive function (of the true and the error), they just focus on the joint distribution of the observed and the true variables $f(X, \theta)$. We do not need to specify any kind of distance between X and θ. E and its relation to X and θ could be anything! E is not equal to $X - \theta$. E could be some kind of distance between the distributions of X and θ.

This leads us naturally to graphical modelling, as presented briefly in the introduction of this chapter. Graphical modelling aims to represent the multidimensional joint distribution of a set of variables by a graph. We will focus on conditional independence graphs. The interpretation of an independence graph is easy. Each multivariate distribution is represented by a graphic, which is composed of nodes and edges between nodes. Nodes represent one-dimensional random variables (observed or latent, i.e., non-observed), whereas a missing edge between two variables means that those two variables are independent conditionally on the rest (all other variables in the multidimensional distribution). Since the pioneering work of Lauritzen and Wermuth (1989), there have been several monographs on graphical modelling, including those by Whittaker (1990), Edwards (2000) and Lauritzen (1996).

The Rasch model in the psychometric context is probably the most popular of modern measurement models. It is defined for the outcome X taking two values (coded for instance 0 or 1):

$$P(X_{ij} = 1/\theta_i, \beta_j) = \frac{\exp(\theta_i - \beta_j)}{1+\exp(\theta_i - \beta_j)}$$

where θ_n is the person parameter that measures the ability of an individual n on the latent trait. It is the true latent variable in a continuous scale. It is the true score that we want to obtain, after the reduction of the k items to 1. The quantity β_j is the item parameter and characterises the level of difficulty of the item (the question). The Rasch model is a member of the item response models (Fisher and Molenaar 1995). The partial credit model (Fisher and Molenaar 1995) is another member of the family of item response model: it is equivalent to the Rasch model for ordinal categorical responses. Let $P_{ijx} = P(X_{ij} = x)$, then

$$P_{ijx} = \frac{\exp\left(x\theta_i - \sum_{l=1}^{x}\beta_{jl}\right)}{\sum_{h=0}^{m_j}\exp\left(h\theta_i - \sum_{l=1}^{h}\beta_{jl}\right)}$$

for $x = 1, 2, \ldots, m_j$ (m_j is the number of levels of item j); $i = 1 \ldots N$ (number of subjects); $j = 1 \ldots k$ (number of items). Under these models a reliability coefficient like the Cronbach alpha coefficient can be derived (Hamon and Mesbah 2002) and used in the same way as in parallel models.

Creating scores: statistical strategy

1. Creating Health scores summarizing Health Conditions such as: Depression, Anxiety, Quality of Life, Accidents, Noise and Allergy scores or indicators using internal analysis and looking for unidimensionality.
2. Exploratory analysis: finding which subsets of items will form a unique dimension and then giving them a unidimensional score. Without any a priori knowledge, factorial analysis (principal component analysis) with varimax rotation (Nunnaly 1978) followed by a cluster analysis is helpful. Common sense can also help as a starting point. It must kept in mind that all items were included in the questionnaire with an a priori latent clustering and with the goal of measuring some specific concepts.
3. More precise analysis of the unidimensionality: build the stepwise Cronbach alpha curve (SCAC) which gives a graphical validation of the parallel model – the model of unidimensionality. Under the parallel model, the reliability of the total is an increasing function of the number of items (Spearman-Brown formula). So, if the SCAC first increases and then decreases when a new item is added (or more exactly, when one is removed), we can suspect the new item to be a bad item:
   (a) the set of remaining items is unidimensional (parallel model), whereas
   (b) the set of remaining items including the new item is not unidimensional.
4. Creating Quality of Housing scores: analysing the relationship between Health and Housing: using each of the Health scores or indicators as response variables in a regression (linear or logistic) model where housing factors will form the set of candidate explanatory variables; select the final model without adjustment on individual factors, as explained above.
5. Deduce from the explanatory part (X part) of these built regression models, Health-Related Quality of Housing scores (H-Q-H)

All computations were made with SAS® software.

Quality of Life-related Housing scores

Results

A total of 6920 valid questionnaires were retained, being those completed by individuals over 18 years old. Various unidimensional scores were derived applying factorial analysis, the stepwise Cronbach alpha curve method (see Figure 12.6, the curve for *defaults* scale) and Rasch model methodology. (Not all details about all built scores are shown.)

The strategy chosen in the Material and Methods section was applied. It was adapted to take account of the huge number of variables in the data, as follows.

As shown in Figure 12.7, instead of analysing a great number of Health scores and relating all these scores to Housing Condition, we focus on creating a score for Quality of Life and showing how this score can be interpreted as the main component of Health, jointly with Anxiety and Depression (Mental Health). These built scores can be interpreted as proportions or estimated probability of Anxiety, good Quality of Life or Depression.

The depression score (SALSA[1]) is clearly a dichotomous (Yes, No) variable, but Quality of Life and Anxiety are percentages of a maximum score (see Appendix 12.1

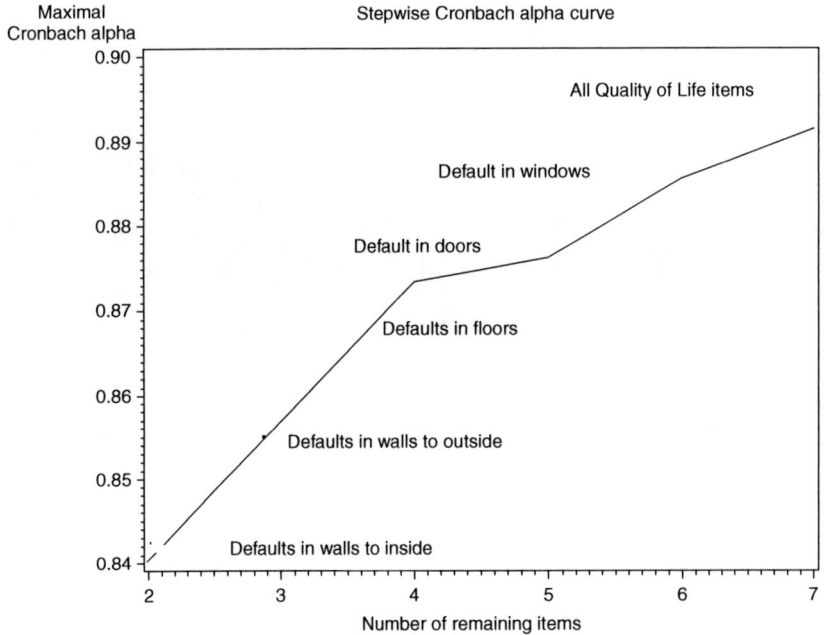

12.6 Cronbach alpha curve for defaults.

---

[1]See Chapter 11 for an explanation of SALSA.

Quality of Life-related Housing scores

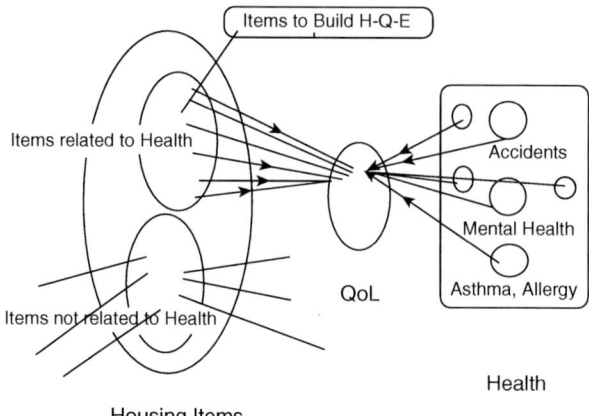

12.7 Analysis of Housing Conditions on Quality of Life as a sufficient outcome for Health.

and Appendix 12.2, respectively). So, we can analyse these scores by multiple logistic regression and present an odds ratio (OR) as a measure of association. These scores are presented and discussed in Chapter 11.

The results shown in Tables 12.1–12.6 set out the evidence that Quality of life is the core of the problem. Because the built score of Quality of Life is strongly related to all health outcomes, if we want to create health-related Quality of Housing scores, the easiest and the simplest way is to create Quality of Life-related Quality of Housing scores. Alternatively, scores could be developed specifically related to any other health variable such as respiratory disease, handicap, mental health, etc. This would probably give different results. But this is of limited practical interest. On the other hand, what we can perform specifically, is, for each part of the health status, an aetiological analysis that will be helpful for the scientist or the policymaker.

Table 12.7 shows ORs for significant Housing Condition factors (non-significant Housing Condition factors are not presented). A OR >1 means that the factor is positively associated with Quality of Life; when the OR is <1 the factor is negatively associated with Quality of Life. Of course, when we change the coding of the factor, we can move from positive to negative association, so the only interest is the distance between the OR and the unit value.

Table 12.1 Scores of Quality of Life and declaration of anxiety and depression

Declared anxiety and depression	Quality of Life		
During the last 12 months	2.879	2.816	2.943
Diagnosed by a physician	2.995	2.914	3.078
Prescribed medicine for this	2.971	2.889	3.056
Think it is related to flat	3.120	2.972	3.276

Quality of Life-related Housing scores

Table 12.2 Score of Quality of Life and chronic illnesses (prescription)

Do not take prescribed medicine for	Quality of Life		
Diabetes	1.628	1.573	1.685
Hypertension (high blood pressure)	1.682	1.652	1.712
Heart attack (myocardial infarction)	1.877	1.801	1.957
Stroke, cerebral haemorrhage	2.586	2.427	2.756
Malignant tumour	1.908	1.797	2.025
Asthma	1.300	1.254	1.348
Chronic bronchitis, emphysema	1.740	1.691	1.792
Arthrosis, (rheumatic) arthritis	1.794	1.759	1.830
Chronic anxiety and depression	2.971	2.889	3.056
Migraine and frequent headache	1.848	1.810	1.886
Serious skin diseases	1.320	1.272	1.370
Allergy (excluding allergic asthma)	1.136	1.111	1.162
Osteoporosis	2.037	1.971	2.105
Cataract	1.789	1.717	1.864
Gastric or duodenal ulcer	1.765	1.710	1.822

Table 12.3 Score of Quality of Life and acute illnesses (prescription)

Do not take prescribed medicine for	Quality of Life		
Cold or a throat illness	1.080	1.065	1.095
Acute bronchitis or pneumonia	1.445	1.406	1.485
Diarrhoeal diseases	1.129	1.101	1.157
Other cited in first	1.258	1.190	1.329
Other cited in second	1.590	1.410	1.793

Table 12.4 Score of Quality of Life and symptoms in last 12 months

Do not take prescribed medicine for	Quality of Life		
Wheezing or whistling in your chest	1.616	1.574	1.660
Attack of asthma	1.533	1.463	1.607
Any nasal allergies, including hay fever	1.130	1.103	1.157
Problem with sneezing	1.237	1.212	1.263
Eczema or any kind of skin allergy	1.174	1.144	1.206
Fatigue	2.334	2.274	2.395
Headache	1.747	1.716	1.779
Watery eyes or eye inflammations	1.544	1.507	1.582
Other cited in first	1.674	1.542	1.817
Other cited in second	2.365	1.963	2.848

Discussion

After investigation, we chose to summarise health by a Quality of Life score, which is well internally validated and strongly associated with all other health outcomes. The incorporated factors in the Quality Housing score were selected by their significant effect on perceived Quality of Life. The final choice was made after a stepwise selection model.

Quality of Life-related Housing scores

Table 12.5 Score of Quality of Life and accidents in dwelling

Accident	Quality of Life		
Falls	0.919	0.899	0.939
Burns	0.880	0.857	0.904
Cuts	0.906	0.888	0.924
Choking/suffocating/drowning	0.789	0.732	0.851
Collision/striking	0.875	0.851	0.900
Poisoning/chemical agents	0.471	0.412	0.539
Gas intoxication	0.168	0.120	0.236
Electrical accident	0.637	0.590	0.687

The ORs obtained were estimated using multiple logistic regression models, after various steps and a specific statistical strategy. When a factor was not significant, it was excluded from the analysis. The strategy used here is similar to that presented in Chapter 11, with a major difference in that here there was no attempt to investigate individual factors. Thus, the ORs presented here are not adjusted on individual profiles, because the goal is not to assess the scientific aetiology of a factor (for health) but its practical and operational probability effect on the Quality of Life whatever the profile of the individual.

Conclusions

Data provided by the LARES study provides environmental scientists with a lot of information about associations between housing and health.

Table 12.6 Score of Quality of Life and other health variables

Other health variable	Quality of Life		
Amount of good health (1 = low to 5 = high)	1.706	1.692	1.720
No physical constraint or handicap	1.899	1.859	1.940
Don't hear	0.609	0.593	0.626
Go up and down a flight of stairs without difficulty	2.093	2.049	2.137
Use fingers to handle a small object without difficulty	1.890	1.822	1.960
Can without difficulty turn a tap on	1.546	1.486	1.609
Can without difficulty bend down and kneel down	2.037	1.999	2.075
Don't feel have problems to make a normal use of the dwelling	1.581	1.549	1.613

Quality of Life-related Housing scores

Table 12.7 Score of Quality of Life and significant Housing Condition factors

Housing Information	
Panel block	0.962 (0.932; 0.993)
Semi-detached housing unit	1.134 (1.077; 1.194)
Multifamily apartment block – up to 6 residential units	1.122 (1.084; 1.162)
In an urban centre close to a busy street	1.095 (1.057; 1.135)
In an urban centre at a less busy street	1.091 (1.050; 1.134)
In the rural area close to a busy street	1.208 (1.113; 1.311)
Housing locations: in the rural area close to a busy street	1.028 (1.002; 1.055)
General aspects	
Window can be opened in flat	1.080; (1.037; 1.124)
Window cannot be closed in flat	0.929 (0.910; 0.947)
Single-glazed windows	1.047 (1.020; 1.075)
Condensation signs at windows	0.937 (0.900; 0.975)
Wallpaper, paint, etc., comes off wall	0.950 (0.924; 0.977)
Faults, disrepair	
Number of faults at several places of the same element > 1	0.755 (0.741; 0.768)
Kitchen	
Hot water available in kitchen	1.188 (1.103; 1.280)
Gas water heater connected to the outside, in the kitchen	0.941 (0.911; 0.972)
Fridge in kitchen	1.368 (1.233; 1.518)
Deep freezer	0.918 (0.885; 0.951)
Kitchen workspace next to the sink	1.051 (1.023; 1.081)
Waste bin without lid	0.945 (0.913; 0.978)
Extract system above the cooker connected to the outside	1.084 (1.056; 1.114)
Extract system above the cooker not connected to the outside	1.061 (1.032; 1.090)
Electricity is energy source for oven	1.086 (1.061; 1.111)
Bathroom	
Hot water is available in the bathroom	1.178 (1.045; 1.327)
The bathroom has a tiled floor	1.088 (1.057; 1.121)
Forced ventilation in toilet	1.072 (1.039; 1.105)
No toilet within dwelling, or for exclusive use	1.438 (1.148; 1.801)
Wash-hand basin in the toilet with cold and warm water	1.586 (1.266; 1.987)
Wash-hand basin with cold water in toilet	1.525 (1.212; 1.918)
No wash-hand basin in the toilet	1.628 (1.297; 2.044)
Number of flush WCs in the dwelling (max.3)	1.134 (1.094; 1.175)
Total number of showers and/or bath tubs (max.3)	0.896 (0.865; 0.927)
Safety, Accessibility	
Doorsteps in the door frames to entrance door	0.921 (0.893; 0.949)
Doorstep in the door frames to bathroom	0.900 (0.874; 0.927)

Continued

Quality of Life-related Housing scores

Table 12.7 (Cont'd)

Doorstep in the door frames to balcony	1.089 (1.062; 1.117)
Most streets or pathways can be overlooked from the dwelling	1.130 (1.101; 1.160)
Spaces can be overlooked through windows	0.974 (0.950; 0.997)
Steps and staircase	
Staircase with handrails	1.126 (1.088; 1.164)
Stairs are perfect and safe	1.298 (1.229; 1.371)
Height difference in steps	0.906 (0.875; 0.938)
Staircase has adequate and sufficient working light equipment	1.177 (1.139; 1.216)
Step or and staircase have handrails	1.121 (1.066; 1.179)
There are many height differences where people can stumble	0.918 (0.893; 0.943)
There are signs of vandalism in the staircase	0.829 (0.803; 0.856)
Lift/elevator in the building	1.108 (1.084; 1.133)
Housing environment	
Shared area belongs to the building	0.941 (0.911; 0.972)
These space are well maintained/taken care of	1.055 (1.027; 1.083)
These space are not maintained and run-down	0.904 (0.854; 0.957)
No graffiti at all	0.954 (0.923; 0.987)
One or two graffiti	0.891 (0.861; 0.923)
Amount of litter	1.030 (1.017; 1.044)
Vegetation/greenery visible on facades/windows/balconies	1.029 (1.006; 1.053)

The LARES database enabled us to derive Quality of Life-related housing scores that can be easily interpreted in term of ORs. Nevertheless, even if the findings obtained here are new and interesting, the fact that the LARES study was transversal, instead of longitudinal and observational, instead of interventional, limit slightly the causal interpretation of housing factors revealed. The criteria for objectively evaluating the relationship between a suspect cause and a chronic disease are (1) probability, (2) time order, (3) strength of association, (4) specificity, (5) consistency on replication, (6) predictive performance and (7) coherence. Thus, establishing evidence of a causal relationship is a more complex work than we were able to undertake.

Here, only housing risk factors that can affect Quality of Life have been assessed. Nevertheless, all of these Housing Condition factors revealed here are, at the least, alarm factors (following the 'precaution principle'). Our method gives an objective hierarchy of the strength of association of all these numerous Housing Condition factors with perceived Quality of Life, summarized by an OR evaluated in a global complex model. We hope that this will be a very useful result for housing policymakers and housing professionals.

References

Bonnefoy X.R., Braubach M., Moissonnier B. *et al* (2004) Habitat et Santé: état des connaissances. Les echos dus logement Octobre No. 4.

Bonnefoy X.R., Braubach M., Moissonnier B., Monolbaev K., Röbbel N. (2003) Housing and health in Europe: preliminary results of a pan-European study. *American Journal of Public Health* 93: 1559–63.

Cronbach L.J. (1951) Coefficient alpha and the internal structure of tests. *Psychometrika* 16: 297–334.

Curt F., Mesbah M., Lellouch J., Dellatolas G. (1997) Handedness scale: how many and which items? *Laterality* 2: 137–54.

Edwards D. (2000) Introduction to Graphical Modelling, 2nd edn. New York: Springer.

Fisher G.H., Molenaar I.W. (1995) Rasch Models, Foundations, Recent Developments and Applications. New York: Springer.

Hamon A., Mesbah M. (2002) Questionnaire reliability under the Rasch model. In: Statistical Methods for Quality of Life Studies. Amsterdam: Kluwer, 155–68.

Kristof W. (1963) The statistical theory of stepped-up reliability coefficients when a test has been divided into several equivalent parts. *Psychometrika* 28: 221–38.

Lauritzen S.L. (1996). Graphical Models. Oxford: Oxford University Press.

Lauritzen S.L., Wermuth N. (1989) Graphical models for association between variables, some of which are qualitative and some quantitative. *Annals of Statistics* 17(1): 31–57.

Moret L., Mesbah M., Chwalow J., Lellouch J. (1993) Validation interne d'une Èchelle de mesure: relation entre analyse en composantes principales, coefficient alpha de Cronbach et coefficient de corrélation intra-classe. *la Revue d'Epidémiologie et de Santé Publique* 41(2): 179–86.

Nunnaly J. (1978) Psychometric Theory, 2nd edn. New York: McGraw-Hill.

Whittaker J. (1990) Graphical Models In Applied Multivariate Statistics, 1st edn. New York: Wiley.

World Health Organization (WHO) (2005) LARES Study (2005): (http://www.euro.who.int/Housing/activities/20020711_1)

Quality of Life-related Housing scores

Appendix 12.1 Quality of Life scoring

Questions included in the Quality of Life scale

H_11	During the past month, have you felt particularly nervous? MHT01
H_12	During the past month, have you felt so down in the dumps nothing could cheer you up? MHT02
H_13	During the past month, have you felt calm and peaceful? MHT01
H_14	During the past month, have you felt downhearted and miserable? MHT04
H_15	During the past month, have you been happy? MHT05
H_16	During the past month, did you have lots of energy? VTT02
H_17	During the past month, did you feel worn out? VTT03
H_18	During the past month, did you feel full of life? VTT01
H_19	During the past month, did you feel tired? VTT04

These items constitute the Vitality (VT) and Mental Health (MT) subscales of the MOS SF36 questionnaire. Below, we derive a validated unidimensional simple score.

All these questions have the same levels of responses:

Response level labels	Original coding
All of the time	1
Most of the time	2
A good bit of the time	3
Some of the time	4
A little of the time	5
None of the time	6

Individual scoring algorithm

For each individual:
Start
Step 1: RH11 = H_11-1; RH12 = H_12-1; RH13 = 7-H_13; RH14 = H_14-1; RH15 = 7-H_15;
RH16 = 7-H_16; RH17 = H_17-1; RH18 = 7-H_18.
Step 2: If H_xx is missing then RHxx = 0. (For all questions between H_11 and H_19)
Step 3: N_MISS = number of missing responses to questions between H_11 and H_19
Step 4: **NumQol** = RH11 + RH12 + RH13 + RH14 + RH15 + RH16 +RH16 + RH17 + RH18 + RH19
Step 5: **DenQol** = 5 x (9-N_MISS)
Step 6: **Qolife** = (NumQol/ DenQol) x 100.
End

Note: Qolife is a score taking values between 0 and 100. A high score means high quality of life.

Quality of Life-related Housing scores

Appendix 12.2 Anxiety scoring

Questions included in the Anxiety scale

H_11	During the past month, have you felt particularly nervous?
H_13	During the past month, have you felt calm and peaceful?
H_19	During the past month, did you feel tired?
H_25	How long did it usually take for you to fall asleep during the past 4 weeks?

The first three questions have the same response level as questions of Quality of Life scale. The last question has the following response level:

Response level labels	Original coding
0–15 minutes	1
16–30 minutes	2
31–45 minutes	3
46–60 minutes	4
More than 60 minutes	5

Individual scoring algorithm

For each individual:
Start
Step 1: RH11 = H_11-1; RH13 = 6-H_13; RH19 = H_19-1; RH25 = .5-H_25;
Step 2: If H_xx is missing then RHxx = 0 (For all questions H_11, H_13, H_19 and H_25.).
Step 3: N_MISS1 = number of missing responses to questions H_11, H_13 and H_19.
Step 4: N_MISS2 = number of missing responses to question H_25.
Step 5: NumAnx = RH11 + RH13 + RH19 + RH25
Step 6: DenAnx = [15– nmiss(h_11rrr, h_13rrr, h_19rrr) x 5] + [4–nmiss(h_25rrr) x 4].
Step 7: Anxiety = 100*NumAnx/DenAnx.
End

Anxiety is a score between 0 and 100. A high score means high anxiety.

Quality of Life-related Housing scores

Appendix 12.3 Depression scoring (SALSA)

Questions included in the Depression scale

H_20	Did you have sleep disturbance every day for a period of 2 weeks or more?
H_21	Did you have loss or decreasing of interest in activities every day for a period of 2 weeks or more?
H_22	Did you have low self-esteem every day for a period of 2 weeks or more?
H_23	Did you have decreased appetite every day for a period of 2 weeks or more?

For each question H_xx:

Response level: labels	Original coding
Yes	1
No	2

Individual scoring algorithm

For each individual:
Start
Step 1: RHxx = H_xx-1 (For all questions between H_20 and H_23)
Step 2: If H_xx is missing then RHxx = 0. (For all questions between H_20 and H_23)
Step 3: DepScore = RH20 + RH21 + RH22 + RH23
Step 4: SALSA = 0; if DepScore is greater or equal to 2, then SALSA = 1.
End

SALSA is a binary score. It takes two values: 0 (not depressed) or 1 (depressed).

Quality of Life-related Housing scores

Appendix 12.4   How to analyse these scores as response variables

Quality of Life and Anxiety are obviously quantitative discrete variables that can be naively analysed by classical linear regression that is available in all general software. Nevertheless, such analyses don't take into account the true nature of the variable analysed, which is, by construction, discrete. In fact, Quality of Life and Anxiety scores are built as observed proportion, ratio of two variables:

- Num, which an integer number corresponding to the sum of all response items.
- Denum, which an integer number corresponding to the maximum possible value of Num.

Thus, one can analyse these scores as independent samples of binomial variables (Event = Num) with different sample sizes (Trial = Denum), using a logistic regression program available in most general statistical software. Nevertheless, one has to take some precautions with interpretation of the model parameters, because the response variable Quality of Life or Anxiety is not an observed dichotomous variable. It is a latent non-observed continuous variable. Consequently, the odds ratio (OR) estimate given by the software can be interpreted as a measure of association between the latent response and the regression variable considered. It can be interpreted similarly to a classical logistic regression situation, assuming that the true binary response variable (Quality of Life or Anxiety) is just not observed. Such a variable could be obtained after dichotomization of the latent score Quality of Life or Anxiety) using a hidden threshold.

The interpretation of an OR is close to a relative risk: it is the ratio of two risks (probabilities). Its value must be compared with 1. When it is significantly larger than 1, it means a positive association and when it is smaller than 1, it means a negative association. For instance, suppose we are interested in investigating the association between probability of good Quality of Life and the variable 'Do not take prescribed medicine for diabetes'. OR = 1.628 means that when someone doesn't take a prescribed medicine for diabetes, his probability of good Quality of Life is increased by 62.8% (in comparison with people taking the prescribed medicine for diabetes).

13 Residential environmental quality and quality of life

Irene van Kamp, Annemarie Ruysbroek and Rebecca Stellato

Introduction – the issue

People spend at least 65% of their time at home or in the near vicinity of their homes (Briggs *et al* 2003). This simple fact justifies the study of health and well-being at the micro level of housing and neighbourhood. A recent pan-European Union (EU) survey (EF 2004[1]) on perceived living conditions showed that good health, sufficient income, having a family and housing quality are perceived as the main factors contributing to a good life for the majority of Europeans. Adequate accommodation is most frequently mentioned in the new member and candidate states of the EU. Finally, satisfaction with the residential environment can contribute to the commitment of people to their environment (Moser and Uzzel 2004).

This chapter addresses the LARES objective to identify and quantify the impact of environmental aspects in the living environment, such as green spaces, safety and perceived environmental quality (indoor and outdoor), on individual residential satisfaction and perceived quality of life/well-being.

The basic questions dealt with are:

- What is the influence of aspects of the physical (indoor and outdoor) environment on the overall judgement people have of their residential situation?
- What is the influence of residential satisfaction on perceived quality of life/well-being?

---

[1] See www.eurofound.com.

Residential environmental quality and quality of life

Residential satisfaction

The environmental components of neighbourhoods that influence the degree of residential satisfaction have been well documented since the 1970s (van Kamp *et al* 2003a, 2003b). From existing evidence (van Poll 1997) it can be concluded that numerous factors determine whether people are satisfied with their living circumstances in a certain area or region. In order to make comparisons between the impact of different components in the social, physical and spatial domain it is necessary to cluster and weigh these components (van Poll 1997).

Several taxonomies can be found in the literature and have resulted in a broad variety of definitions and models referring to environmental quality, residential satisfaction, housing satisfaction, quality of life and well-being (van Kamp *et al* 2003a).

Research (Connerly and Marans 1988; van Poll 1997, Bonaiuto *et al* 1999, 2003; Ellaway *et al* 2001) into residential satisfaction indicates that residents' perceptions of urban environmental quality and satisfaction with their residential situation are determined by a large number of different residential aspects in the physical, social and spatial domain. The most important residential quality aspects appearing in the literature are social ties in the neighbourhood, safety risks (crime, traffic), environmental aspects such as noise pollution, air pollution and the presence of facilities (shops, green areas). Personal characteristics such as age, gender and socio-economic status (SES) appear to influence quality judgements only marginally. Woudenberg (2000) concludes that Dutch research in the past has consistently shown that some aspects are more important than others in the total evaluation of the environment. Table 13.1 organises environmental aspects as perceived by Dutch residents, from most important to least important.

However, it is not only the measurable, 'objective' aspects of the living environment that determine whether people are satisfied but also – and sometimes

Table 13.1 Types of indicator ordered by importance

MOST IMPORTANT ↓ LEAST IMPORTANT	Housing size and quality
	Social safety
	Social cohesion
	Appearance
	Space
	Green area
	Noise pollution
	Amenities
	Playgrounds
	Air pollution
	Reachability of amenities

Adapted from Woudenberg 2000.

primarily – the perceptions of these aspects; these do not necessarily parallel each other. Seldom are objective and subjective aspects studied in conjunction (Pacione 2003). Empirical evidence is still limited and there is no integrated model yet available; and most studies are data-driven. However, consensus exists that the field requires an interdisciplinary approach that integrates physical, spatial, social and environmental aspects (van Kamp *et al* 2003a).

Quality of life

Quality of life (QoL) can be defined as the factual material and immaterial equipment of life and its perceptions pertaining to different aspects from the social, spatial and physical domain (RIVM 2000). A distinction should be made between health-related quality of life and quality of life in the broader sense. Subjective aspects of QoL are often referred to as well-being at the individual level. Environmental quality is an essential part of the broader concept of QoL, and residential satisfaction can be considered its subjective counterpart.

QoL is a concept that has inspired much research in the past decades and has claimed a strong position on local, national and EU agendas (André and Bitondi 2002). The concept has also had a strong influence on social and political trends and has been applied to a vast number of fields, such as urban and regional planning, health promotion, disability, social indicators research and economic and mental health research. The strengthening position of the quality of life discussion is also due to its strong relation to sustainability, equity and social cohesion agendas.

Why was QoL adopted as an important topic on the political agenda? According to Pacione (1993) a major reason for this growing interest in issues relating to QoL is the fact that people in developed countries have come to realise that quality of life is not necessarily a simple function of material wealth. Growing awareness of the importance of other social well-being factors, including the social, political and environmental health of a nation, has led to a search for indicators that reflect the overall health of a nation and the well-being of its citizens more adequately than simple gross national product (GNP)-based indicators. Central to this developing interest in quality of life is research into the relationship between people and their everyday living environment.

Choice of indicators: objective versus subjective

There appears to be general consensus in the literature that objective as well as subjective indicators are necessary in the study of the person–environment relationship. In the choice of indicators, research goals play an important role. If the aim is primarily scientific, different indicators will be chosen than if the aim is primarily policy-oriented. In general, a combination of objective and subjective

Residential environmental quality and quality of life

indicators is considered preferable. Where objective data are often used in the planning process, subjective data shed light on what people consider important in their environment and give insight into the well-being/satisfaction of a person (van Kamp *et al* 2003a). MacIntyre and Ellaway (2000) warn against a strictly perceptual approach, since perceptions of the environment might be contaminated with health outcomes (particularly mental health/well-being) and possibly confounding of area and individual characteristics (see also Chapter 14). Although we (strongly) endorse the notion that objective as well as subjective indicators should be included in the analyses, due to data availability the analyses in this chapter are restricted to subjective and observational data (Housing Inspection Survey Sheets).

Framework

The literature provides a broad variety of definitions and models referring to environmental quality, residential satisfaction, housing satisfaction, quality of life and well-being. Of the broad variety of models in the field, the model of Marans and Couper (2000) is shown here as an example (Figure 13.1). The model focuses primarily on residential satisfaction and distinguishes the domains dwelling, neighbourhood, city and community; as such it serves as a good base for the LARES analyses of environmental quality and well-being/satisfaction.

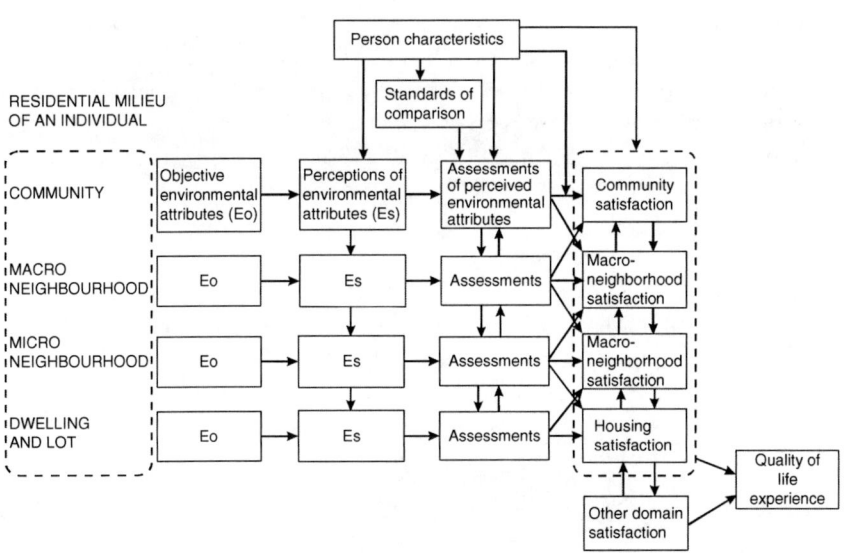

13.1 Model showing the relationships between residential domain satisfactions and quality of life. (From Marans and Couper, 2000).

Residential environmental quality and quality of life

The model assumes that the perceptions of the different residential domains mutually affect each other. Residential satisfaction, at the level of housing and neighbourhood, in conjunction with other life domains form the ingredients of quality of life.

Method

A full description of the LARES study is given in Chapter 1 (see also Bonnefoy *et al* 2003). Most studies into environmental quality and residential satisfaction have been performed at local/neighbourhood level, and on rare occasions using aggregated measurements, e.g. type of neighbourhood, type of housing and age of buildings (RIVM 2000). The LARES dataset enables us to make comparisons at different scale levels.

Choice of variables and datasets

The analysis in this chapter was based on a variety of characteristics of the indoor and outdoor residential quality, such as the amount and quality of green areas in the immediate surroundings, visual appearance and cleanliness/maintenance issues such as litter and graffiti (taken from the Housing Inspection Survey Sheet). Data on the age of building, neighbourhood and housing type, and location were also taken from the Housing Inspection Survey Sheet. Data on noise exposure, perceived indoor quality (view, light, dampness, air quality and dust), as well as satisfaction with dwelling and perceived quality of life, were collected from the Housing and Health Questionnaire. Satisfaction with the area was only available for the principal interviewee and was based on the Inhabitant Questionnaire. Personal characteristics (age, gender, SES and length of residency) were obtained through the Housing and Health Questionnaire as well. In Table 13.2 an overview is given of the variables and indices that have been used in the analyses.

In Figure 13.2 the residential satisfaction model of Marans and Couper is adapted at the measurement level for the LARES data available for analysis. Most of the information from LARES is available only at the dwelling/lot level or the micro level; very little information is available at the macro level. The environmental indicators pertain primarily to indoor environment/climate, and most are subjective or observational: few truly 'objective' data are available.

Statistical analysis

In order to reduce the number of quality of life and residential satisfaction indicators, and thus increase the robustness of the analysis, a factor analysis and item

Residential environmental quality and quality of life

analysis were performed. Initial analysis was carried out to study the correlational patterns between the variables related to residential satisfaction and quality of life. Once scales for the outcome measures (satisfaction with dwelling, satisfaction with area and well-being) were developed, differences of means were

Table 13.2 Review of instruments used to measure environmental quality and quality of life

INPUT	OUTPUT	CONFOUNDERS
VISUAL APPEARANCE	SATISFACTION HOUSE	CITY PERSONAL
graffiti	evaluation dwelling	ASPECTS
lack of green space	privacy	age
litter	getting away from it all	gender
dog droppings	can do what I want at home	length of residency
	most people would like my	SES
	home	TYPOLOGY OF
GREEN AREA	feeling in control at home	NEIGHBOURHOOD
Vegetation, in immediate	home makes me feel doing	building age
housing environment	well in life	urbanisation
Vegetation, private	my home feels safe	type of
grounds	my home expresses my	neighbourhood
Vegetation, on balconies	personality	
Indoor AIR QUALITY	SATISFACTION AREA	
Indoor DAMPNESS	evaluation of area as a place	
Indoor VIEW	to live	
Indoor DUST	area evaluated by others	
Indoor LIGHT	satisfaction with parking	
Outdoor # NOISE	UNWELL-BEING (SF-10/ SALSA)	
SOURCES	nervous	
traffic	down in dumps	
air traffic	not calm and peaceful	
train	unhappy	
parking	lack of energy	
	worn out	
	not full of life	
	tired	
	sleep disturbance	
	decreased interest + low	
	self-esteem	
	lack of appetite	

Residential environmental quality and quality of life

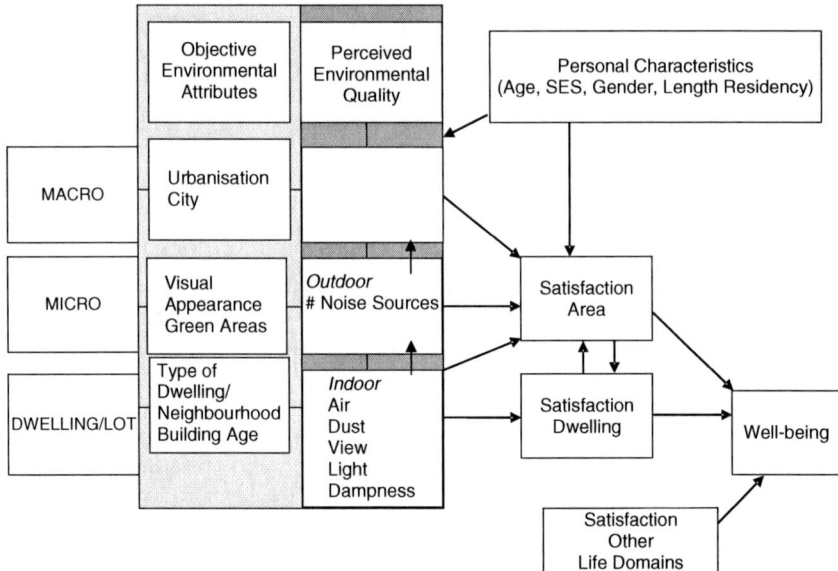

13.2 Measurement model concerning environmental quality, residential satisfaction and quality of life, based on Marans and Couper (2000).

studied between groups based on city, neighbourhood/housing type, level of urbanisation, building age and a combination of building age and level of urbanisation.

Analyses to predict satisfaction with the dwelling, satisfaction with the area and well-being were conducted separately, whereby three linear regression models were run for each outcome measure. In Model 1, the association between environmental quality and the outcome measure was tested. Housing-related variables were added in Model 2. In Model 3, potentially confounding personal characteristics were taken into account. Additionally, a fourth model (Model 4) was estimated for the prediction of well-being. In this last Model, satisfaction with the dwelling was added to the model.

- Model 1: visual appearance, presence and quality of green areas, noise (number of sources), and indoor climate (view, light, dampness, air quality, dust)
- Model 2: + building age, level of urbanisation and type of neighbourhood[2]

---

[2] Because of high levels of association between these aspects and City it was decided not to include city in the models. Neighbourhood features are considered as more relevant in terms of policymaking and planning.

- Model 3: + age, gender, length of residency, SES (potential confounders)
- Model 4: + satisfaction with the dwelling (only for the outcome well-being).

Satisfaction with the area was one of the variables available only for the first interviewee in the household, as mentioned previously. Therefore simple linear regression analysis was used to determine the environmental and personal attributes that were related to satisfaction with the area, and analyses included only the prime interviewees.

Information on satisfaction with the dwelling and well-being was obtained for all individuals within a household. These two outcome measures were analysed using multilevel linear regression models. Multilevel modelling enables the simultaneous use of data from the household level (e.g. housing type or visual appearance of the dwelling) and the individual level (e.g. demographic characteristics such as age and gender) in the same statistical model.

Results

Value of instruments

Factor analysis revealed seven interpretable factors, on the basis of which five scales were constructed and the reliability was tested in terms of internal consistency (see Table 13.3). It was decided to include aspects of the indoor climate

Table 13.3 Review of instruments to measure environmental quality and quality of life

Subject	Content	Coefficient alpha
OUTCOME		
	Dissatisfaction house	0.82
	Dissatisfaction area	0.75
	Unwell-being	0.87
PREDICTOR		
Vegetation	Number and quality of green areas	0.58
Appearance	Visual appearance of neighbourhood	0.62
Safety	Feeling safe after dark	1 item
NOISE	Number of outdoor noise sources	1 item
LIGHT	Dissatisfaction light	1 item
VIEW	Dissatisfaction view from window	1 item
DAMP	Dissatisfaction dampness	1 item
AIR	Dissatisfaction air quality	1 item
DUST	Dissatisfaction dust	1 item

All scales transformed into 10–100 scale.
NB: In all cases a high score = unfavourable.

Residential environmental quality and quality of life

at the items level, since the two factors with items referring to aspects such as dampness, dust, view, light, etc., were not easy to interpret.

The reliability of the outcome measures was strong, with internal consistency coefficients varying between 0.75 and 0.87. The reliability of the two observant scales – visual appearance of the immediate housing environment and the number and quality of green areas – is moderate (the alpha coefficients in range from 0.60 to 0.75) but is sufficient to allow for further analysis.

Correlational pattern

Dissatisfaction with the dwelling and with the area are interrelated, while unwell-being shows only very weak associations with the residential dissatisfaction indicators in the pooled data (Table 13.4). This supports the assumption that there is only partial overlap between these different concepts.

Dissatisfaction with the dwelling and area are both associated with indicators of indoor climate, number of noise sources, visual appearance of the neighbourhood and the presence and quality of green areas in the neighbourhood (Table 13.5). Overall, the associations are stronger for dissatisfaction with the area.

Table 13.4 Pearson correlations between outcome variables

	Dissatisfaction dwelling	Unwell-being	Dissatisfaction area
Dissatisfaction dwelling	1.00		
Unwell-being	0.13 (**)	1.00	
Dissatisfaction area	0.44 (**)	0.08 (**)	1.00

Table 13.5 Pearson correlations between environmental quality and outcome variables

	Dissatisfaction dwelling	Dissatisfaction area	Unwell-being
LIGHT	0.154 (**)	0.211 (**)	0.071 (**)
VIEW	0.236 (**)	0.401 (**)	0.061 (**)
AIR	0.313 (**)	0.413 (**)	0.080 (**)
DUST	0.134 (**)	0.222 (**)	0.070 (**)
DAMP	0.183 (**)	0.233 (**)	0.115 (**)
Number of noise sources	0.160 (**)	0.188 (**)	−0.005
Visual appearance	0.207 (**)	0.340 (**)	0.054 (**)
Green area*	0.160 (**)	0.239 (**)	0.120 (**)

Residential environmental quality and quality of life

This is somewhat surprising since most environmental aspects included in the analysis pertain to the indoor environment. It might be, as often stated regarding noise annoyance, that people judge their satisfaction with the housing environment 'as if standing on their doorsteps'. Although most environmental aspects are also significantly associated with well-being, the strength of the correlations is systematically weaker, showing that environmental quality is only one of the many domains that influence well-being. Finally, there is a relatively strong association between the number of perceived (transport-related) noise sources and perceived air quality, indicating again that it is hard to distinguish between perceived indoor and outdoor quality when measured in a survey.

Differences between groups

It can be assumed that the association between environmental quality and satisfaction with the dwelling and area is influenced by geographical aspects, quality of the housing stock and levels of urbanisation. Before including these aspects in multi-level analysis, the influence of these factors was studied separately. Hereto groups were made based on the following aspects: city, level of urbanisation, neighbourhood type and a combination of building age and level of urbanisation. Overall, results show that the environmental quality indicators, satisfaction with the dwelling and well-being differ significantly between the different groups. Below some examples of distributions over the identified groups are presented for the three outcome measures and for some environmental indoor and outdoor aspects separately.

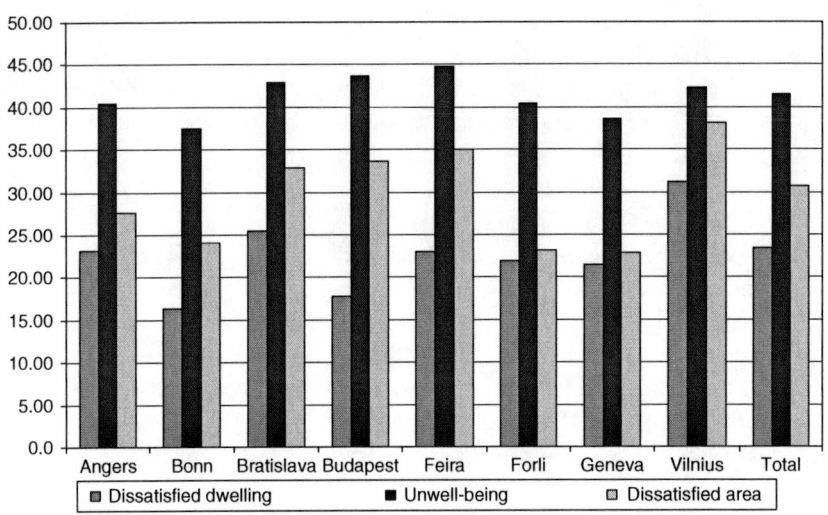

13.3 Difference of means between cities on dissatisfaction dwelling, area and unwell-being.

Residential environmental quality and quality of life

There is a strong and significant city effect for all aspects included in the analysis. However, the effect is not consistent. In other words, the different cities score unfavourably on different aspects. In Figure 13.3, the mean scores (all ranging from 0 to 100) are presented for dissatisfaction with the dwelling, dissatisfaction with the area and unwell-being.

Figure 13.4 illustrates that the differences between cities are quite specific, with a favourable score on one aspect and an extremely high score on the other. We see, for example, a high score of dampness and a lack of green space in Ferreira do Alentejo, but a favourable score regarding exposure to traffic noise, on which the cities of Vilnius, Bratislava but also Bonn score higher than the other five cities. A last example concerns feeling unsafe, which has the highest scores in Vilnius, Bratislava and Budapest.

Level of urbanisation shows a mixed picture. People living in urban centres and suburban areas are least satisfied with their dwelling and living area. People in the more rural areas are more satisfied with their dwellings and neighbourhood, but score unfavourably on the well-being scale. The differences between urban centres and suburban areas are only marginal (Figure 13.5).

Figure 13.6 shows that city centres score unfavourably on visual appearance, green areas and view from the home (data not shown), whereas suburban areas score higher on the number of noise sources and unsafety (data not shown). Most aspects pertaining to the indoor environment score better in the peripheral (semi-rural) city areas, with the exception of dust and dampness.

As has been reported earlier (Bonnefoy et al 2003), analysis of **type of neighbourhood and housing** reveals that neighbourhoods with primarily panel block housing overall score unfavourably on satisfaction with the dwelling and the area, Whereas well-being is lowest in semi-detached/terraced housing areas (Figure 13.7).

Figure 13.8 shows that visual appearance, feeling unsafe, the number of traffic-related noise sources (data not shown) and dissatisfaction with air quality also follow this pattern. Aspects of indoor climate as well as the amount and quality of green area score more highly (unfavourably) in areas with primarily semi-detached or terraced housing.

Building age: differences in residential satisfaction and well-being do not clearly differ between periods when the dwellings were built (Figure 13.9).

In general (Figure 13.10) people in housing built before 1950 (pre- and early post-World War II) are less satisfied with the indoor conditions such as light, view, dampness, air quality and dust. Satisfaction with green areas is also lower in areas built before the 1960s. As we saw above (Figure 13.9), this is not clearly reflected in unwell-being or dissatisfaction with the dwelling or area.

Residential environmental quality and quality of life

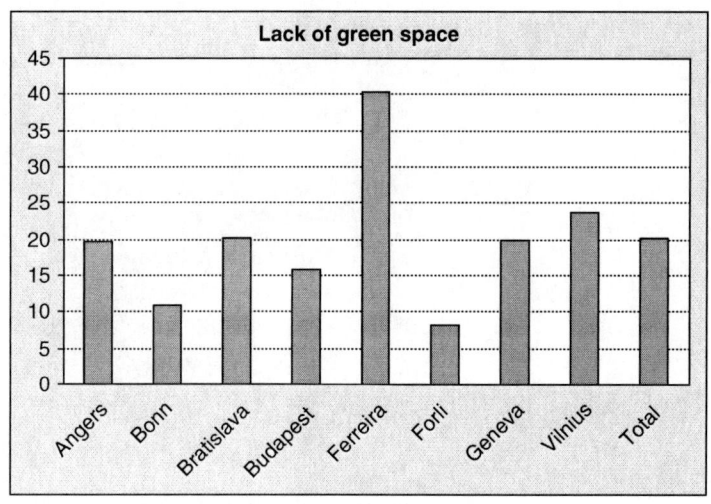

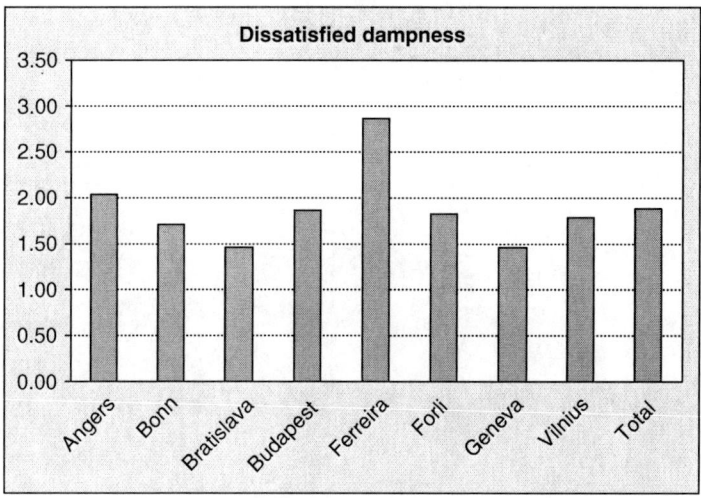

13.4 Selected aspects of environmental quality per city (means).

Residential environmental quality and quality of life

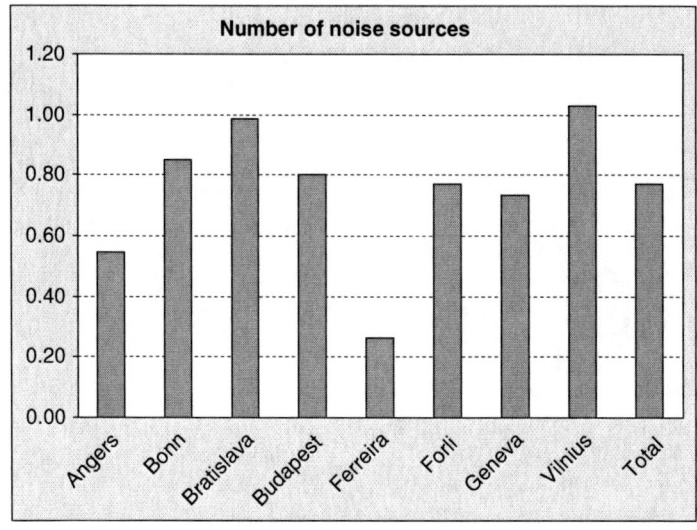

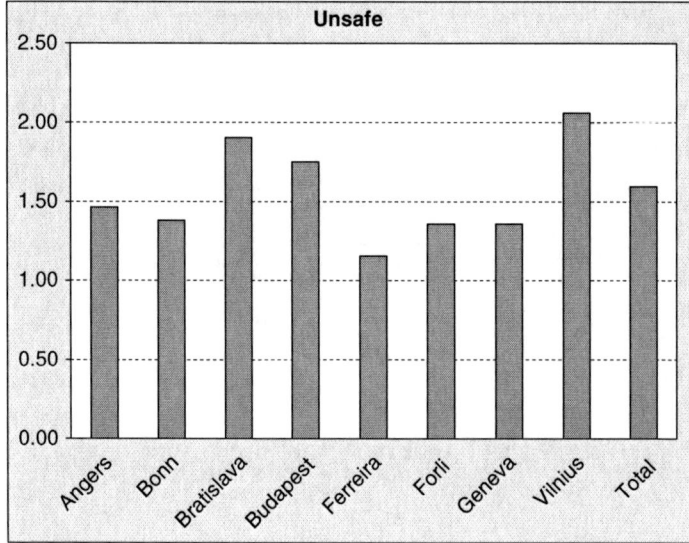

13.4 (Cont'd).

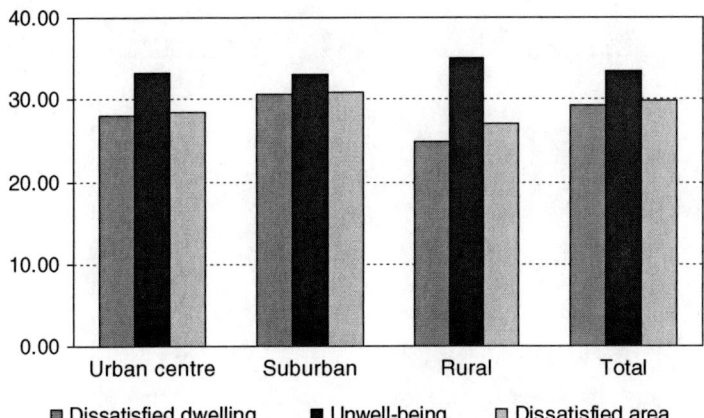

13.5 Difference of means by level of urbanisation on dissatisfaction dwelling, area and unwell-being.

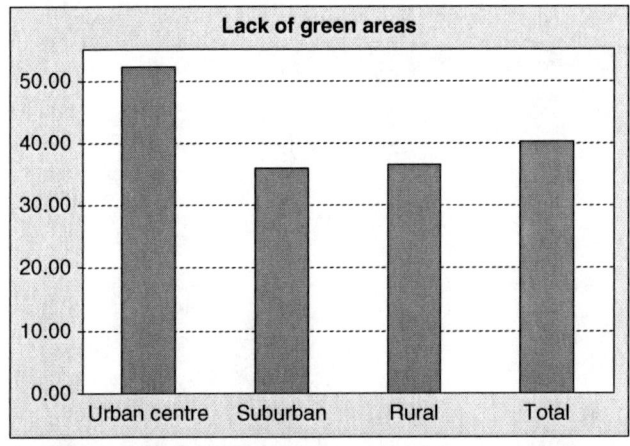

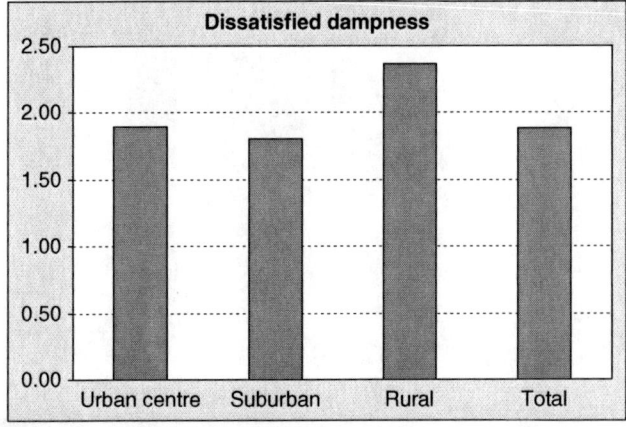

13.6 Selected aspects of environmental quality by level of urbanisation (means).

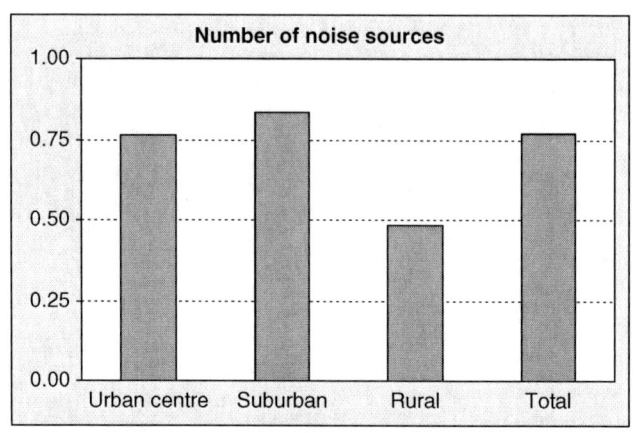

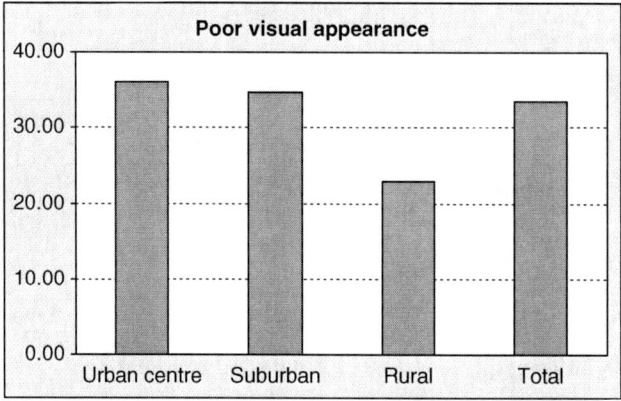

13.6 (Cont'd)

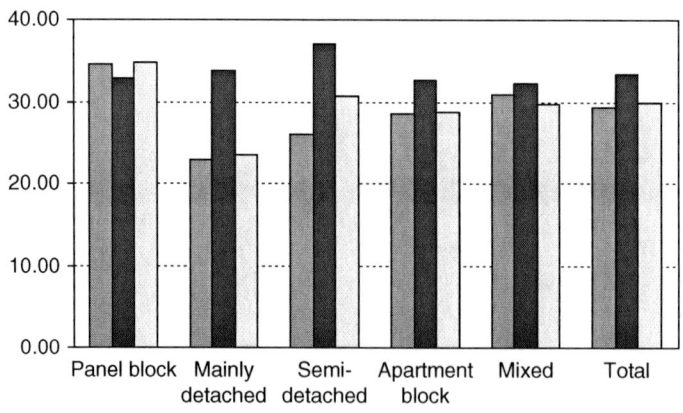

13.7 Difference of means by neighbourhood type on dissatisfaction dwelling, area and unwell-being.

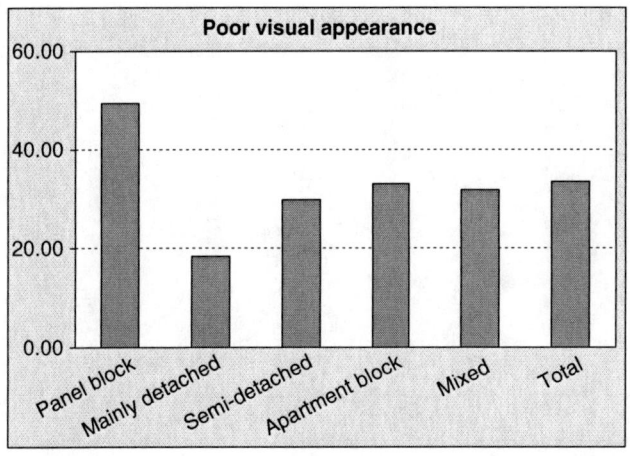
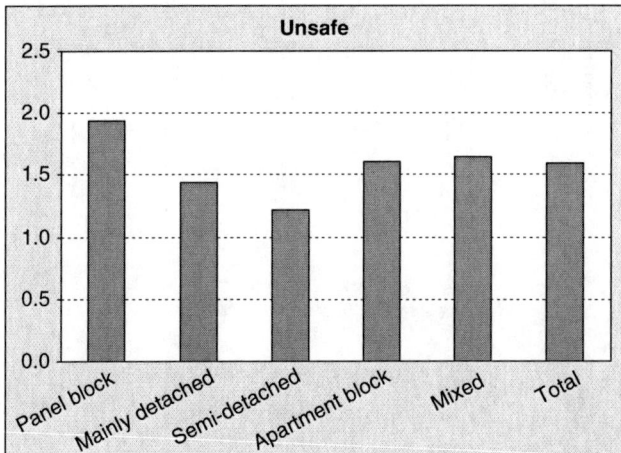

13.8 Selected aspects of environmental quality by neighbourhood type (means).

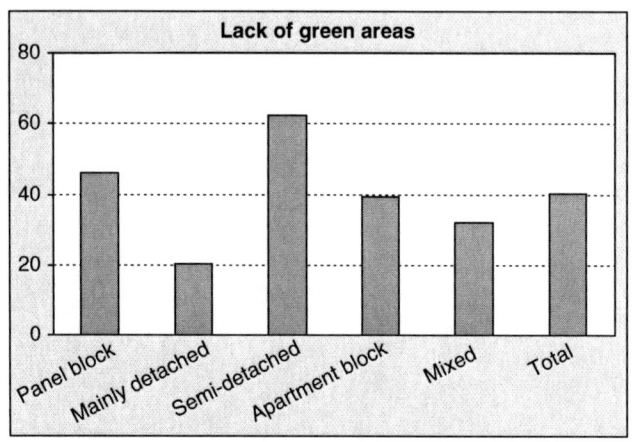

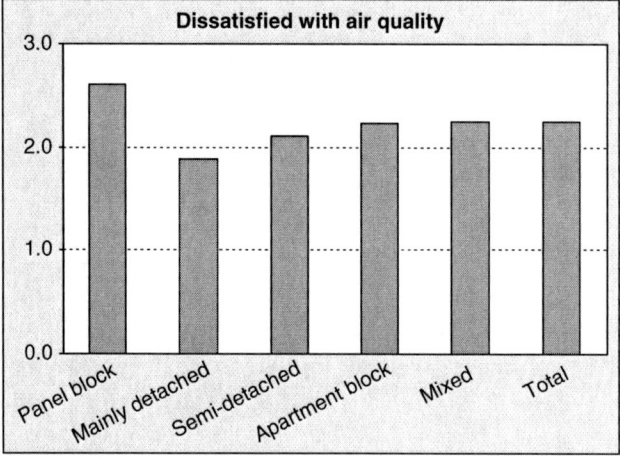

13.8 (Cont'd)

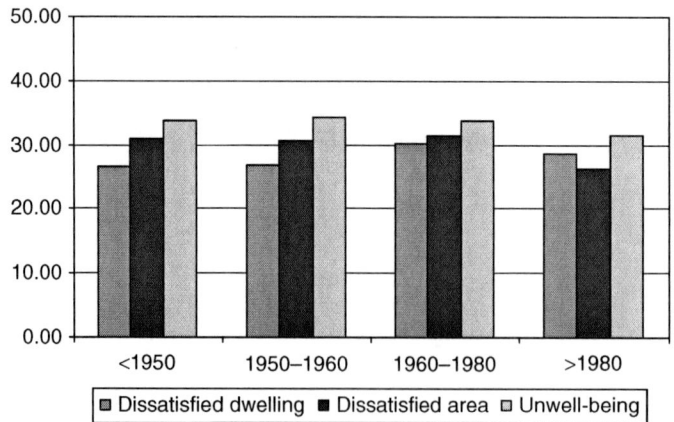

13.9 Difference of means by building age on dissatisfaction house, area and unwell-being.

Residential environmental quality and quality of life

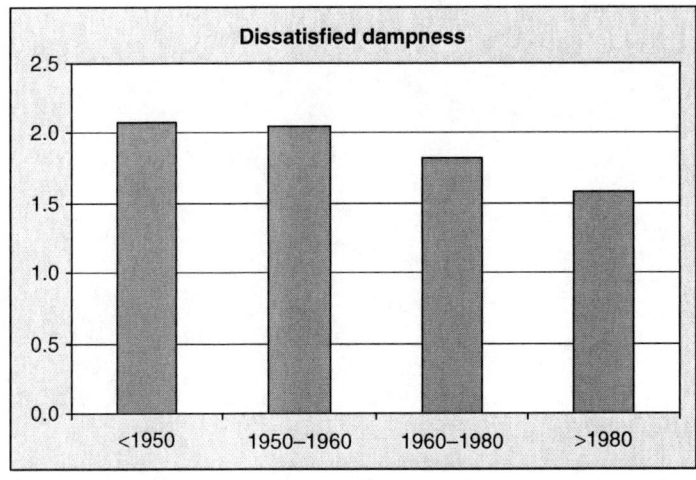

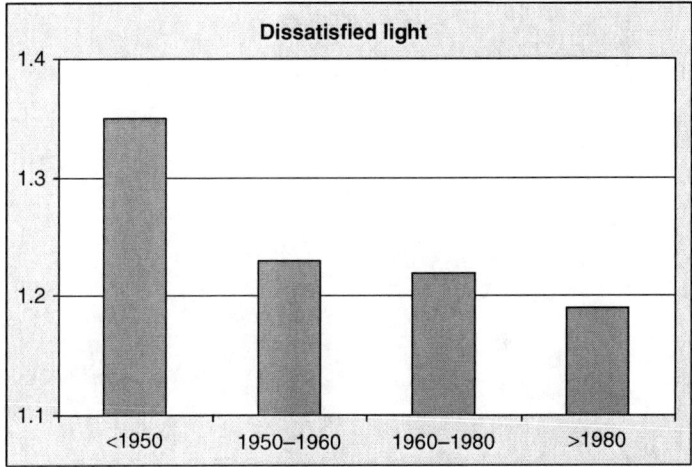

13.10 Selected aspects of environmental quality by building age (means).

Residential environmental quality and quality of life

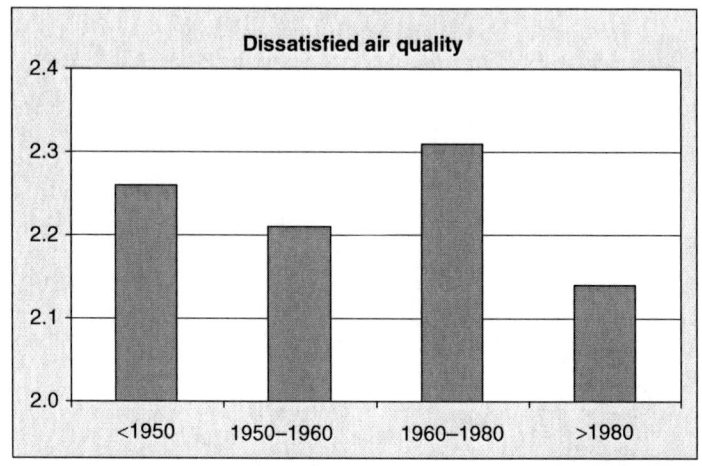

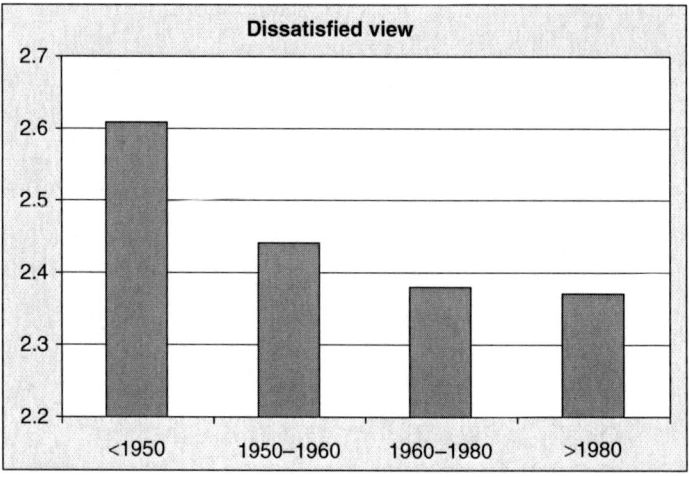

13.10 (Cont'd).

Residential environmental quality and quality of life

Results of linear regression analysis

Satisfaction with area

Satisfaction with the area could only be studied in a part of the sample for reasons mentioned above. Linear regression was therefore used to predict satisfaction with the area using environmental quality characteristics. Analogue to the multilevel analysis, three models were tested stepwise: including environmental quality indicators first; then, building age level of urbanisation and neighbourhood type; and in the last step, including demographic features. Table 13.6 displays the results of the linear regression models.

Environmental quality characteristics (with the exception of light) appear to be important predictors of satisfaction with the area. This pattern remains after adjustment for type of neighbourhood, building age and degree of urbanisation and aspects such as age, gender, SES and length of residency.

Table 13.6 The regression models for dissatisfaction with area on observed and perceived environmental quality (pooled data)

$N = 1,861$	STEP I: not adjusted for background characteristics B (SE)	STEP III: adjusted for background characteristics[1] B (SE)
Appearance	0.17 (0.02)***	0.16 (0.02)***
Vegetation	0.05 (0.01)**	0.06 (0.01)***
Number of traffic noise sources	1.70 (0.42)***	1.69 (0.43)***
Indoor climate: light	2.07 (0.86)	2.17 (0.86)
Indoor climate: view	2.88 (0.41)***	2.98 (0.41)***
Indoor climate: dampness	1.81 (0.29)***	1.60 (0.30)***
Indoor climate: air quality	4.50 (0.43)***	4.47 (0.44)***
Indoor climate: dust	2.36 (0.79)*	2.51 (0.79)*
Feel safe in neighbourhood:		
safe	0.69 (0.91)	0.69 (0.93)
relatively safe	−0.25 (1.08)	−0.15 (1.09)
unsafe	(ref)	(ref)

*$p < 0.01$, **$p < 0.001$, ***$p < 0.0001$.
[1]Adjusted for age of building, degree of urbanisation, type of neighbourhood, gender, age, length of residency and SES.

Results of multilevel analysis

Multilevel analysis of housing satisfaction and well-being overall shows that indicators of environmental quality (indoor and outdoor) are strongly associated

Residential environmental quality and quality of life

with the satisfaction with home and to a lesser extent with well-being, with and without adjustment for demographic characteristics, age of building, level of urbanisation and neighbourhood type.

Satisfaction with the dwelling

Most environmental quality characteristics (with the exception of dust) are significantly associated with satisfaction with the dwelling both before and after adjustment for building age, neighbourhood type, urbanisation and demographic aspects (Table 13.7). Appearance of the neighbourhood is significantly associated with dissatisfaction before, but not after adjustment, primarily because of the strong association between type of neighbourhood and appearance. Age, gender and SES are also significantly associated with satisfaction with dwelling. One remarkable finding is that younger adults and men are less satisfied with their homes than middle-aged and older adults and females, respectively (data not shown).

Table 13.7 The multilevel models for dissatisfaction with the dwelling on observed and perceived environmental quality (pooled data)

$N = 5,710$	STEP I: not adjusted for background characteristics B (SE)	STEP III: adjusted for background characteristics[1] B (SE)
Intercept	3.11 (1.29)	−3.38 (1.71)
Appearance	0.07 (0.01)***	0.03 (0.01)
Vegetation	0.04 (0.01)**	0.05 (0.01)***
Number of traffic noise sources	2.00 (0.33)***	1.50 (0.31)***
Indoor climate: light	2.71 (0.72)**	2.91 (0.69)***
Indoor climate: view	1.88 (0.26)***	1.75 (0.25)***
Indoor climate: dampness	1.55 (0.24)***	1.76 (0.24)***
Indoor climate: air quality	3.52 (0.34)***	3.05 (0.33)***
Indoor climate: dust	0.42 (0.62)	0.36 (0.59)

*$p <0.01$, **$p <0.001$, ***$p <0.0001$,
[1]Adjusted for age of building, degree of urbanisation, type of neighbourhood, gender, age, length of residency and SES.

Well-being

Only a few of the indoor and outdoor environmental indicators are associated with unwell-being, before and after adjustment for confounders

Table 13.8 The multilevel models for unwell-being on observed and perceived environmental quality (pooled data)

N = 5,535	STEP I: not adjusted for background characteristics B (SE)	STEP III: adjusted for background characteristics[1] B (SE)
Intercept	24.42 (0.99)	26.77 (1.32)
Appearance	0.00 (0.01)	0.00 (0.01)
Vegetation	0.04 (0.01)***	0.03 (0.01)**
Number of traffic noise sources	−0.15 (0.25)	−0.09 (0.24)
Indoor climate: light	1.71 (0.54)*	1.46 (0.52)*
Indoor climate: view	0.26 (0.20)	0.11 (0.19)
Indoor climate: dampness	0.87 (0.18)***	0.62 (0.18)**
Indoor climate: air quality	0.45 (0.26)	0.17 (0.26)
Indoor climate: dust	1.13 (0.47)	1.31 (0.45)*
Dissatisfaction with dwelling		0.12 (0.01)***

*$p < 0.01$, **$p < 0.001$, ***$p < 0.0001$,
[1]Adjusted for age of building, degree of urbanisation, type of neighbourhood, gender, age, length of residency and SES.

(Table 13.8). The most important are dampness and dissatisfaction with the light in the home. Women and the elderly and the bottom 40th percentile of SES score significantly lower on the well-being index (data not shown). Finally, satisfaction with the dwelling adds considerably to our explanation of the variance in unwell-being and diminishes the importance of dissatisfaction with dampness and light as predictors of unwell-being somewhat, although it is still significant.

Figure 13.11 summarises the findings on satisfaction with the neighbourhood in relation to indoor and outdoor factors, thereby accounting for objective attributes as well as some personal characteristics.

Figure 13.12 summarises the findings on residential dissatisfaction and unwell-being in relation to indoor and outdoor factors, thereby accounting for objective attributes as well as some personal characteristics. The diagram shows that some aspects (vegetation, and indoor lack of a view and air quality) indirectly influence well-being via dissatisfaction, whereas other indoor environmental qualities (lack of light, dampness and dust) also have a direct link with levels of well-being.

Residential environmental quality and quality of life

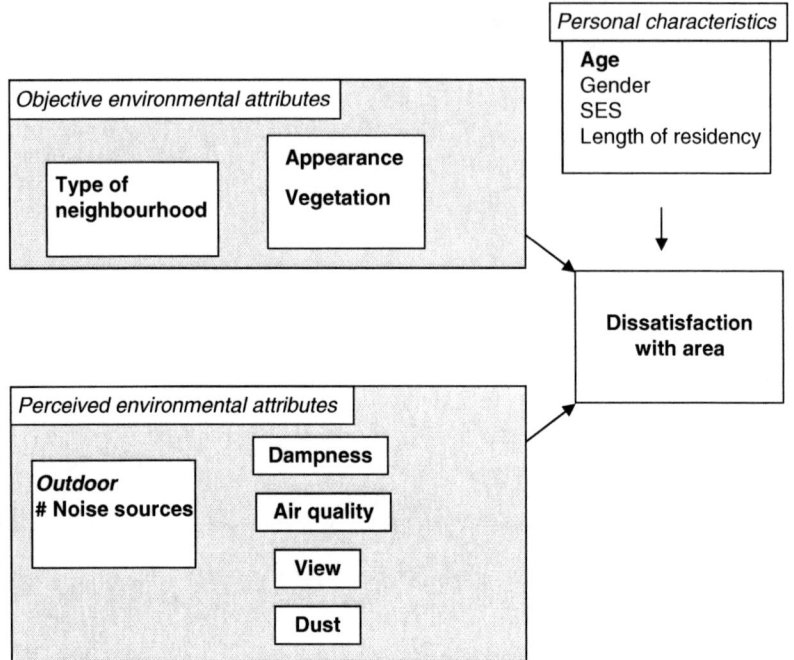

13.11 Outcome model concerning environmental quality and satisfaction with the living area (not significant shown in grey).

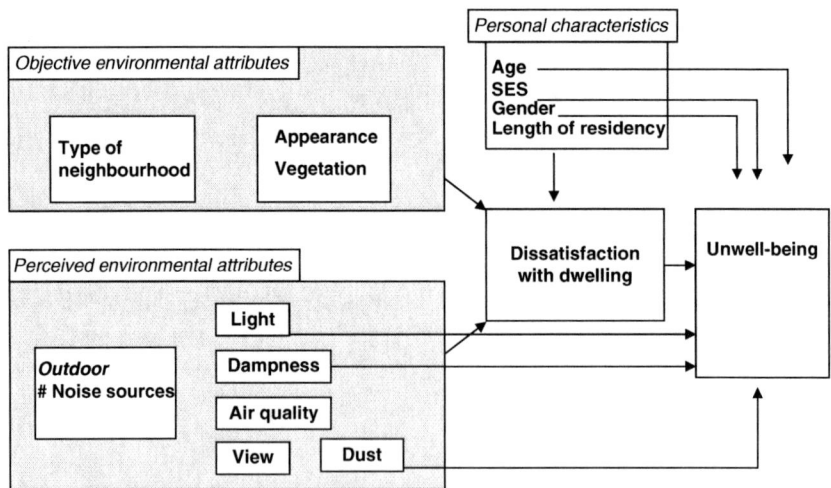

13.12 Outcome model concerning environmental quality, dissatisfaction with the dwelling and unwell-being (not significant shown in grey).

Conclusion and discussion

The results from regression analysis and multilevel analysis in broad lines support previous findings (see Introduction) that environmental quality is strongly associated with residential satisfaction (dwelling and neighbourhood) and, be it to a lesser degree, well-being. Results indicate that housing conditions and aspects of the immediate environment strongly influence satisfaction with the dwelling and the area. The condition and age of the housing stock and demographic features explain differences between cities to a considerable degree. Still it is possible that differences found are artefacts of the choice of cities in the sample. However, we do not expect a change in the strength or direction of the associations when other cities are studied. Even though there are strong regional variations in mean level of well-being and satisfaction, the direction and strength of the associations is comparable over all the cities that were included in the survey. Indoor and outdoor environmental characteristics remain important predictors of well-being and residential satisfaction after adjustment for potentially confounding factors (such as level of urbanisation, type of neighbourhood, age, gender and SES), indicating that these relations are generalisable across different types of urban environments. The drawback of this approach is that typical city effects and aspects which are strongly associated with the type of neighbourhood are not visible in the pooled analysis. This is particularly the case for visual appearance in terms of graffiti, litter and dog droppings and perceived safety. Both aspects strongly vary between type of neighbourhood and city, respectively, as shown in Figures 13.4 and Figures 13.8.

The results in broad lines confirm the already known residential determinants of satisfaction and well-being. New is the notion that, although there are some clear differences between cities and regions, the patterns of correlations are rather stable across them. The influence of indoor climate, light and the number and quality of green areas on well-being is noteworthy, as is the strong influence of housing satisfaction on well-being. An important finding is also that the variation in well-being between the cities included in the LARES survey cannot be exclusively explained by SES. However, it is possible that an overall SES index, as opposed to a country-specific index, cannot grasp the SES-related differences.

The analysis was limited to perceived environmental quality and environmental quality observed by the surveyors (appearance and number and quality of green areas) and it cannot fully be ruled out that the relations between the determinant (perceived environmental quality) and the outcome variables of satisfaction and well-being are contaminated. Strong arguments against this are (1) the relatively weak interrelations between the outcome variables, (2) the association between the observed (by the surveyors) environmental quality through the inspection sheet and satisfaction/well-being and (3) the differential associations between the environmental indicators and outcome variables. The fact that satisfaction with housing and the area is clearly influenced by indoor and outdoor quality (perceived as well as observed), building age and level of urbanisation makes the conclusions more solid.

The results confirm that a cross-EU approach to the issue of housing condition, environmental quality and well-being is feasible and justifiable. Despite regional differences, which can to some degree be explained by demographic variables, SES and housing stock, the direction and strength of associations is comparable across the different regions. However, more in-depth studies performed at a local level might allow for more specific anchors for interventions aimed at improving the environmental and housing conditions. The slogan of the Rio de Janeiro Summit on sustainable development (1999) – 'think globally act locally' – is also applicable here. Specific attention should be given to the influence of green areas and indoor climate and to the visual appearance of the neighbourhood.

The correlational pattern between the outcome variables and the differential patterns in the multilevel analysis confirm that the findings are solid and justify pooled analysis. However, there are four clear-cut restrictions to this analysis:

- The environmental indicators pertain primarily to indoor environment/climate.
- Only subjective and some observational data are available for the environmental indicators. Therefore, we still cannot fully rule out contamination, even though the observer data do associate with residents' perceptions.
- Aspects of perceived environmental quality are only complete for the prime interviewee. For the other respondents, those values had to be estimated on the basis of answers per household and checklists.
- Satisfaction with the area is also only available for the first interviewee. Because this is an outcome variable, it was not possible to perform multilevel analysis on this variable. Instead, simple regression analysis was performed, including only those people who filled out both the housing and health questions.

Further research should include more indicators of outdoor environmental quality and combine objective area data (preferably at grid level) with perception data. Objective data and self-reported evaluations can be seen as complementary, and their importance varies along the environmental issues studied and the objectives of the study. The implications of using different measurement strategies or of using residents' subjective reports, compared with objective measures of neighbourhood environments, are largely unknown (Van Kamp *et al* 2003b). The synthesis of datasets on physical, spatial and environmental characteristics with data derived from social surveys would be the next step to further this field.

References

André P., Bitondo D. (2002) Quality of life and EIA: a conceptual and methodological framework for an integrated approach in linear infrastructure projects. Paper presented to the 22nd Annual Meeting of the International Association for Impact Assessment, The Hague, 15–21 June 2002.

Bonaiuto M., Aiello A., Perugini M., Bonnes M., Ercoloni A.P. (1999) Multidimensional perception of residential environment quality and neighbourhood attachment in the urban environment. *J Environ Psychol* 19: 331–52.

Bonaiuto M., Fornara F., Bonnes M. (2003) Indexes of perceived residential environment quality and neighbourhood attachment in urban environments: a confirmation study on the city of Rome. *Landscape and Urban Planning* 65: 41–52.

Bonnefoy X.R., Braubach M., Moissonnier B., Monolbaer K., Röbbel N. (2003) Housing and health in Europe: preliminary results of a pan-European study. *Am J Public Health* 93(9): 1559–63.

Briggs D.J., Denman A.R., Gulliver J. et al (2003) Time activity modelling of domestic exposures to radon. *J Environ Manage*: 107–20.

Brody D.S., Hahn S.R., Spitzer R.L. et al (1998). Identifying patients with depression in the primary care setting: a more efficient method. *Arch Int Med* 158(22): 2469–75.

Connerly C.E., Marans R.W. (1988) Neighborhood quality: a description and analysis of indicators. In: Huttman E., van Vliet W. (eds) Handbook of Housing and the Built Environment in the United States. New York: Greenwood Press, pp 37–61.

EF (2004) European Foundation for the Improvement of Living and Working Conditions Perceptions of living conditions in an enlarged Europe. Luxembourg: Office for Official Publications of the European Communities.

Ellaway A., Macintyre S. (2000) Social capital self rated health: support for a contextual mechanism. *Am J Public Health* 90: 988.

Ellaway A., Macintyre S., Kearns A. (2001) Perceptions of place and health in socially contrasting neighbourhoods. *Urban Studies* 38(12): 2299–316.

Marans R.W., Couper M. (2000) Measuring the quality of community life: a program for longitudinal and comparative international research. In: Proceedings of the Second International Conference on Quality of Life in Cities, Volume 2, Singapore.

Moser G., Uzzell D. (2004) Editorial for psychology and the challenge of global environmental change. Newsletter of the International Human Dimensions Programme on Global Environmental Change.

Pacione M. (1993) The quality of the urban lifespace – a geographical perspective. In: Bonnes M. (ed.) Perception and Evaluation of Urban Environmental Quality. UNESCO, pp 17–42.

Pacione M. (2003) Urban environmental quality and human wellbeing – a social geographical perspective. *Landscape and Urban Planning* 65: 19–30.

RIVM (2000), de Hollander A.E.M. *et al*, National Outlook, English Summary.

van Kamp I., Leidelmeyer K., Marsman G., de Hollander A.E.M. (2003a) Urban environmental quality and human well-being; towards a conceptual framework and demarcation of concepts; a literature study. *Landscape and Urban Planning* 65: 5–18.

van Kamp I., van Loon J., Droomers M. (2003b) Augustinus de Hollander Residential Environment and Health: a review of methodological and conceptual issues. *REH* 19: Nos 3–4.

van Poll R. (1997) The perceived quality of the urban residential environment. A multi-attribute evaluation academic thesis. Roermond: Westrom.

Woudenberg F. (2000) Leefbaarheid in de Rijnmond. Municipal Health Service, Rotterdam.

14 The health relevance of the immediate housing environment
Matthias Braubach

Introduction

Urban settings, housing environments and health effects

Urban settings show considerable differences in health measures which may partially be caused or influenced by the conditions in the different housing neighbourhoods. Empirical research has shown that, within cities and neighbourhoods, health differences can be extreme (e.g. Mackenbach and Howden-Chapman, 2002; Cohen *et al* 2003; Macintyre *et al* 2003; Stafford and Marmot 2003). It has been argued that

> ... individual or household level socio-economic factors can explain most of these area differences in health. On the other hand, other studies hypothesise that ecological or environmental effects on health exist, independent of individual or household level factors (Chandola 2001, p 105).

One of the main concerns in current research on the relationship between neighbourhood quality and health effects is therefore to identify the association between quality and perception of physical and social characteristics of the residential area and the health status of residents (Wilson *et al* 2004). This is supported by various research projects and publications showing that, next to the housing quality, the impact of the immediate environment is a relevant health determinant (van Poll 1997). In addition to the mere physical and architectural quality, the neighbourhood is also affected by social and community-level parameters such as social cohesion or safety, and is used commonly by all neighbourhood residents.

Housing environment and health

Neighbourhood quality and health: empirical findings

Recent work provides accumulating evidence that the health status of residents is affected by the quality of the housing environment (Ellaway and Macintyre 2000; Cattell 2001; Dunn 2002; Evans 2003; Latkin and Curry 2003; Stafford and Marmot 2003).

Neighbourhood effects on health and well-being can be of varying nature. Urban and residential health research deals with all kinds of physical, mental and social effects of physical and built environments (Evans 2003; Jackson 2003; Twiss 2003). In urban planning and landscape architecture, numerous publications also emphasise the meaning and importance of public and social places (Thompson 2002), of green and open spaces and of vegetation in urban settings (Botkin and Beveridge 1997; Attwell 2000). Urban ecology is a major field within urban planning, and concepts such as the urban green structure aim at improving the liveability of cities (Bergen Jensen *et al* 2000), including ecological as well as urban and recreational functions. Urban design discusses issues of accessibility and participation while trying to make cities integrative spaces for all groups of society (Imrie 2000). Healthy city networks focus on the health effects of urban conditions. Evidence from various studies indicates that the view of natural scenery positively affects mental capacity and physiological indicators such as mood states and stress hormones (Ulrich *et al* 1991; Kaplan 1995).

The availability and quality of green open spaces and places for physical exercise have been associated with the arising epidemic of obesity (Emery *et al* 2003). In addition to the decreased use of neighbourhood amenities in unsafe and deteriorated areas, the perception of insecurity has been identified as a health threat per se (Chandola 2001; Austin *et al* 2002; Green *et al* 2002; Latkin and Curry 2003) that is capable of strongly affecting the life of residents and impacting on their mental health.

Litter, bad smells and fumes, and animal excrements in the neighbourhood, limit not only the aesthetic value of the neighbourhood and its usability (van Poll 1997) but also threaten physical and mental health by posing the risk of infectious diseases, allergies, respiratory effects and general discomfort and irritation. Annoyance and disturbance from exposure to noise, probably the largest component of environmental pollution in urban settings, is increasing in most European cities (Sharp 2002) and has been linked with sleep disturbance, emotional and hormonal effects, and an increased risk for cardiovascular effects (Stansfeld and Matheson 2003; Niemann *et al* 2005). Studies on children also found cognitive and social effects of night noise exposure, e.g. expressed by an impaired ability for learning in school.

Analytical objectives and data selection

The analyses of the LARES dataset presented in this chapter attempt to identify the impact of the immediate housing environment on the health perceptions and on the health status of residents. The analysis was based on a variety of characteristics of the housing environment, such as greenery, playgrounds, security, and cleanliness and maintenance issues from the Inhabitant Questionnaire and the Housing Inspection Survey Sheet. Data on the building and neighbourhood types, and their location, were taken from the Housing Inspection Survey Sheet, whereas data on noise exposure, subjective health perceptions, mental health, sleep disturbance and the prevalence of reported diagnosed diseases such as cardiovascular symptoms were collected from the Housing and Health Questionnaire, as were personal characteristics (age, gender, socio-economic status (SES), functional limitations).

The database therefore enables a variety of investigations linking the quality of the immediate housing environment with a number of health outcomes while adjusting for individual characteristics of the residents. Although the results of this cross-sectional study cannot be interpreted as providing causal evidence, they are capable of providing important indications on the existence and the strength of associations between the immediate housing environment and the health and health problems of the residents.

Methods

The results presented are based on (a) bivariate cross-tabulations and (b) multivariate logistic regression models. The cross-tabulations were done between neighbourhood types and housing environment problems and between housing environment problems and self-rated health. The regression models used various residential environment characteristics as independent variables, which were selected on the basis of a literature review on residential environments and health, and the results of a correlation test using the Spearman rank correlation coefficient. The chosen independent variables were related to the aspects identified as some of the most relevant residential and urban stressors (see Table 14.1). For the analysis, all variables were transferred into a dichotomous format.

As the dependent outcome variables, self-rated health and three specific health outcomes (sleep disturbance, depression and cardiovascular symptoms) were selected. For each outcome variable, an individual regression model was computed. All regression models included the variable 'city' as a fixed effect in order to control for the variation of the eight cities included in the database and to make sure that identified differences could not be related to city differences with little relation to residential conditions.

To adjust for the confounding influences of known health determinants related to individual characteristics, the four variables 'age group' (child–adult–senior),

Table 14.1 Variables used for analysis

Environment category	Independent variable	Original variable format
Greenery, public spaces and play areas	Vegetation along streets	Binary variable (Yes–No)
	Play areas for children	3-point scale (Yes–to some extent–no)
	Place to sit and relax outside of dwelling	Binary variable (Yes–No)
Noise exposure	Traffic noise	5-point scale (not at all–extreme)
	Surrounding area noise	5-point scale (not at all–extreme)
Public safety	Safety perception in residential area at night	3-point scale (Yes–to some extent–no)
	Feeling of safety in the dwelling	5-point scale (Strongly agree–strongly disagree)
Upkeep and maintenance	Graffiti on residential buildings	4-point scale (no–one or two–three to five–six and more)
	Litter and trash in residential environment	5-point scale (Very dirty / littered–not at all dirty / littered)

Health outcome	Dependent variable	Original variable format
Health	Self-rated health status	5-point scale (very good–very bad)
Sleep	Sleep disturbance	Binary variable (Yes–No)
Mental health	Depression screening tool SALSA	Four aggregated binary variables (Yes–No) based on sleep, motivation, self esteem and appetite)
Circulatory system	Cardiovascular symptom index	Three aggregated binary variables (Yes–No) based on diagnosed hypertension, heart attacks and strokes

Personal characteristic	Confounding variable	Original variable format(s)
Socio-economic status	SES score	Aggregated score based on housing size, social benefits, education of household, and ratio of residents being unemployed / employed
Gender	Gender	Binary variable (male–female)
Age	Age groups (child, adult, senior)	Year of age
Functional limitation	Functional limitation	Binary variable (Yes–No)

Housing environment and health

'gender' (male–female), 'SES score'[1] (high–low) and 'functional limitations' (yes–no) were selected as potential confounding variables to be tested for.

Each regression model was run in two steps. With the first step, the association between the selected residential environment characteristics and the four selected health outcomes was tested. The second step included the four confounder variables, testing the stability of the associations found by the first step.

Bivariate results

Immediate housing environment problems and neighbourhood types

In general terms, the major immediate housing environment issues identified by the LARES survey can be defined as (1) lack of greenery and park-like spaces (2) lack of recreational places and (3) traffic noise exposure. All three problems were prevalent in all neighbourhood types and affected more than one-third of all sampled residents. Other variables showed large variations of residential problems by neighbourhood type: for example, for the perception of not being safe when out at night, which is valid for almost one-fifth of the whole sample but is very different in regard to the neighbourhood type.

Compared to all other neighbourhood types, 'one-family house areas' (detached, semi-detached and terraced houses) had a low availability of public recreational areas for children, teenagers, or the elderly, although this was compensated by the high percentage of private gardens (64.5% of all one-family houses have private gardens). On the other hand, one-family housing areas scored best on matters such as noise, cleanliness of the housing area and the feeling of safety (Table 14.2A).

In 'panel block areas', noise (especially from traffic, ranging to as high as 42.8%) and parking were high on the problem agenda, as was the presence of graffiti. The lack of private outside areas, however, was compensated for by a greater provision with recreational places and public parks for the residential population: only around one-third of the residents reported a lack of recreation options within their residential area. Another problem is the relatively high prevalence of dog droppings and litter, and the fact that almost each third resident (30.9%) said that they felt unsafe when out during the hours of darkness.

'Apartment block areas' had some similar problems to panel block areas. Problems with noise were at the same level as in panel block neighbourhoods and represented one of the main challenges. Although there was a greater provision of public recreational places, there was also a lack of greenery and vegetation on public grounds, and a lack of parks or green spaces around the buildings.

---

[1] The socio-economic status score developed by M Davidson (see Chapter 5).

Table 14.2A Bivariate analysis for neighbourhood types and problems with the housing environment

Residential problem reported by the residents (in per cent)	Total population (varying number of responses)	Panel block neighbour- hoods (n = 1636)	Mainly apartment blocks (n = 2577)	Mixed neighbour- hoods (n = 1942)	Mainly one-family houses (n = 2338)	χ^2 p value
Frequent residential noise exposure	20.9	25.7	25.1	23.1	10.8	***
Frequent traffic noise exposure	38.0	42.8	42.5	41.5	26.8	***
Sleep disturbed by noise	23.3	29.4	25.3	23.5	16.5	***
Dissatisfaction with parking situation	30.9	47.3	37.7	28.2	14.7	***
Annoyance by trash / litter (residents)	28.1	40.4	30.8	30.7	14.3	***
Large amount of litter (surveyor rating)	9.0	17.2	9.7	7.6	3.6	***
Lack of recreational places for children	32.2	26.8	25.3	28.3	46.8	***
Lack of recreational places for teens	43.6	35.7	38.1	39.3	58.5	***

Lack of recreational places for elderly	38.5	33.5	32.4	32.1	53.4	***
Not feeling safe outside in the darkness	19.0	30.9	19.8	20.4	8.8	***
Lack of feeling of safety in the dwelling	8.7	13.1	7.7	11.1	4.4	***
Existence of graffiti	31.5	64.7	35.3	31.4	4.2	***
Large amount of dog droppings	11.1	26.0	11.1	7.7	3.5	***
No vegetation on public grounds	47.1	12.1	46.4	39.5	78.7	***
No vegetation on private grounds	56.2	92.1	56.9	42.0	42.0	***
No private garden	68.9	98.2	81.2	68.2	35.5	***
No private garden and no commonly shared area around the residential building	26.8	21.9	32.6	17.2	31.7	***
No park / green space close to residence	43.7	28.2	38.6	38.1	64.9	***

***Significant at 0.001 level.

Housing environment and health

Table 14.2B Bivariate analysis for self-rated health

Characteristic	N	Percentage with low self-rated health	χ^2 p value
FULL SAMPLE OF RESIDENTS	**8,519**	**38.1**	
Gender			***
Male	3,927	34.9	
Female	4,473	41	
Functional limitation			***
Yes	846	76.7	
No	7466	33.6	
SES			***
Low SES score	3,687	49.6	
High SES score	4,403	28.7	
Age group			***
Child (<18)	1,569	11.1	
Adult (18–65)	5,555	37.1	
Senior (>65)	1,296	75	
Play areas for children			***
Not enough play areas	3,811	43	
Enough play areas	4,465	34	
Place to sit and relax outside of dwelling			***
No such place exists	2,656	46.7	
Place exists	5,544	34.1	
Vegetation along streets			***
Not present	3,062	43.5	
Present	5,358	35	
Traffic noise			***
Reported as relevant annoyance	1,731	43.8	
Not reported as relevant annoyance	6,202	36.2	
Surrounding area noise			***
Reported as relevant annoyance	545	47.3	
Not reported as relevant annoyance	7,348	37	
Graffiti on residential buildings			*
Graffiti exist	2,636	39.8	
No graffiti	5,723	37.2	
Litter and trash in residential environment			***
Rather dirty and littered	3,058	43.5	
No litter and trash	5,273	34.9	
Feeling of safety in residential area at night			***
Not feeling safe at night	3,411	44.3	
Feeling safe at night	4,891	33.3	
Feeling of safety in the dwelling			***
Not feeling safe in dwelling	1,772	48.9	
Feeling safe in dwelling	6,134	35	

*Significant at 0.05 level; ***Significant at 0.001 level.

Housing environment and health

Finally, while 'mixed neighbourhoods' balance both advantages and disadvantages, once more the greatest problems were traffic noise and the lack of open, green and recreational spaces.

This quantitative comparison showed that neighbourhood types provide different residential conditions that come with specific advantages and specific problems; however, there is a general pattern that seems quite stable – noise, greenery and recreational places kept coming up as the most relevant problems, whatever the neighbourhood type.

Immediate housing environment problems and self-rated health

Table 14.2B presents the results of descriptive cross-tabulations, showing the essential features of the population sample and the ratio of residents reporting low self-rated health for each independent variable of the residential problems discussed here. Self-rated health is taken as a composite indicator on health status in this analysis (Gold *et al* 1996; Dunn 2002), aggregating the general perception of a resident on his or her health status. It is thereby different than defined diseases or health symptoms, and provides information on a more general level on the health status and the quality of life of the residents.

The cross-tabulations show that individual characteristics such as age, gender, SES or functional limitations were more strongly associated with self-rated health than the residential environment characteristics. The strongest health variation of these individual characteristics is found for functional limitations and age. Still, all residential environment characteristics were significantly associated with self-rated health status. The strongest associations with low self-rated health were found for those residents reporting a perception of not being safe in the dwelling (48.9%) and those reporting exposure to surrounding area noise (47.3%), while the existence of graffiti on the residential buildings seems to have had the lowest impact on self-rated health (39.8%).

Table 14.2B provides descriptive data on the impact of the residential environment on self-rated health, showing strong statistical associations. However, these data do not account for potentially confounding influences of city, age or SES, and they do not explain the mechanisms of how residential environments can affect the health of the residents. Multivariate logistic regression models were therefore applied to elucidate in more detail the relationship between the quality of the residential environment, and the four selected health outcomes: self-rated health, sleep disturbance, depression and cardiovascular symptoms.

Multivariate results

Four independent regression models were adopted using diverse health outcomes (self-rated health, sleep disturbance, depression and cardiovascular symptoms)

Housing environment and health

as the criterion variable. Each regression model was done in two steps: Step 1 covers the neighbourhood characteristics only and Step 2 covers both the neighbourhood and personal characteristics of the residents (see Table 14.3). The results are shown in Tables 14.4A and 14.4B.

Table 14.3 Overview of models

Model	Effect	Step 1	Step 2
1	Self-rated health	Nine selected neighbourhood characteristics (plus: city)	Nine selected neighbourhood characteristics plus four personal characteristics (plus: city)
2	Sleep disturbance	Nine selected neighbourhood characteristics (plus: city)	Nine selected neighbourhood characteristics plus four personal characteristics (plus: city)
3	Depression	Nine selected neighbourhood characteristics (plus: city)	Nine selected neighbourhood characteristics plus four personal characteristics (plus: city)
4	Cardiovascular symptoms	Nine selected neighbourhood characteristics (plus: city)	Nine selected neighbourhood characteristics plus four personal characteristics (plus: city)

Self-rated health (Model 1)

The results for Step 1 indicated that four out of the nine residential environment variables failed to provide a significant influence on the variation of self-rated health status ('play areas for children', 'place to sit and relax outside of dwelling', 'graffiti on residential buildings' and 'litter and trash in residential environment'). For the five variables with a significant increase of likelihood for low self-rated health, the two safety perception variables ('safety perception in residential area at night' and 'feeling of safety in the dwelling') showed the strongest impact, followed by the two noise exposure variables ('traffic noise' and 'surrounding area noise') and 'vegetation along streets'.

Table 14.4A Logistic regression results – examining the impact of the neighbourhood on health outcomes for self-rated health and sleep disturbance

	Model 'self-rated health'				Model 'sleep disturbance'			
	Step 1		Step 2		Step 1		Step 2	
Residential environment characteristic	OR for low health	CI	OR for low health	CI	OR for sleep disturbance	CI	OR for sleep disturbance	CI
Play areas for children								
Enough play areas	1		1		1		1	
Not enough play areas	0.98	0.85–1.12	1.07	0.91–1.25	**1.3**		**1.28**	1.09–1.51
Place to sit and relax outside of dwelling								
Place exists	1		1		1		1	
No such place exists	1.08	0.95–1.22	1.05	0.91–1.21	**1.16**		**1.17**	1.01–1.37
Vegetation along streets								
Present	1		1		1		1	
Not present	**1.22**	1.08–1.38	1.07	0.93–1.23	0.99		0.98	0.84–1.13
Traffic noise								
No annoying traffic noise	1		1		1		1	
Yes – traffic noise is annoying	**1.4**	1.17–1.68	**1.34**	1.10–1.65	**6.52**	5.41–7.86	**6.42**	5.31–7.77
Surrounding area noise								
No surrounding area annoying noise	1		1		1		1	
Yes – surrounding area noise is annoying	**1.4**	1.08–1.82	1.32	0.98–1.76	**6.39**	4.45–9.17	**6.03**	4.19–8.7

Continued

Table 14.4A (Cont'd)

Residential environment characteristic	Model 'self-rated health'				Model 'sleep disturbance'			
	Step 1		Step 2		Step 1		Step 2	
	OR for low health	CI	OR for low health	CI	OR for sleep disturbance	CI	OR for sleep disturbance	CI
Graffiti on residential buildings								
No graffiti	1		1		1		1	
Graffiti exist	0.83	0.66–1.04	0.85	0.65–1.10	**1.13**		0.88–1.46	1.18	0.91–1.53
Litter and trash in residential environment								
No litter and trash	1		1		1		1	
Dirty and littered area	1.19	0.98–1.43	**1.26**	1.02–1.56	**1.19**		1.03–1.38	**1.17**	1.01–1.36
Safety perception in residential area at night								

	OR	95% CI	OR	95% CI	OR	95% CI	OR	95% CI
Feeling safe at night								
Feeling safe at night	1		1		1		1	
Not feeling safe at night	**1.64**	1.41–1.90	**1.58**	1.33–1.87	**1.22**	1.03–1.45	**1.22**	1.02–1.46
Feeling of safety in the dwelling								
Feeling safe in dwelling	1		1		1		1	
Not feeling safe in dwelling	**1.75**	1.43–2.13	**1.6**	1.28–2.00	**2.53**	2.03–3.14	**2.43**	1.94–3.03
Socio-economic status								
Higher SES			1				1	
Lower SES			**1.43**	1.25–1.63			1.11	0.96–1.27
Age group								
Seniors			1				1	
Adults			**0.19**	0.16–0.23			**1.23**	1.01–1.50
Children			**0.04**	0.03–0.05			0.92	0.71–1.18
Gender								
Female			1				1	
Male			**0.73**	0.65–0.83			0.98	0.87–1.12
Functional limitation								
Does not exist			1				1	
Exists			**6.36**	5.06–7.98			1.18	0.95–1.46

OR, odds, ratio; CI, confidence interval.
Step 1 only including REC (residential environment characteristics).
Step 2 including REC and individual characteristics of residents.
Bold figures are significant at 95% level.

Table 14.4B Logistic regression results – examining the impact of the neighbourhood on four health outcomes

Residential environment characteristic	Model 'depression'				Model 'cv symptoms'			
	Step 1		Step 2		Step 1		Step 2	
	OR for depression	CI	OR for depression	CI	OR for CV symptoms	CI	OR for CV symptoms	CI
Play areas for children								
Enough play areas	1		1		1		1	
Not enough play areas	1.06	0.9–1.26	1.15	0.96–1.38	0.94	0.78–1.14	0.95	0.79–1.14
Place to sit and relax outside of dwelling								
Place exists	1		1		1		1	
No such place exists	1.16	0.99–1.36	1.13	0.96–1.33	1.03	0.89–1.2	0.96	0.82–1.14
Vegetation along streets								
Present	1		1		1		1	
Not present	1.14	0.97–1.33	1.06	0.9–1.25	**1.24**	1.07–1.43	1.06	0.90–1.25
Traffic noise								
No annoying traffic noise	1		1		1		1	
Yes-traffic noise is annoying	**1.56**	1.26–1.92	**1.41**	1.13–1.76	**1.34**	1.09–1.66	1.24	0.98–1.57
Surrounding area noise								
No surrounding area annoying noise	1		1		1		1	
Yes – surrounding area noise is annoying	**2.15**	1.54–3	**2.13**	1.46–3.05	1.06	0.73–1.54	1	0.66–1.53
Graffiti on residential buildings								
No graffiti	1		1		1		1	
Graffiti exist	0.95	0.72–1.26	1.02	0.76–1.38	1	0.77–1.31	1.09	0.81–1.46

Variable	OR	95% CI	OR	95% CI	OR	95% CI	OR	95% CI
Litter and trash in residential environment								
No litter and trash	1		1		1		1	
Dirty and littered area	1.22	0.97–1.53	1.22	0.96–1.55	0.98	0.78–1.23	0.99	0.77–1.28
Safety perception in residential area at night								
Feeling safe at night	1		1		1		1	
Not feeling safe at night	**1.42**	**1.18–1.71**	**1.3**	**1.07–1.58**	**1.24**	**1.04–1.48**	**1.22**	**1.02–1.45**
Feeling of safety in the dwelling								
Feeling safe in dwelling	1		1		1		1	
Not feeling safe in dwelling	**2.3**	**1.84–2.88**	**2.11**	**1.66–2.67**	1.07	0.85–1.35	0.95	0.73–1.23
Socio-economic status								
Higher SES			1				1	
Lower SES			**1.42**	**1.22–1.66**			**1.48**	**1.27–1.73**
Age group								
Seniors			1				1	
Adults			**0.8**	**0.66–0.96**			**0.23**	**0.2–0.28**
Children			**0.34**	**0.25–0.45**			**0.01**	**0.01–0.02**
Gender								
Female			1				1	
Male			**0.59**	**0.51–0.68**			**0.85**	**0.74–0.98**
Functional limitation								
Does not exist			1				1	
Exists			**2.6**	**2.14–3.17**			**2.31**	**1.9–2.81**

OR, odds, ratio; CI, confidence interval; CV, cardiovascular.
Step 1 only including REC (residential environment characteristics).
Step 2 including REC and individual characteristics of residents.
Bold figures are significant at 95% level.

The integration of individual characteristics, Step 2, strongly modifies the impact of the residential environment variables. Two of the significant variables of Step 1 ('vegetation along streets' and 'surrounding area noise') were no longer significant after controlling for the confounding influence of the personal characteristics, although 'surrounding area noise' almost remained significant (confidence interval [CI] 0.98–1.76). On the other hand, 'litter and trash in residential environment' became a significant contributor after adjusting for the confounders (odds ratio [OR] = 1.26). 'Feeling of safety in the dwelling' and 'safety perception in residential area at night' still provided the largest influence on self-rated health (OR = 1.60 and 1.58, respectively), although their ORs decreased slightly in comparison to Step 1. Finally, exposure to 'traffic noise' remained the only significant noise variable (OR = 1.34), showing a stable association with low self-rated health.

Sleep disturbance (Model 2)

The impact of the residential environment on sleep disturbance is dominated by the impact of the two noise variables – 'traffic noise' and 'surrounding area noise'. In Step 1, all residential environment variables except 'vegetation along streets' and 'graffiti on residential buildings' showed a significant association with reported sleep disturbance, but only for three variables were there strongly increased ORs: 'traffic noise' and 'surrounding area noise' with ORs >6 and 'feeling of safety in the dwelling' with an OR of 2.53.

In Step 2 there was a very modest impact of the individual characteristics of the residents. All seven significant variables remained significant, and there were only extremely small changes for the OR and CI values. This is especially valid for 'traffic noise', which was identified as the most relevant predictor of sleep disturbance in Step 1, and only showed an OR decrease from 6.52 to 6.42 after the inclusion of the confounders. Similarly, 'surrounding area noise' and 'feeling of safety in the dwelling' remained much more relevant than any of the other significant residential characteristics.

Compared with the strong influence of the environmental variables, there was almost no significant impact of any personal characteristics except for 'age group', in which adults are slightly more likely to suffer from sleep disturbance than the elderly (OR = 1.23).

Depression (Model 3)

Step 1 of this model identified four environment variables that were significantly associated with depression: 'traffic noise', 'surrounding area noise', 'safety perception in residential area at night' and 'feeling of safety in the dwelling', with

Housing environment and health

'surrounding area noise' being more relevant than 'traffic noise' and 'feeling of safety in the dwelling' being more relevant than 'safety perception in residential area at night'.

The integration of the confounding factors in Step 2 did not provide any significant change to the association between the environment and depression. 'Surrounding area noise' (OR reduction from 2.15 to 2.13) and 'feeling of safety in the dwelling' (OR reduction from 2.3 to 2.11) remained the most relevant environmental predictors for depression, and 'traffic noise' (OR reduction from 1.56 to 1.41) and 'safety perception in residential area at night' (OR reduction from 1.42 to 1.3) remained significant. All other environment variables were not significant, although recreational factors ('play areas for children' and 'place to sit and relax outside of dwelling') and 'litter and trash in residential environment' show increased ORs for depression as well but have lower CI values of 0.96 only.

However, all individual characteristics provided a significant influence on depression – especially 'age group' (OR = 0.34 for children compared with elderly) and 'functional limitations' (OR = 2.6 for handicapped persons). SES (OR = 1.42) and gender (OR = 0.59) show OR values that are less strong than those of 'surrounding area noise' or 'feeling of safety in dwelling', suggesting that the impact of environment conditions matched or even exceeded the impact of SES on depression.

Cardiovascular symptoms (Model 4)

This model reviewed the effect of the residential environment on the circulatory system based on research findings that have shown the impact of neighbourhood conditions and cardiovascular health (Diez Roux 2001). Step 1 identified three significant residential environment variables ('vegetation along streets', 'traffic noise', and 'safety perception in residential area at night'), but the OR values were low (ranging from 1.24 to 1.34).

The integration of the individual characteristics changed the results to a large extent. 'Safety perception in residential area at night' (OR = 1.22) was the only environment variable that remained significant. 'Traffic noise', the residential environment variable with the highest OR (1.24), was not significant because of the lower CI level of 0.98. All other environmental variables showed very little influence, as their ORs ranged closely around 1 (0.95–1.09).

However, all individual characteristics provided a significant influence on cardiovascular symptoms, although 'age group' showed by far the largest OR variation. 'Socio-economic status' (OR = 1.48 for low SES) and 'gender' (OR = 0.85 for males) provided relatively little influence on the prevalence of cardiovascular symptoms.

Discussion

Self-rated health

Despite the strong health relevance of individual level factors, there are still four environment characteristics with an independent impact on self-rated health – 'traffic noise', 'litter and trash in residential environment', 'safety perception in residential area at night' and 'feeling of safety in the dwelling'. The impact of 'traffic noise', which was only slightly affected by the inclusion of the confounding variables, indicates that exposure to noise is capable of influencing the self-rated health status of the residents, which is supported by both empirical evidence and by biological mechanisms linking noise exposure with health outcomes such as sleep disturbance, mental health symptoms and hormonal changes (Stansfeld and Matheson 2003). The fact that traffic noise provided higher ORs than neighbourhood noise for the selected health effects supports the view that noise should be defined as one of the few directly health-relevant neighbourhood characteristics – traffic noise shows a significant association with self-rated health while surrounding area noise (although with an OR of 1.32) fails to be significant.[2]

Dirty and littered neighbourhoods were associated with decreased health perceptions. Although direct links cannot be ruled out, and may be especially relevant for mental health effects, the association may be a result of less privileged and therefore less healthy population groups inhabiting littered areas with low levels of maintenance. This would define housing conditions as a health inequality parameter, as suggested by Evans and Kantrowitz (2002) and may lead to an aggravation of pre-existing health problems.

Issues of safety are the most important residential features for health perception. Fear and perceived residential danger, representing a very personal and emotional threat to health, are more closely linked with perceived health than any other residential feature. Although there are a variety of mechanisms linking the perception of safety problems and fear of crime with health (Chandola 2001; Green *et al* 2002), it cannot be ruled out that some of those reporting 'not feeling safe' suffer from a decreased health status that makes them more vulnerable, leading to a higher perception of fear.[3]

In summary, the results showed that the immediate housing environment has an impact on self-rated health, although this is only valid for some of the selected variables. It is especially true for the relative impact of environment variables in relation to 'SES' (OR = 1.43 for residents with low SES) and 'gender' (OR = 0.73 for males): the results for the four significant environment characteristics (ORs ranging from 1.26 to 1.60) are of the same magnitude and are therefore identified

---

[2]See also Chapter 15.
[3]See also Chapter 10.

as being as relevant. This suggests that various health outcomes, although most often seen as a product of individual determinants, can be partially influenced and modified by environmental conditions (Macintyre *et al* 2002). In this context, the results presented are in line with previous research in relation to noise, maintenance and safety issues which have been already defined as powerful indicators for residential quality.

Sleep disturbance

The results for sleep disturbance support the view that the environment can be the most dominant factor. The more a specific health outcome is related to the environmental conditions, the less relevant is the impact of the individual characteristics. For sleep disturbance, only age had some measurable but limited impact, whereas gender, functional limitations and SES (considered one of the most influential parameters) provided no significant change to the results. The fact that those residents exposed to noise were over six times more likely to report disturbed sleep shows that noise exposure must be seen as one of the major public health problems in urban settings. The significant associations with 'play areas for children', 'place to sit and relax outside of dwelling' and 'litter and trash in residential environment' showed that noise exposure is most likely partially linked to the general quality of the urban setting. These results support the view that urban planning can considerably improve the degree of noise exposure, if noise is actively considered and mitigated.

The environment variables suggest that sleep disturbance is also a psycho-social phenomenon. The perception of safety, and especially the feeling of being protected from the outside influences when being at home, is strongly associated with sleep disturbance independent of gender, age or SES. Sleep disturbance may be one of the consequences of compromised psycho-social benefits of the home.

Depression

The results for depression further support the argument that bad housing and inadequate residential environments can strongly affect the mental well-being of residents. The fact that, before and after the integration of the confounders, the two noise variables as well as the two safety variables are significantly associated with depression shows that these factors have an independent and stable influence that, compared to some of the individual characteristics, is rather strong. This suggests that noise and safety constraints may represent relevant aspects for depression, and provides another piece of evidence for a psycho-social link between housing and health. On the other hand, those residents with psycho-social problems may have

---

[4]See also Chapter 11.

had a more negative perception of their residential surroundings, which could have affected the evaluation of the noise or safety aspects.[4]

Cardiovascular symptoms

For cardiovascular symptoms, the data clearly showed that they are mostly independent from the residential environment parameters selected for the regression models, as only one of the contextual variables ('safety perception in residential area at night') proved significantly associated at all. In addition, the OR was lower than the OR changes for three of the confounders, and roughly on the same level as the lowest confounder ('gender' with an OR of 0.85). As expected, age turned out as the dominant parameter that remains unchallenged by any other factor.

However, on noise exposure and the increased risk for heart attacks and infarcts, the OR of 1.24 for 'traffic noise' is remarkable as it corresponds to the findings provided by various other studies. Stansfeld and Matheson (2003) suggested that, with noise exposure, there is a 20% increased likelihood for heart attacks and myocardial infarction. Although the applied regression model did not provide a significant result in the LARES study, it is noteworthy that 'traffic noise' shows the highest OR increase of all residential environment variables.[5] This is supported by the results of Niemann *et al* (2005), who have – using a more detailed approach that distinguished between (a) age groups and (b) severity of exposure – successfully identified significantly increased ORs for cardiovascular symptoms and high blood pressure for adults being exposed to traffic noise as well as neighbourhood noise.

General

In general terms, it was obvious that several variables (especially noise and safety) showed associations with more than one health outcome (see Table 14.5).

It is interesting to note that 'traffic noise', in comparison to 'surrounding area noise' provided the higher OR for the prevalence of sleep disturbance, but is much less relevant for depression: it shows an increased OR of 1.41 only, while 'surrounding area noise' increases the likelihood for depression more than twofold (OR = 2.13). This suggests that noise sources may have a varying impact on different health outcomes, and possibly the perception and the characteristics of

---

[5]There is reason for assuming that a larger sample size could have provided a similar but significant result. More detailed analyses of the original five-point noise exposure ranking scale show that for the highest exposure level (permanent exposure), the OR is as high as 1.5. However, there are only 249 residents that belong to this exposure group, leading to large CI intervals that require strongly increased OR values to be statistically significant.

Housing environment and health

Table 14.5 Overview of significant associations (95% level)

Effect	Significant associations (controlling for age, gender, socio-economic status, functional limitation and city)
Self-rated health	Traffic noise; litter and trash in residential environment; safety perception in residential area at night; feeling of safety in the dwelling
Sleep disturbance	Play areas for children; place to sit and relax outside of dwelling; traffic noise, surrounding area noise; litter and trash in residential environment; safety perception in residential area at night; feeling of safety in the dwelling
Depression	Traffic noise, surrounding area noise; safety perception in residential area at night; feeling of safety in the dwelling
Cardiovascular symptoms	Safety perception in residential area at night

the noise exposure explain the reaction. Traffic noise may be more easy to accept, as most likely every resident has a self-interest in functional traffic (transport) systems. Traffic noise may be a major source of sleep problems, but less relevant for mental health effects as they are evaluated as an unavoidable characteristic of urban living, and so subjectively accepted and justified. Neighbourhood noise from other sources, such as playgrounds and other outside areas, may have a more devastating effect on mental health, as the perception of such noise may have a more emotional dimension and may contain some social characteristics. Such noise is often the reason for social conflicts, even leading to legal cases. Because of to this psycho-social dimension, it seems natural that the effects of residential noise exposure are more strongly expressed in the mental health domain.

A different pattern, however, appears for the safety parameters, for which 'feeling of safety in the dwelling' shows the higher relevance for both sleep disturbance and depression. Here, 'safety perception in residential area at night' is less important. A possible explanation would be that a resident has a number of options to avoid or reduce the feeling of being exposed to threats in the residential area by his or her behavioural choices (not going out at night, not going alone, taking a taxi, etc.). Such a choice does not exist when being in a home that does not provide the feeling of total security and protection from outside threats.

However, any interpretation of the results must keep in mind that the LARES data is cross-sectional. Therefore, it cannot be excluded that those residents suffering from depression have a more negative assessment of their residential environment (or tend to live in less healthy neighbourhoods owing to some

Housing environment and health

socio-economic selection mechanisms), which will inevitably result in statistical associations between the residential environment variables and depression.

For cardiovascular symptoms, 'safety perception in residential area at night' was the only significant environment variable. This may surprise, as for sleep disturbance and depression, the 'feeling of safety in the dwelling' was more influential. However, it has been argued above that the perception of security in the home may be more functional on a mental or psycho-social level, while the perception of not being safe in the neighbourhood, based on these findings, could be more effective for physical health effects such as cardiovascular symptoms.

Based on the two core problems of noise exposure and perceived safety, the major health impact of the immediate housing environment is likely to occur through a psycho-social pathway, triggering feelings of fear and/or aggression and the recognition that as a resident one is not always in full control of the environment. This lack of influence is a typical characteristic for all those environment variables that are identified as the core problems – they are a part of the residential experience that cannot be avoided, and therefore are most powerful to initiate effects on health and well-being. This is further complemented by the fact that 'litter and trash in residential environment' is the second-most important characteristic. Other characteristics, such as recreational areas or the presence of greenery, could to some extent be complemented by visits to playgrounds and leisure walks in other neighbourhoods, or in nearby parks and forests. This would require some transportation needs, but it is definitely possible to cover the residential needs and demands in this way. This option, however, does not exist for safety issues, noise exposure and, to some extent, low levels of maintenance in the immediate area. A quiet, clean or safe neighbourhood close by cannot compensate for the perception of living in a noisy, dirty or unsafe area, the disadvantages of which are perceived every day. Even worse, exposure to noise, lack of safety and dirtiness may be outside the influence or control of the residents. This external locus of control, paired with the feeling of being exposed to outside sources intruding one's home, provides a psycho-social burden that may easily translate into mental health effects as well as into social conflicts. Therefore, the multivariate analyses suggest that the main health effects of residential environments lie within the psycho-social and mental health area and are much less expressed as physical health limitations.

Conclusion

Self-rated health, taken as a composite indicator of health and well-being, was significantly associated with nine selected environment variables. Many of these

Housing environment and health

nine variables proved significant in the multivariate logistic regression models identifying the impact of the neighbourhood quality on the health outcomes of self-rated health, sleep disturbance, depression and cardiovascular symptoms. Adjustment for confounding factors such as age, gender and SES changed this result only to a limited extent.

The multivariate analyses identified two key problems that showed the highest and most consistent impact on the likelihood to suffer from the four analysed health outcomes. These two problem areas were noise exposure and perceived safety; both were significantly associated with self-rated health, sleep disturbance and depression. For cardiovascular symptoms, only perceived safety aspects were significant, but the traffic noise variable provided an even higher OR of 1.24 just below the significance level. Except these two core problem areas, a relevant residential environment characteristic was 'litter and trash in residential environment', which was significantly associated with self-rated health and sleep disturbance and provided a not significant OR of 1.22 for depression. Recreational characteristics ('play areas for children' and 'place to sit and relax outside of dwelling') were associated with sleep disturbance and provided slightly increased but not significant OR values for depression (1.15 and 1.13, respectively).

In concrete terms, the results support the argument that the quality of the immediate housing environment is significantly associated with a variety of health outcomes and therefore has a direct impact on the health and the health-related quality of life of the residents. This finding, based on data from eight European cities, corresponds to the results of other research on the health impact of neighbourhood conditions (Dunn 2002; Drukker *et al* 2003; Howden-Chapman 2004). The study thereby suggests that, irrespective of the city, the relationship between the selected environment factors and the selected health outcomes seems to be universal. Based on the results presented, it can thus be concluded that – at least – 'neighbourhoods have a small but consistent impact on health status' (Howden-Chapman 2004, p 165), and it can be added that the larger part of this impact may be based on psycho-social mechanisms.

Although urban planning and neighbourhood development projects are often based on a variety of health-relevant objectives, they have yet to develop an improved understanding of how their practices can impact on human well-being (Dannenmaier 1995), and of how physical features of neighbourhoods (traffic system, density, recreational facilities, greenery and physical incivilities such as trash), together with the social components (residential behaviours and social incivilities), can translate into non-physical effects and shape the general feeling of well-being and the health-related quality of life of a residential area. In this context, it remains

> ... one of the major challenges ... to bridge the divide between the environmental quality/wellbeing/quality-of-life specialists and the players who

make urban policy and who shape our physical and social environments – in other words the engineers, planners, architects, service delivery specialists, etc.

(Brown 2003, p 85)

Urban and neighbourhood planning has both the capacity and the mandate for developing health-supportive settings, promoting and supporting the health status of individuals. The empirical results presented show that in residential settings there are a variety of health-relevant elements, such as public greenery and recreational areas, cleanliness and maintenance, noise exposure and public safety. Well-designed neighbourhoods and housing environments are able to reduce or compensate health-relevant exposures to physical, social and mental challenges. If adequately considered and located, many neighbourhood features could improve the health-related quality of life of the residents and represent a strong and preventive contribution to the health of the population.

Acknowledgements

The author would like to acknowledge the comments and advice given by Philippa Howden-Chapman, Irene van Kamp and David Ormandy during the development of this paper.

References

Attwell K. (2000) Urban land resources and urban planting – case studies from Denmark. *Landscape and Urban Planning* 52: 145–63.

Austin D.M., Furr A.L., Spine M. (2002) The effects of neighborhood conditions on perceptions of safety. *Journal of Criminal Justice* 30: 417–27.

Bergen Jensen M., Persson B., Guldager S., Reeh U., Nilsson K. (2000) Green structure and sustainability: developing a tool for local planning. *Landscape and Urban Planning* 52: 117–33.

Botkin D.B. and Beveridge C.E. (1997) Cities as environments. Urban Ecosystems 1: 3–19.

Brown A.L. (2003) Increasing the utility of urban environmental quality information. *Journal of Landscape and Urban Planning* 65: 85–93.

Cattell V. (2001) Poor people, poor places, and poor health: the mediating role of social networks and social capital. *Social Science and Medicine* 52: 1501–16.

Chandola T. (2001) The fear of crime and area differences in health. *Health and Place* 7: 105–16.

Cohen D.A., Mason K., Bedinio A. et al (2003) Neighborhood physical conditions and health. *American Journal of Public Health* (93)3: 467–71.

Dannenmaier M. (1995) Healing gardens. *Landscape Architecture* 85/01: 56–8.

Diez Roux A.V. (2001) Investigating neighbourhood and area effects on health. *American Journal of Public Health* 91(11): 1783–9.

Drukker M., Kaplan C., Feron F., von Os J. (2003) Children's health-related quality of life, neighbourhood socio-economic deprivation and social capital. A contextual analysis. *Social Science and Medicine* 57: 825–41.

Dunn J.R. (2002) Housing and inequalities in health: a study of socio-economic dimensions of housing and self reported health from a survey of Vancouver residents. *Journal of Epidemiology and Community Health* 56: 671–81.

Ellaway A., and Macintyre S. (2000) Social capital and self-rated health: support for a contextual mechanism. *American Journal of Public Health* 90: 988.

Emery J., Crump C., Bors P. (2003) Reliability and validity of two instruments designed to assess the walking and bicycling suitability of sidewalks and roads. *American Journal of Health Promotion* 18(1): 38–46.

Evans G.W. (2003) The built environment and mental health. *Journal of Urban Health* 80(4): 536–55.

Evans G.W., Kantrowitz E. (2002) Socioeconomic status and health: the potential role of environmental risk exposure. *Annual Reviews of Public Health* 23: 303–31.

Gold M., Franks P., Erickson P. (1996) Assessing the health of a nation. The predictive validity of a preference-based measure and self-rated health. *Medical Care* 34: 163–77.

Green G., Gilbertson J.M., Grinstey M.F. (2002) Fear of crime and health in residential tower blocks. A case study in Liverpool, UK. *European Journal of Public Health* 12: 10–15.

Howden-Chapman P. (2004) Housing standards: a glossary of housing and health. *Journal of Epidemiology and Community Health* 58: 162–8.

Imrie R. (2000) Responding to the design needs of disabled people. *Journal of Urban Design* 5(2): 199–220.

Jackson R.J. (2003) The impact of the built environment on health: an emerging field [editorial.]. *American Journal of Public Health* 93(9): 1382–3.

Kaplan S. (1995) The restorative benefits of nature: towards an integrative framework. *Journal of Environmental Psychology* 15: 169–82.

Latkin C.A., Curry A.D. (2003) Stressful neighbourhoods and depression: a prospective study of the impact of neighbourhood disorder. *Journal of Health and Social Behaviour* 44: 34–44.

Macintyre S., Ellaway A., Cummins S. (2002) Place effects on health: how can we conceptualise, operationalise and measure them? *Social Science and Medicine* 55: 125–39.

Macintyre S., Ellaway A., Hiscock R. *et al* (2003) What features of the home and the area might help to explain observed relationships between housing tenure and health? Evidence from the West of Scotland. *Health and Place* 9: 207–18.

Mackenbach J.P., Howden-Chapman P. (2002) Houses, neighbourhoods and health. *European Journal of Public Health* 12: 161–2.

Niemann H., Maschke C., Hecht K. (2005) Lärmbedingte Belästigung und Erkrankungsrisiko. Ergebnisse des paneuropäischen LARES-Survey. *Bundesgesundheitsblatt* 48: 315–28

Sharp D. (2002) Silencing cities. *Journal of Urban Health* 79(2): 162.

Stafford M., Marmot M. (2003) Neighbourhood deprivation and health: does it affect us all equally? *International Journal of Epidemiology* 32: 357–66.

Stansfeld S.A., Matheson M.P. (2003) Noise pollution: non-auditory effects on health. *British Medical Bulletin* 68: 243–57.

Thompson C.W. (2002) Urban open space in the 21st century. *Landscape and Urban Planning* 60: 59–72.

Twiss J. (2003) Community gardens: lessons learned from California Healthy Cities and Communities. *American Journal of Public Health* 93(9): 1435–38.

Ulrich R.S., Simons R.V., Losito B.D. *et al* (1991) Stress recovery during exposure to natural and urban environments. *Journal of Environmental Psychology* 11: 201–30.

van Poll R. (1997) The Perceived Quality of the Urban Residential Environment. A Multi-attribute Evaluation. Roermond: Westrom.

Wilson K., Elliott S., Law M. *et al* (2004) Linking perceptions of neighbourhood to health in Hamilton, Canada. *Journal of Epidemiology and Community Health* 58: 192–8.

Further Reading

Amerigo M. and Aragones J.I. (1997) A theoretical and methodological approach to the study of residential satisfaction. *Journal of Environmental Psychology* 17: 47–57.

Anderson, J.R. and Weidemann S. (1997) Developing and utilizing models of resident satisfaction. In: Moore G.T., Marans R.W. (eds), Advances in Environment, Behavior, and Design, Vol. 4. New York: Plenum Press, pp 287–314.

Antonovsky A. (1987) Unraveling the Mystery of Health. How People Manage Stress and Stay Well. San Francisco: Jossey Bass.

Bistrup M.L. (1991) Housing and community environments – how they support health. Briefing book for the Sundsvall Conference on Supportive Environments 1991. National Board of Health, Copenhagen.

Bonnefoy X.R., Braubach M., Moissonnier B., Monolbaer K., Röbbel N. (2003) Housing and health in Europe: preliminary results of a pan-European study. *American Journal of Public Health* 93(9): 1559–63.
Dieckmann F. *et al* (eds) Psychologie und gebaute Umwelt. Konzepte, Methoden, Anwendungsbeispiele. Darmstadt: Institut Wohnen und Umwelt.
Gatrell A.C. (1997) Structures of geographical and social space and their consequences for human health. *Geografiska Annaler* 79B(3): 141–54.
Halpern D. (1995) Mental Health and the Built Environment: More than Bricks and Mortar? London: Taylor & Francis.
Herzog T.R., Magnire C.P., Nebel M.B. (2003) Assessing the restorative components of environments. *Journal of Environmental Psychology* 23: 159–70.
Keane C. (1998) Evaluating the influence of fear of crime as an environmental mobility restrictor on women's routine activities. *Environment and Behavior* 30(1): 60–74.
Ley D. (1981) Behavioral geography and the philosophies of meaning. In: Cox K.R., Golledge R.C. (eds), Behavioral Problems in Geography Revisited. New York: Methuen, pp 209–30.
Macintyre S., Ellaway A. (2000) Ecological approaches: rediscovering the role of the physical and social environment. In: Berkman L.F., Kawachi I. (eds), Social Epidemiology. Oxford: Oxford University Press.
McMichael A.J., Beaglehole R. (2000) The changing global context of public health. *Lancet* 356: 495–9.
Rapoport A. (1982) The Meaning of the Built Environment. A Nonverbal Communication Approach. London: Sage Publications.
Sime J.D. (1986) Creating places or designing spaces? *Journal of Environmental Psychology* 6: 49–63.
Stokols D., Grzywacz J.G., McMahan S., Phillips K. (2003) Increasing the health promotive capacity of human environments. *American Journal of Health Promotion* 18(1): 4–13.
Thomson H., Keams A., Petticrew M. (2003) Assessing the health impact of local amenities: a qualitative study of contrasting experiences of local swimming pool and leisure provision in two areas of Glasgow. *Journal of Epidemiology and Community Health* 57: 663–7.
Türkoglu H.D. (1997) Resident's satisfaction of housing environments: the case of Istanbul, Turkey. *Landscape and Urban Planning* 39: 55–67.
Van den Berg A.E., Kode S.L., van der Wulp N.Y. (2003) Environmental preference and restoration: (How) are they related? *Journal of Environmental Psychology* 23: 135–46.
van Kamp I., Leidelmeijer K., Morsman G., De Hollander A. (2003) Urban environmental quality and human well-being: towards a conceptual framework and demarcation of concepts; a literature study. *Landscape and Urban Planning* 65: 5–18.

Wainwright N.W.J., Surtees P.G. (2003) Places, people, and their physical and mental functional health. *Journal of Epidemiology and Community Health* 58: 333–9.

Warner S.B. (1995) Restorative landscapes. *Landscape Architecture* 85(1): 128.

WHO (1986) Ottawa Charter for Health Promotion. World Health Organization, Health and Welfare Canada, Canadian Public Health Association. Geneva: World Health Organization.

15 Noise effects and morbidity

Hildegard Niemann and Christian Maschke

Introduction

Environmental noise, irrespective of its source – traffic, leisure or neighbourhood activities – is an important issue in most European countries. The predominant health effect of noise is auditory damage, which includes hearing loss. This is frequently caused by loud noise at the work site or by loud music (i.e. from continuous high exposure to personal stereos and discotheques) as well as by fireworks. But, in addition to auditory damage, non-auditory health effects can be caused by noise at levels far below those required to damage the hearing organ.

Environmental noise acts as a stressor at night by disturbing sleep and as an annoyance during the day; and long-term stress can trigger or aggravate diseases. It is therefore necessary to test what health dangers in the residential environment are linked to sleep disturbances caused by noise. The repercussions on health have been only marginally looked at in studies examining the relationship between traffic noise and health. Studies that examine night noise have indeed documented that elevated health risks due to sleep disturbances from traffic noise are very probable.

The health effects of annoyance and sleep disturbance caused by noise include effects on the cardiovascular, the respiratory, and the musculoskeletal systems. The biological plausibility for these effects has been shown in experimental examinations. With central nervous processes, noise stress influences the neuroendocrine system either directly or indirectly through emotional experience (disturbances, annoyance) or disturbed sleep (chronobiological stress). In this way exposure to noise can lead to an inadequate neuroendocrine reaction pattern and finally to regulation diseases (Frankenhäuser and Lundberg 1976). Pathological changes can manifest themselves in the cardiovascular system (Babisch and Ising 2001), in the respiratory system (Langewitz and Soler 2003)

effects and morbidity

as well as in the musculoskeletal system (Eich 2003) or can appear as psychological disturbances (Maschke *et al* 2003).

Pathological changes can affect mental well-being and therefore may increase the susceptibility to noise. From this point of view the epidemiological association between annoyance and health endpoints could be interpreted as being caused by the diseases. For the association between sleep disturbances and health endpoints it is nearly the same. Sleep could be disturbed by diseases such as bronchitis or asthma.

The LARES study included information on various sources of environmental noise and their effects on sleep and annoyance. It also included data on several morbidities. This chapter examines the strength of the association between noise-induced annoyances and noise-induced sleep disturbances with stress-mediated diseases.

Annoyance, sleep disturbances and chronic illnesses in the LARES study

The LARES study provided information on annoyance from different noise sources through the question, 'In the last 12 months, were you bothered or annoyed in your residence by noise from the following sources?' The intensity of the noise was registered with the five-level ICBEN scale from 'not at all' to 'extreme' (see Figure 15.1).

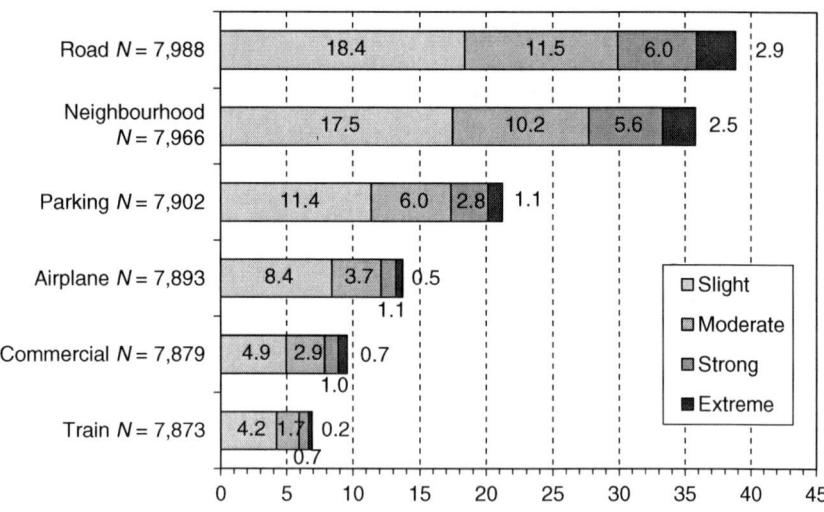

15.1 Frequency of occurrence of annoyance (and intensity levels from slight to extreme; 'not at all' completes to 100%) in the LARES study for six selected sources of noise – adults, children and elderly $N = 8{,}519$.

The results showed that about 39% of those surveyed were troubled in their residence by road traffic noise (9% rated the intensity of road traffic noise 'strong' to 'extreme'). Following closely behind, 36% of the respondents cited disturbances from neighbourhood noise. Perhaps surprisingly, 21% felt disturbed by the noise vehicles made when parking. Aircraft noise was reported by 13% of the respondents, and 6.8% reported railway noise.[1]

The individual annoyances from road traffic noise, aircraft noise and rail noise, as well as the annoyance caused by parking vehicles were summarised under the term 'traffic noise.' This was because traffic noise represented the dominant noise factor in the residential surroundings, and the majority of respondents indicated that they were troubled by more than one source of traffic noise. The second largest source of noise in the residential surroundings was neighbourhood noise. The individual annoyances by noise from a neighbour's residence, a common stairwell, children playing, as well as the annoyance from noises within the dwelling itself were summarised under the term 'neighbourhood noise'. Both road traffic noise and neighbourhood noise were divided into categories (slight, moderate and strong). All results were based on these three variables.

Information on sleep disturbance from different noise sources was gained through the questions, 'Has your sleep been disturbed by noise during the past 4 weeks?' and 'If yes, what was/were the source(s) of noise?' The results showed that about 10% of the respondents reported that their sleep had been disturbed by road traffic noise, closely followed by neighbourhood noise (9.5%). Noise made by parking vehicles was cited by approximately 5% of the respondents. The proportional distribution of six selected noise-related causes of sleep disturbances is shown in Figure 15.2.

The questions, 'Have you had one of the following diseases in the last 12 months?' and 'Was the illness diagnosed by a physician?' were used in the LARES study to obtain the period prevalence[2] of medically diagnosed illnesses. The prevalence of selected illnesses in adults, in the elderly and in children is represented in Figure 15.3. Hypertension and allergies were the most frequently diagnosed illnesses for adults (12.1% and 11%, respectively), followed by arthritis and migraines (9.6% and 9.5%, respectively). Depression was reported by 6.1% of the respondents.

In the elderly participants in the LARES study, hypertension and arthritis were the most frequently diagnosed illnesses, with a prevalence of 41.7% and 37.5%, respectively. This was much higher than for the adults group. Bronchitis (11.4%),

---

[1]Note that the field of data acquisition included airport and railway areas, but did not concentrate on areas specifically troubled by flight patterns or railway noise.
[2]Period prevalence is the number of medical cases that arose in a defined time period, related to the total population.

Noise effects and morbidity

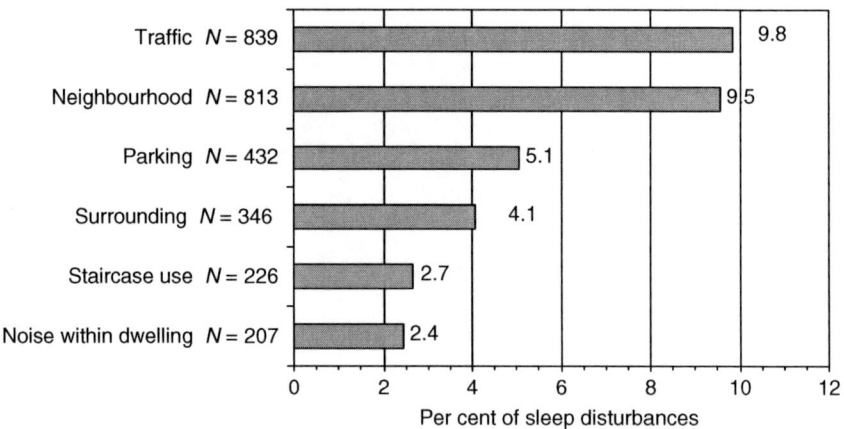

15.2 Frequency of occurrence of sleep disturbances in the LARES study for six selected sources of noise – adults, children and elderly, N = 8,519.

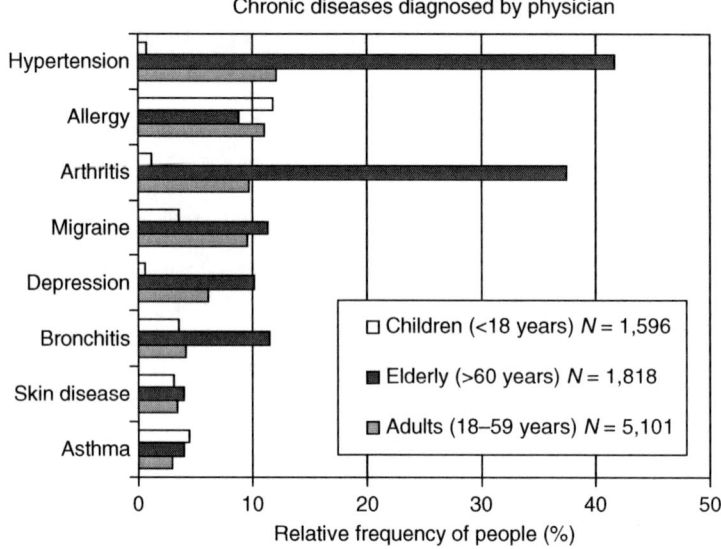

15.3 A comparison of the prevalence of selected medically diagnosed illnesses in adults (18–59 years of age), elderly and children in the LARES study.

migraines (11.3%) and depression (10.1%) followed; the prevalence of these illnesses was again markedly higher than for the adults group.

The results for children show clear differences from the adults and elderly groups. The most frequently diagnosed illnesses for children were allergies (11.7%), followed by asthma (4.4%), bronchitis (3.6%) and migraines (3.6%).

Noise effects and morbidity

With the exceptions of allergies, bronchitis and skin diseases, the prevalence of illnesses in children were markedly less than in adults.

Method

An examination of the statistical association between noise annoyance as well as noise-induced sleep disturbances and diseases must take account of the fact that both diseases and risk factors are affected by many other factors than noise. A meaningful statistical analysis of multiple methods must be applied. In total, 13 control variables were included block-wise in the logistic regression, which, in the case of the diseases, are assumed to influence the result. Odds ratios (ORs) were calculated as an estimator of the relative risk (RR).

Furthermore, the different European cities in the LARES study (control variable 'city') were taken into account in the basic model as well as in neighbourhood annoyance if traffic noise-induced annoyance was evaluated. If neighbourhood annoyance was evaluated, traffic noise-induced annoyance was taken into account in the basic model (Block 1). Similarly, for traffic noise-induced annoyance, the annoyance by neighbourhood noise was taken into account as an additional control variable in the basic model (Block 1) – see Table 15.1.

Table 15.1 Control variables divided into five analysis blocks

Block	Label	Control variables
Block 1	Basic model	Age, gender, city
Block 2	Socio-economic status	Socio-economic status
Block 3	Risk factors	Consumption of alcohol, smoking behaviour, sports activity, body mass index
Block 4	General environment	Satisfaction with residential areas, green areas
Block 5	Housing factors	The perception of: dampness in dwelling, air quality in dwelling, temperature and heating in winter, daylight in dwelling

Results for noise annoyance

Annoyance is defined as a feeling of discomfort that is related to an adverse influence upon an individual or a group by any substances or circumstances. Annoyance expresses itself, for example, by malaise, fear, threat, feeling troubled, uncertainty, restricted liberty experience, excitability or defencelessness. In this sense, annoyance is emotional stress.

Noise effects and morbidity

In the following figures, the RR, including a 95% confidence interval (CI), is represented for people who have felt annoyed by traffic or neighbourhood noise in the last 12 months. This is compared with people who did not indicate any annoyance from the analysed noise source (comparison group). In addition, the level of significance is recorded for a linear trend (1 d.f.) above the intensity levels. The results were adjusted for 'age', 'gender', 'city', 'neighbourhood noise' (Block 1); 'socio-economic status' (Block 2); 'consumption of alcohol', 'smoking behaviour', 'sports activity', 'body mass index' (Block 3); 'satisfaction with residential areas' and 'green areas' (Block 4); and 'dampness in dwelling', 'air quality in dwelling', 'winter temperature in dwelling', 'daylight in dwelling' (Block 5).

Traffic noise – adults

In each case the relative risk of diseases (ORs) are represented for 18- to 59-year-old subjects.

The analysis of the LARES data showed a close relationship between chronic annoyance by traffic noise and a higher risk to the cardiovascular system in adults. Significantly increased risks appeared for cardiovascular symptoms as well as for hypertension, which exhibited a positive trend over the intensity stages (see top of Figure 15.4). The significant trend supports the assumption of a dose–effect relationship. On the other hand, there was no recognisable increased risk for a medically diagnosed heart attack. Strong chronic annoyance by traffic noise showed significantly increased RR for respiratory symptoms and bronchitis alike (see Figure 15.4, centre).

On the other hand, a trend over the intensity stages could not be determined for asthma illnesses. For psychological illnesses and chronic annoyance by traffic noise the relationship was very pronounced (see Figure 15.4, bottom). Medically diagnosed 'depressions' as well as the 'trend to depression' (SALSA[3]) appeared significantly more frequently with chronic annoyance by traffic noise.

In addition, an increased risk of migraines was associated with strong chronic annoyance.

The increased risk of illness due to a strong annoyance by traffic noise demonstrates that a highly noisy residential environment should be classified as a serious danger to health for adults.

Neighbourhood noise – adults

Analysis of the data suggests that an increased risk of hypertension and cardiovascular illness is connected to chronic annoyance by neighbourhood noise

---

[3] See Chapter 11 for explanation of SALSA.

Noise effects and morbidity

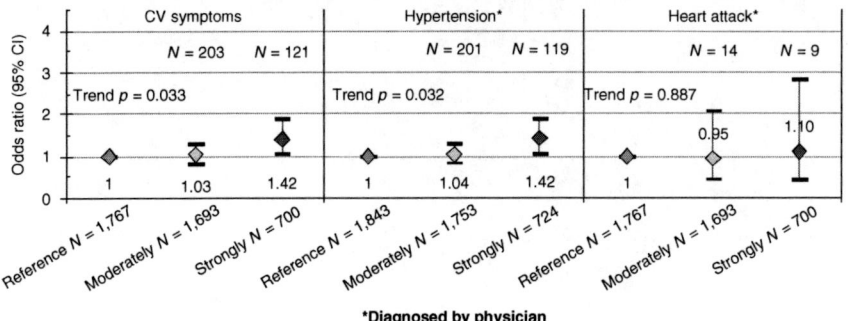

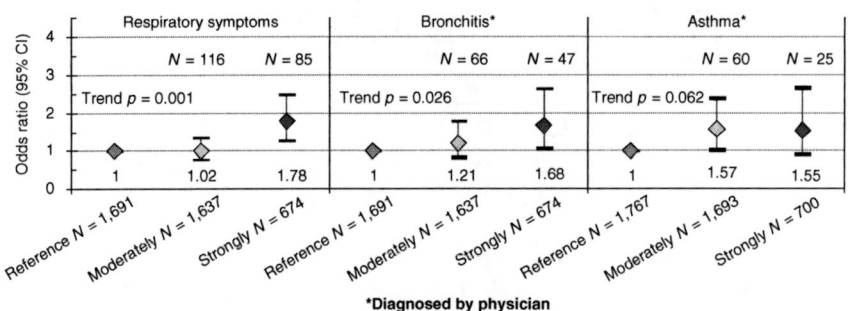

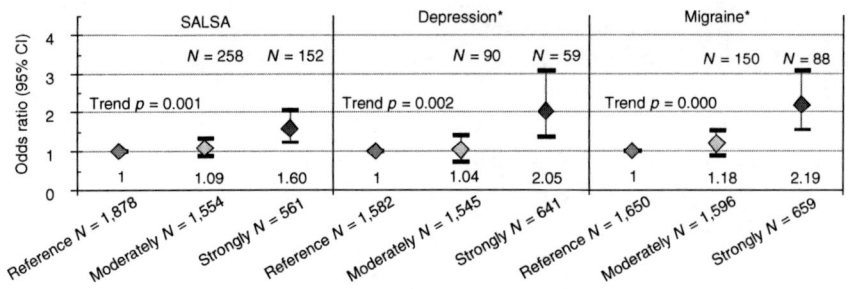

15.4 Relative disease risks for adults who indicated noise-induced annoyance by general traffic noise within the last 12 months, compared to adults without traffic noise-induced annoyance.

Noise effects and morbidity

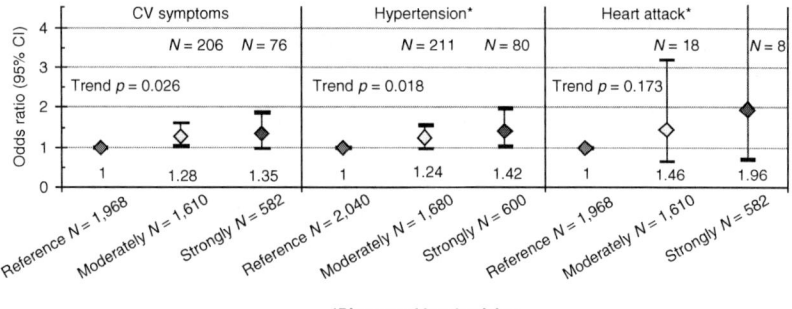

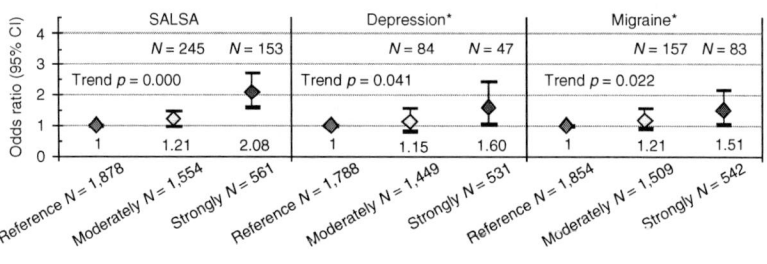

15.5 Relative disease risks for adults who indicated noise-induced annoyance by general neighbourhood noise within the last 12 months, in comparison with adults without neighbourhood noise-induced annoyance.

(see Figure 15.5, top). However, an increased risk of heart attacks could not be confirmed.

For the respiratory system, the impact of a chronic annoyance by neighbourhood noise was less clear than that of chronic annoyance by traffic noise. Only the risk of bronchitis appeared significantly increased.

Pronounced effects were noted in the psychological system (see Figure 15.5, bottom). Strong, chronic annoyance by neighbourhood noise raised significantly the occurrence of medically diagnosed 'trend to depression' (SALSA) and depression. In addition, a higher risk of migraines was associated with strong, chronic annoyance by neighbourhood noise.

The evaluation of the effect of noise-induced annoyance from the general neighbourhood suggests that it has an influence on health, and that the risk pattern for strong neighbourhood noise annoyance is nearly the same as for traffic noise annoyance.

Noise effects and morbidity

Traffic noise – children

Many systems of small children, such as the nervous system and the cognitive system, are subject to rapid growth and development. The development of the child is not designed to compensate for high environmental noise exposure. Beyond that, with early exposure to environmental influences, children have significantly more time to develop chronic illness. Against this backdrop, children can be regarded as a separate risk group.

The following figures represent the RRs for 1 to 17 year olds. Health conditions such a hypertension, heart attack, gastric ulcer, malignant tumour and stroke appear only rarely in children, with their prevalence increasing with age. This meant that the low number of cases in the data did not allow a meaningful analysis.

A second problem is the reliability of the annoyance rating from younger children. We assumed that the annoyance rating by children is meaningful for children ≥10 years old (Herdman et al 2002; Kamtsiuris et al 2002). Therefore, for the younger children we use the averaged annoyance rating of all adults in the household.

The results of the analyses show a close relationship between a chronically strong annoyance by traffic noise and increased risk for impairments of the respiratory system and bronchitis in children (see Figure 15.6).

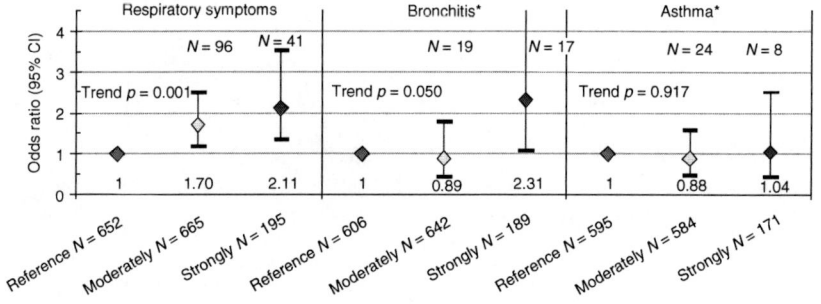

15.6 Relative disease risks for children who indicated noise-induced annoyance by general traffic noise within the last 12 months, compared to children without traffic noise-induced annoyance.

Neighbourhood noise – children

A chronic annoyance through neighbourhood noise also showed a strong effect on children's respiratory systems and the risk of bronchitis (see Figure 15.7). With an indication of strong chronic annoyance, a significantly higher risk was registered for respiratory systems as well as for bronchitis. For children who

Noise effects and morbidity

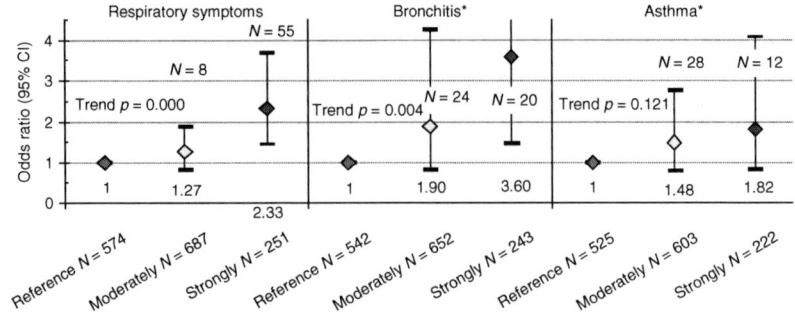

15.7 Relative disease risks for children who indicated noise-induced annoyance by general neighbourhood noise within the last 12 months, compared to children without neighbourhood noise-induced annoyance.

reported a strong annoyance, the RR of respiratory illness and bronchitis was 2.3% and 3.6%, respectively, a markedly higher RR than in adults.

The strongly increased illness risks in the respiratory system support the acceptance that in regards to neighbourhood noise annoyance, children can be classified as a risk group.

Traffic noise – elderly

It is well known from general stress research that the ability to cope with noise decreases in the elderly. Therefore, elderly people, those ≥60 years old, could be a risk group regarding noise annoyance and health.

The results of the analyses of the LARES data cannot confirm an increased illness risk for the elderly, and no statistical association could be shown between chronic annoyance by traffic noise and an increased risk of cardiovascular conditions. The same applies for the respiratory and neuro-psychological systems. For the elderly, chronic annoyance by traffic noise only affected the musculoskeletal system, and a significantly increased risk of arthritis symptoms as well as arthritis was associated with strong chronic annoyance by traffic noise (see Figure 15.8).

Neighbourhood noise – elderly

As in the case of traffic noise annoyance, the only impact of chronic annoyance by neighbourhood noise was upon the musculoskeletal system (see Figure 15.9), with a significantly increased risk of arthritis symptoms.

Noise effects and morbidity

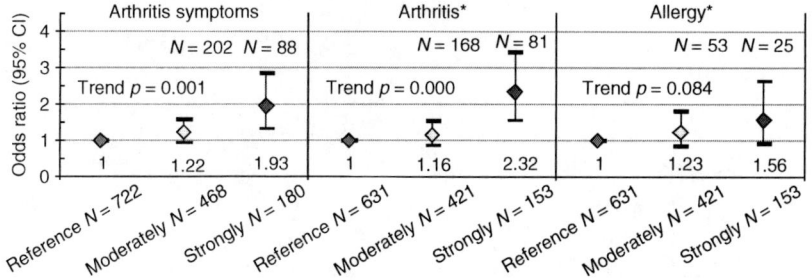

15.8 Relative disease risks for elderly people who indicated noise-induced annoyance by traffic noise within the last 12 months, in comparison with elderly people without traffic noise-induced annoyance.

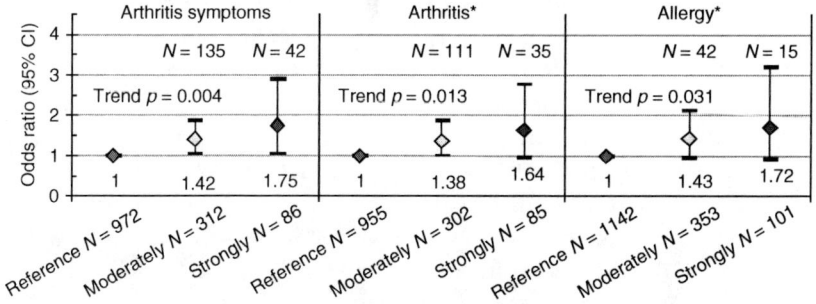

15.9 Relative disease risks for elderly people who indicated noise-induced annoyance by neighbourhood noise within the last 12 months, in comparison with elderly people without neighbourhood noise-induced annoyance.

For annoyance by neighbourhood noise, the analyses could not categorize the elderly as a risk group.

Effect of noise-induced disturbed sleep

Sleep is an essential condition for humans and can be severely disturbed by noise. Acute sleep disturbances affect the subjective well-being and, with an individual

Adults

In Figure 15.10, the RRs are represented for adults (18–59 years of age) who indicated noise-induced sleep disturbances. Noise-induced sleep disturbances are associated in this study with significantly increased risks for the vast majority of diseases in adults. Only for diabetes, heart attack, malignant tumour, skin disease, asthma and stroke were there no remarkable associations found.

The results suggest that chronic noise-induced sleep disturbances can be classified as a meaningful risk factor to the health of adults.

Children

In Figure 15.11, the RR is represented for 1 to 17 year olds who indicated noise-induced sleep disturbances.

With children, noise-induced sleep disturbances are statistically associated with a highly increased risk of medical conditions such as bronchitis (RR = 3.9) as well as an increased risk for respiratory symptoms (RR = 2.1). Because a physician is consulted only rarely for headaches and migraines in children, noise-induced sleep disturbances with self-reported migraines were further examined. The amount of self-reported migraines was more than double the migraines diagnosed by a physician. Children with noise-induced sleep disturbances who self-reported migraines fall ill 2.3 times more often.

The structure and quality of sleep change significantly in the course of childhood, and the finding of a high increased risk of illness associated with noise-induced sleep disturbances supports the view that children are a risk group.

Elderly

In Figure 15.12, the RR of diseases is represented for elderly people ≥ 60 years old who indicated noise-induced sleep disturbances.

In elderly people, noise-induced sleep disturbances are associated with allergies (RR = 1.6), arthritic symptoms (RR = 1.6), arthritis (RR = 1.6), asthma (RR = 2.0), gastric and duodenal ulcer (RR = 2.0), migraines (RR = 1.8) and SALSA (RR = 1.6).

Sleep quality decreases strongly in the elderly and, therefore, the elderly could be a risk group. However, the results of the analyses of the LARES data showed that while elderly people are affected by sleep disturbances, the results cannot confirm that they should be classified as a risk group.

Noise effects and morbidity

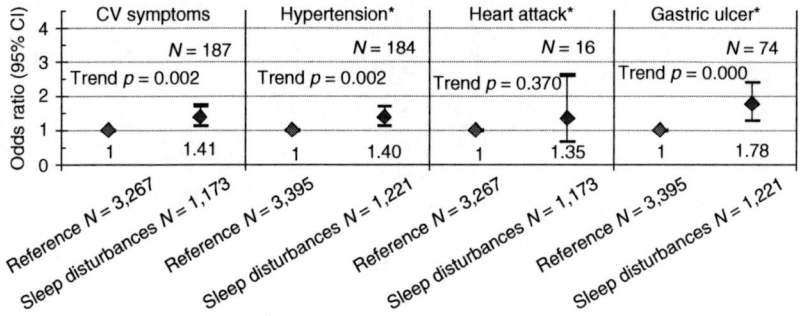

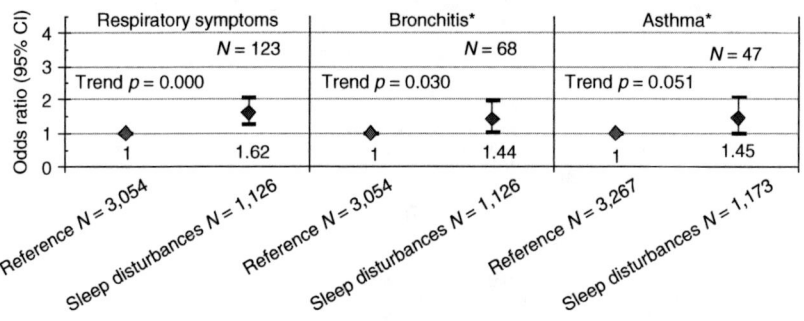

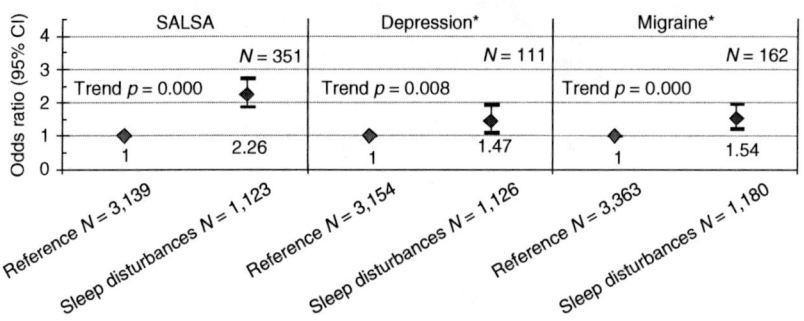

15.10 Relative disease risks for adults who indicated noise-induced sleep disturbances within the last 12 months, in comparison with adults without noise-induced sleep disturbances.

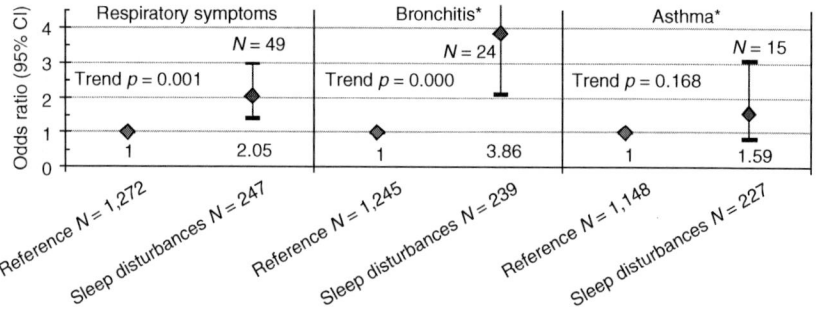

15.11 Relative disease risks for children who indicated noise-induced sleep disturbances within the last 12 months, in comparison with children without noise-induced sleep disturbances.

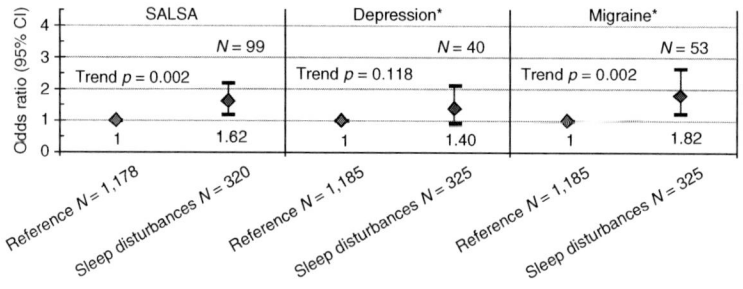

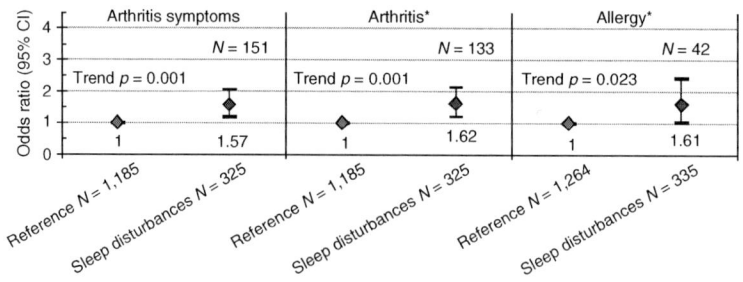

15.12 Relative disease risks for elderly people who indicated noise-induced sleep disturbances within the last 12 months, in comparison with elderly people without noise-induced sleep disturbances.

Discussion

In the investigation of the connection between noise and health, it must be acknowledged that everyday health is influenced by many factors. The evaluation of the LARES data was therefore carried out with an extensive set of control variables, taking into account the influence on health of housing conditions and the housing environment. With regard to the variety of the examined diseases, the large control variable set was not always to be considered complete. Furthermore, well-known control variables are missing, such as family history and occupational noise exposure.

Air pollution, such as fine dust, which has the same origin as traffic noise, could have a confounding impact on the results, but the effect should not differ essentially, because the risk pattern for traffic noise and neighbourhood noise does not differ significantly (except in the respiratory system for adults), and neighbourhood noise is hardly ever correlated with air pollutants.

That well-being as well as sleep could be influenced by the individual's state of health is well known, but the thesis that the associations in the LARES data are essentially caused by the state of health is not very probable. Most of the examined diseases are heavily dependent on age, with a considerably higher occurrence among the elderly (with the exception of allergies). If the epidemiological associations are essentially caused by diseases, the relative frequency of annoyance as well as sleep disturbance in elderly people must be considerably higher than in adults: that is not the case for annoyance and not the case for noise-induced sleep disturbances. The relative frequencies of annoyance as well as of sleep disturbance in elderly people are remarkably less than in adults. Therefore, while acknowledging the state of health of the individual, we assume that the associations are essentially caused by noise annoyance as well as by noise-induced sleep disturbances.

This assumption of a causal relation between noise-induced annoyance and health endpoints is supported by dose–effect considerations. The relative risks for pathological changes in the cardiovascular system (hypertension, CV-symptoms) were clearly increased in adults reporting chronically strong annoyance compared to adults indicating moderate annoyance. At moderate annoyance the relative risks are no different from, or only slightly higher than, the reference group. This also applies to pathological changes in the respiratory system (bronchitis, respiratory symptom), to arthritis and to depression.

To summarise, the data from the LARES study support the proposition that there are increased health risks from chronically strong noise annoyance as well as from noise-induced sleep disturbances.

The analysis shows that the health risks are dependent on the age groups. Few differences can be recognised within an age group regarding the pathogenesis mechanism of annoyance and sleep disturbances. At strong annoyance the risk patterns between general traffic noise and general neighbourhood noise are very similar within the age groups. As noted above, with children, we assumed that the annoyance rating by children is meaningful if children are ≥10 years old, but for younger children we used the averaged annoyance rating of all adults in the household.

Pathological changes appear in adults in the cardiovascular system, the respiratory system, the musculoskeletal system and the psychological system (depression). Unlike adults (18–59 years old), the elderly experienced significantly increased risks from annoyance only in the musculoskeletal system (arthritic symptoms), independent of the noise source. The results of the analyses do not confirm the thesis that elderly people are subject to a noise-induced increased risk to health. Similar results were found in a study by Maschke *et al* (2003), with a stronger association between treatments for hypertension and the nightly noise level for adults < 60 years old than for elderly people.

Age-related hardness of hearing is often cited as a possible reason for the difference between the age groups, a condition that could not be controlled for in the LARES study. This notion presumes that the elderly hear more poorly, sense noise as less loud and therefore have a weaker reaction to it. However, this assumption applies only for very pronounced hearing loss. Normal age-related hardness of hearing cannot be compared with an ear plug that altogether muffles the perception of sound; instead, age-related hardness of hearing is characterized by so-called 'recruitment'. Quiet noises are heard poorly or not at all; however, loud noises are perceived at the same volume as those with normal healthy hearing. Because loud noises crop up abruptly for the elderly who are hard of hearing, they often perceive loud noises as more disturbing than those with a normal sense of hearing do. Hence, the normal loss of hearing that comes with age is no protection against noise.

This was also shown in the Spandau Health Survey (see Maschke *et al* 2003), in which hardness of hearing due to age was controlled for and a relevant connection between age-related hardness of hearing and treatments for hypertension due to noise conditions was not found.

For children, the effects of noise are seen primarily in the respiratory system. Strongly annoyed children were found to suffer respiratory diseases twice as often as non-noise-annoyed children do. The same effect exists for noise-disturbed sleep, with approximately the same range of risk. In contrast, allergy, one of the most frequent illnesses of children, does not seem to respond to noise. According to the results, children have to be classified as particularly sensitive to noise with regard to the respiratory system.

This connection was also identified in a study by Ising *et al* (2003). In the so-called Harz study, the frequency of respiratory problems was determined in addition to the release of stress hormones in the first and second halves of the night. The children experiencing greatest strain lived along a German federal highway, on which a truck with L_{max} >80 dB(A) passed by every 2 mins on average, including at night. The reference group was composed of children from the same localities but who lived on less-trafficked streets. The occurrence of allergies and/or bronchial asthma in the Harz study had a significant correlation with the noise annoyance. It also showed significantly increased health risks for skin and respiratory diseases from long-term annoyance through traffic emissions (noise, exhaust gases), the diseases increasing as the noise pollution did.

Analysis of data from the LARES study showed there was a strong relationship between strong annoyance and respiratory illnesses for both street traffic noise and neighbourhood noise (see Table 15.2). This is informative, since for neighbourhood noise, as opposed to traffic noise, no correlation with traffic-dependent air pollutants is assumed. The occurrence of bronchitis in children seems to be caused not only by the provocation of air pollutants, but also – as seen in the case of neighbourhood noise – through emotional stress.

Table 15.2 Relative risks for illnesses/disease symptoms in children experiencing chronic annoyance through traffic noise and neighbourhood noise

Illnesses	Traffic noise			Neighbourhood noise		
	Annoyance moderately	Annoyance strong	Trd	Annoyance moderately	Annoyance strong	Trd
Respiratory symptoms	1.70	2.11	s	1.27	2.33	s
Bronchitis	0.89	2.31	s	1.90	3.60	s
Asthma	0.88	1.04	ns	1.48	1.82	ns

Trd = trend over the intensity levels; s = significant; ns = not significant.

Conclusions

The LARES study gives an overview of the close relationship between strong noise annoyance, noise-induced sleep disturbances and the health of people in the eight European cities. The evaluation of the data took place with an extensive set of control variables, and for the first time also took into comprehensive consideration the influences of living and residential conditions.

However, it would have been advantageous if further control variables had been available, such as inherited predispositions to diseases; exposure to noise in one's profession; and also information on hearing ability (audiograms, hearing-aid users, etc.). On the other hand, in spite of the lack of these uncontrolled influencing variables in the LARES study, the results are comparable with findings from studies such as the Noise and Risk of Myocardial Infarction Study (Willich *et al* 2006), which included data on hereditary predisposition and exposure to noise at work, and the Spandau Health Survey, which included data on hearing ability. Even the existing uncertainties regarding the reliability of the LARES study's resulting data – particularly concerning the self-reported illnesses and information regarding medically diagnosed illnesses – do not call the results into question. The uncertainties are no greater than those in recognized national health surveys (for e.g. the German Federal Health Survey). In future studies, it would be useful if the self-reported data could be checked with random sampling to determine the reliability.

Beyond that, the causality problem must be considered. For a causal correlation to be determined, the exposure of the illness must take place first, which cannot be documented in a cross-section study such as the LARES study. If the results are looked at with regards to noise problems, it can be determined that the necessary causality criteria have been fulfilled. The intended causality interpretation of the results is therefore a gradual one based on the collection of indices (in view of the evidence).

The results support the thesis that for chronic strong annoyance, a causal chain exists between three steps: health, strong annoyance and increased morbidity.

For adults with strong annoyance, significantly increased risks exist in the cardiovascular system, the respiratory system and the musculoskeletal system as well as in the psychological system (depression). Elderly people with strong annoyance show less illness effects than adults do. With children, the effects of noise are seen primarily in the respiratory system. The respiratory system also reacts to neighbourhood noise with increased relative risks. In contrast to traffic noise, for neighbourhood noise, air pollution cannot be responsible as an alternative reason for the increased health risks in the respiratory system. The noise has to be classified as an independent risk factor for the respiratory system.

A further effect of noise is sleep disturbances. Acute sleep disturbances affect performance and, in the long run, health. For adults, significantly increased relative risks to the cardiovascular, respiratory and musculoskeletal systems, as well as to depression, occur with noise-induced sleep disturbances. Many of these diseases increase with age and therefore appear only rarely in children. For children, significantly increased relative risks to the respiratory system, as well as to migraines (self-reported), are of great significance. Therefore, particular attention must be paid to nightly environmental noise exposure.

Until now, little attention has been paid to neighbourhood noise annoyance as regards the development of diseases, and therefore pathological effects have been considerably underestimated. The health effect of neighbourhood noise-induced annoyance is approximately in the same range as the health effect of traffic noise-induced annoyance. The results suggest that improving sound insulation in residential buildings will have positive health benefits.

In view of the connection between noise-induced annoyance and noise-induced sleep disturbances and illness risks, there is a need for further research. In future studies on the health effects of noise-induced annoyance, the causality should be confirmed with the implementation of cohort studies. Noise-induced sleep disturbances call for sleep studies that not only register the subjective statements about night-time sleep but also document objective, measurable sleep parameters. The innovative and comprehensive LARES study should be the starting point for further noise effect studies in the area of housing and health studies.

References

Babisch W., Ising H. (2001) Noise induced stress is a risk factor in cardiovascular disease. The 2001 International Congress on Noise Control Engineering. The Hague, The Netherlands.

Eich W. (2003) Chronische polyarthritis and fibromyalgie [Chronic polyarthritis and fibromyalgia]. In: Adler R.H., Herrmann J.M., Köhle K. et al (eds), Uexküll Psychosomatische Medizin – Modelle ärztlichen Handelns, 6 Munich: Urban & Fischer, pp 941–6.

Frankenhäuser M., Lundberg U. (1976) Psychological reactions to noise as modified by personal control. Reports from the Department of Psychology, University of Stockholm, Vol. 471.

Hecht K., Engfer A., Peter J.H., Poppei M. (eds) (1993) Schlaf, Gesundheit, Leistungsfähigkeit [Sleep, Health, Efficiency] Berlin: Springer.

Herdman M., Rajmil L., Ravens-Sieberer U. et al and the European Kidscreen Group Disabkids Group (2002) Expert consensus in the development of a European health-related quality of life measure for children and adolescents: a Delphi study. *Acta Pediatrica* 91(12): 1385–90.

Ising H., Lange-Asschenfeldt H., Lieber G.F., Weinhold H., Eits M. (2003) *Noise and Health*, 5(19): 41–50.

Kamtsiuris P., Bergmann K.E., Dippelhofer A. et al (2002): Der Pretest des Kinder – und Jugendgesundheitssurveys: Methodische Aspekte und Durchführung. Gesundheitswesen 64 Stuttgart: Georg Theme, pp 99–106.

Langewitz W., Solèr M. (2003) Asthma bronchiale [Bronchial asthma]. In: Adler R.H., Herrmann J.M., Köhle K. et al (eds), Uexküll Psychosomatische Medizin-Modelle ärztlichen Handelns. 6. Auflage. Munich: Urban & Fischer, pp 891–907.

Maschke C., Wolf U., Leitmann T. (2003) Epidemiologische Untersuchungen zum Einfluss von Lärmstress auf das Immunsystem und die Entstehung von Arteriosklerose [Epidemiological examinations of the influence of noise stress on the immune system and the emergence of arteriosclerosis]. Umwelt-forschungsplan des Bundesministeriums für Umwelt, Naturschutz und

Reaktorsicherheit, Abschlussbericht des Forschungsvorhabens Z.2.2-60424/107 im Aktionsprogramm 'Umwelt und Gesundheit' (UFOPLAN) 298 62 515, WaBoLu-Hefte 01/03, Umweltbundesamt Berlin.

Willich S.N., Wegscheider K., Stallmann M., Keil T. (2006) Noise burden and the risk of myocardial infarction. *Eur Heart J* 27(3): 276–82.

16 Domestic accidents
Richard Moore

Introduction

Accidents in the home are a serious public health problem. In 1998, it was estimated that home and leisure accidents resulted in around 20 million injuries requiring medical treatment in the European Union. About 2 million of these led to hospital admissions, and around 83,000 resulted in death. Over half of these accidents occurred in or around the home (EHLASS 1998).

In the UK, home accidents in 1999 resulted in 2.8 million injuries requiring medical treatment (that is over 7,600 a day), and official estimates (DTI 2002) put the cost to the UK at around £25,000 million per year. It has been estimated that the total cost to the United States of unintentional home injuries is at least $217 billion; $1.74 million per fatal injury and $288,000 for each hospital-admitted non-fatal injury (Zaloshnja et al 2005).

Causes of home accidents

There are various factors contributing to home accidents, but human behaviour and the design and maintenance of the dwelling appear to be the main causes.

Human behaviour can contribute, to a greater or lesser extent, to a home accident or it can be the sole cause. Very young children lack the knowledge and experience to recognise danger, but are inquisitive by nature. The mobility and sight of the elderly may be impaired. A person may be distracted by something, such as an unexpected noise. Some people, perhaps in a hurry, will take risks, whereas others may be dyspraxic, unskilled or just plain careless. In addition, occupiers may introduce and create hazards – for example, by leaving electric cables over floors, obstacles on stairs, loose carpets, and medicines and cleaning products easily accessible to young children.

Dwellings contain a number of physical dangers, many of which society considers necessary or desirable, such as gas and electricity supplies, steps and stairs, and balconies. Most of these can be made relatively, but perhaps not completely, safe. However, some structural features may clearly increase the risk of an accident. For example, horizontal bars to a balcony guarding will provide a climbing frame for small children, a small change in levels in unexpected locations can be a trip hazard and non-safety glass at the base of stairs will increase the severity of an injury if there is a fall.

Individuals who spend more time in and around the home are exposed to dangers for longer than others. This may be one of the factors why the elderly and the very young are high-risk groups, but the lifestyle and activities of a person when at home (e.g., frequent DIY) are as, if not more, important. Socio-economic factors also affect home accidents, and accident and injury rates are generally higher in areas of social deprivation.

The LARES project facilitated a comparison of the types of accidents and injuries and an investigation of some of the possible causal factors.

The analyses

The analyses covered:

1. Accidents and outcomes – analyses the most frequent type and combination of accidents and the health outcomes from those accidents.
2. Accidents in eight cities – the accidents reported in each of the eight cities.
3. Psycho-social factors – the main psycho-social factors affecting the prevalence of accidents.
4. Exposure to home accidents – factors which increase the exposure to the risk of accidents.
5. Housing factors – the main housing factors affecting the accident rates.
6. Detailed analyses of falls – more detail on falls in general and stair falls in particular.
7. Housing hazards and accidents – accidents related to particular hazards identified in the home.
8. Influence of each factor – analyses the independent influence of psycho-social and housing factors on the various accident rates.

Finally, the conclusions discuss the relative importance of housing conditions in accidents.

Accidents and outcomes

The most frequent accidents and combinations of accidents

In the Housing and Health Questionnaire, 2,082 respondents (or nearly 1 in 4 of the total sample of 8,519 persons) reported accidents during the last 12 months.

Domestic accidents

Of these, some 63% reported just one type of accident, 24% two types and the remaining 13% between 3 and 7 types, giving a total of 3,205 accident cases. However, as multiple accidents of the same type are not generally recorded by the survey, the total number of accidents is likely to be even greater.

Figure 16.1(a) illustrates the percentage of the total sample population reporting accidents and the proportion having more than one type of accident. Figure 16.1(b) gives the percentage of all reported accidents for each particular type, with just four types (cuts, falls, burns and collisions) accounting for nearly 94% of all accidents. With the combination of types, these four types affect 96% of all accident victims and 24% of the total population.

Cuts and falls are the most common accidents, but are less likely to be reported with other accidents. Under 44% of fall victims report other types of accident, compared with 77% of persons reporting burns. The eight specific types of accident are found combined in 67 different ways. However, the top 20 most frequent accident combinations account for nearly 95% of all accidents. These include all single accident cases, excluding gas intoxication, and all 16 ways that the four most common types (cuts, falls, burns and collisions) can be combined. (Table 16.1).

Because of their prominence and larger samples, the rest of this chapter focuses on cuts, falls, burns and collision accidents. However, wherever accidents are referred to generally or totals for all accident types are given, the estimates also include the less frequent types of choking, electrocution, poisoning and gas intoxication, as well as other unspecified types.

Accident outcomes

For those cases where accidents are reported, nearly 4 out of 5 victims reporting one or more accidents treat all of the injuries themselves (71%), seek rest or some other 'non-medical' outcome (3%) or have no treatment at all (6%). Over 5% are

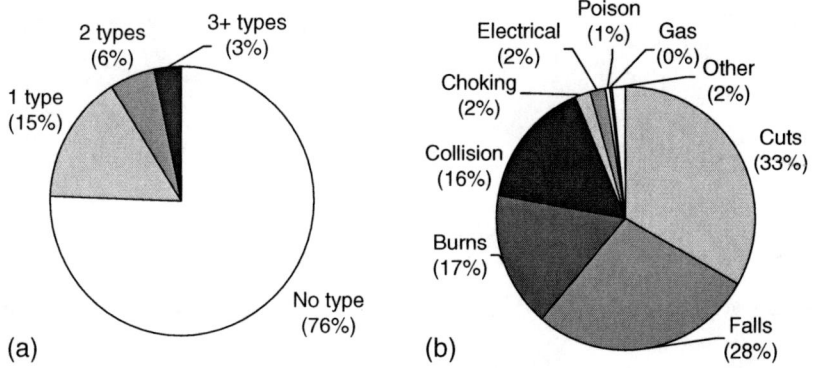

16.1 Sample proportions of number and types of accident reported. (a) Number of types of accident reported. (b) Types of accident reported.

Domestic accidents

Table 16.1 The 20 most frequently recorded accident combinations

	Accident(s) reported	Number	Percent of accidents	Percent of population
	No accident recorded	6,470		75.9
1	Falls	503	24.2	5.9
2	Cuts	464	22.3	5.4
3	Cuts and burns	170	8.2	2.0
4	Collisions	151	7.3	1.8
5	Burns	129	6.2	1.5
6	Cuts and falls	92	4.4	1.1
7	Cuts and collisions	85	4.1	1.0
8	Cuts, burns and collisions	60	2.9	0.7
9	Falls and collisions	58	2.8	0.7
10	Cuts, falls and collisions	56	2.7	0.7
11	Cuts, falls and burns	49	2.4	0.6
12	Falls and burns	36	1.7	0.4
13	Cuts, falls, burns and collisions	34	1.6	0.4
14	Choking	20	1.0	0.2
15=	Electrics	16	0.8	0.2
15=	Burns and collisions	16	0.7	0.2
17=	Falls, burns and collisions	12	0.6	0.1
17=	Falls and choking	12	0.6	0.1
19=	Cuts, falls and electrics	5	0.2	0.1
19=	Poisoning	5	0.2	0.1
Totals of above 20 combinations		**1,973**	**94.7**	**99.1**
Total accident victims/population		**8,519**	**2,082**	**100.0**

examined by a doctor, without treatment, and 9% are treated by a doctor, without being referred to or kept in hospital. Only the remaining 6% are hospitalised.

The range of outcomes, however, varies substantially with the type of accident. Based on single accident cases, falls are the only main type where a substantial proportion of the accidents (35%) result in medical treatment being sought or obtained. For all of the other main types, the number of accidents where medical help is sought is under 12%. Only in the case of falls do more than 1 in 10 of reported accidents result in hospitalisation.

Accidents in eight cities

Type and frequency of all reported accidents by city

For all accidents, both Bonn and Bratislava report a significantly higher rate than the other six cities, but while Bonn records a higher proportion of accident victims (33%), Bratislava records a higher proportion of accidents (55%), having

Domestic accidents

more multi-accident cases. Forlì and Geneva have the lowest rate in terms of both accident victims (both 20%) and proportion of accidents recorded (27 and 31%, respectively). However, these differences may, at least in part, reflect differences in reporting rather than any absolute difference in accident rates.

In most cities, the rank order of accident types is similar to that for the total sample, Bratislava and Budapest showing the greatest variation from the norm. However, the reported accident rates by type vary significantly. Bratislava records the highest proportion of cuts (nearly 21%) and Forlì the lowest (8%). Falls are most frequent in Bonn (nearly 16%) and again lowest in Forlì (under 8%). By comparison, burn accidents generally show less variation by city, although Bratislava has the highest proportion (over 9%) and Budapest the smallest (3%). In contrast, reports of collision accidents are particularly frequent in Bratislava (over 14%) and particularly infrequent in Ferreira (under 1%).

Type and frequency of serious accidents by city

If only serious accidents are considered, that is those in which treatment is sought or obtained from a doctor or hospital, the rank order of both accidents and the cities changes significantly. Falls are the most frequent accident and cuts the second most frequent in all eight cities. Ferreira, rather than Bonn, has the highest rate of serious falls (4.4%) and Bratislava, rather than Forlì, the lowest proportion (2.1%). Ferreira is also highest for serious cuts (2.0%), but the lowest rate remains with Forlì (0.7%). Vilnius has the largest proportion of collision accidents and Ferreira the smallest, whereas for serious burns the highest and lowest rates can now be found in Ferreira and Budapest, respectively.

Psycho-social factors

Age of accident victims

In the total sample, the distribution of accidents amongst different age groups varies substantially with the type of accident. (No accidents were reported for the four infants in the survey, the sample size being clearly insufficient for this youngest group).

For cuts, the accident rate increases up to the age of young adults, 21% of whom report such accidents; the number thereafter decreases, to under 5% for older seniors. In contrast, young children have the most falls (nearly 32%); the rate then decreases to under 6% in older adults, but increases again to more than 20% for those aged ≥80 years old. Burns shows a similar but less pronounced distribution pattern to cuts, with young adults again having the highest rate (11%)

Domestic accidents

and those aged 65–79 years old the lowest (3%). Between 9 and 11% of respondents in all four of the youngest age groups report collision accidents, but the rate then progressively declines with age to under 2% and only increases again (to over 5%) for the oldest seniors.

Overall, for any type of accident, very young children have the highest accident rate (over 37%), followed by older children and young adults, with over 33%, and the very elderly with 27%. Young seniors have the lowest rate, with below 17% reporting accidents in the last 12 months. Nearly a half of teenage accident victims have more than one accident type, but amongst young seniors only a little over 1 in 5 report multiple accidents.

Health outcomes and age

For young children <5 years old, the most important outcome is relatively minor in over 4 out of 5 cases; under 20% of outcomes involve professional medical treatment and under 5% result in hospitalisation. The importance of the outcome then further decreases with age, only 12% of accidents by adults receiving medical help. After that, the frequency of a major outcome progressively increases with age. For the oldest age group, over half (54%) of accidents receive medical treatment and 28% result in hospitalisation.

Gender and age

Overall, women have a significantly higher accident rate than men, but in part this difference can be attributed to the fact that there are significantly more elderly women than elderly men.

Under the age of 25 years old, there is relatively little difference in the accident rate for males and females, although young females appear more likely to suffer burns. The differences between the sexes are much greater for adults and older adults (25–64 years old). Here, women suffer over half as many more cuts, up to double the rate of falls and over three times the frequency of burns than men. Over all age groups, women have over double the rate of burns than men and this can probably be attributed to the traditional roles of women in the home and kitchen. The less pronounced differences in accident rates between younger men and women may result from these traditional roles being less rigid amongst younger adults (Figure 16.2).

For persons aged ≥65 years old, there is little difference for cuts, but women still suffer a higher rate of burns, collisions and (particularly) falls. However, these differences are again due, in part, to variation in the age distribution, 22% of women over 65 years old being over 80 years old compared with 17% of men.

Domestic accidents

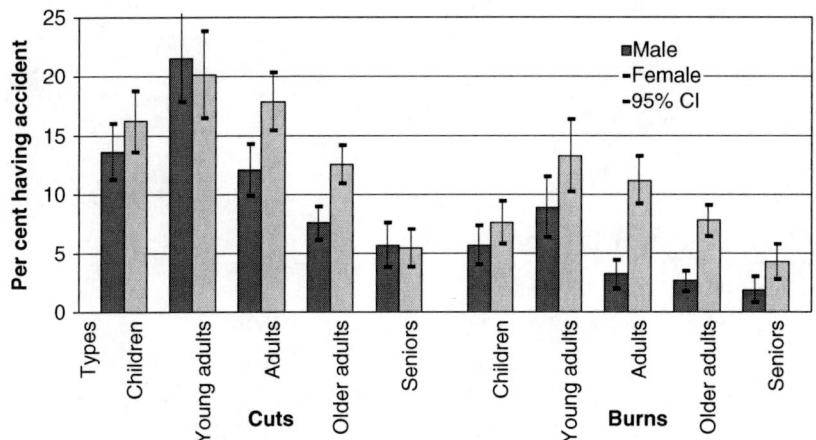

16.2 Accident rates for cuts and burns by age group and gender.

Physical constraints and handicaps

Respondents were asked if they had any particular kind of physical constraint or handicap. Perhaps, not surprisingly, persons with physical constraints and handicaps are much more likely to have suffered a fall in the last 12 months than those with no such complaint. Over 19% of persons reporting difficulty with stairs have had some kind of fall, compared with only 9% of those who have no difficulty in climbing or descending stairs. However, in contrast, the other main types of accident – cuts, burns and collisions – show little or no relationship to these 'handicaps'.

Tiredness

As with traffic accidents, tiredness can increase the risk of an accident in the home. For all main accident types, the incident of an accident is significantly greater where the respondent reported that they feel tired all or most of the time, than where they say they rarely feel tired – the total percentages being 31% and 23%, respectively. The correlation is particularly strong in the case of burns and collisions (Table 16.2).

Nervousness

Residents who are nervous, for whatever reason, have a significantly higher accident rate than those who report that they are not particularly nervous. For cuts, the accident rate for those who say they are nervous 'all of the time'

301

Domestic accidents

Table 16.2 Percentage of persons reporting accidents by degree of tiredness

Feel tired	Cuts	Falls	Burns	Collisions	All accidents	Sample
All/most of time	14.7	15.6	8.6	8.4	31.3	900
Bit/some of time	13.5	9.1	7.0	6.0	24.5	4,583
Little/none of time	11.0	10.8	5.0	5.3	22.9	2,842
Totals	**12.5**	**10.4**	**6.3**	**5.9**	**24.4**	**8,519**

Excludes non-response.

or 'most of the time' (16%) is double that of residents who say they are not nervous at all (8%). The picture is similar for both burns and collisions, where again rates for the most nervous are double those for the least nervous. The decrease with falls is less clear cut, the equivalent accident rates being some 17% and 11%, respectively.

Depression

Like tiredness and nervousness, depression may also increase the risk of accidents by making people less attentive while they are undertaking domestic tasks. A 'depression screening tool' has been derived from four questions in the health survey using the SALSA methodology.[1] For all main types of accident, the accident rate appears higher where a person suffers from depression, and this is particularly the case for falls. For all accidents, the overall rate for persons assessed as 'depressed' is some 30% higher than for those where no depression is indicated.

Alcohol consumption

Alcohol consumption can affect accident rates and the survey included a question on this topic. However, as not all respondents may have answered this question truthfully, the results need to be treated with caution. The incidence of cuts is greatest amongst those who drink occasionally – who may temporarily be more affected by alcohol than regular drinkers. The most falls clearly occur amongst very heavy drinkers, but it is also high amongst persons answering 'never been drinking', who may possibly include some heavy drinkers in denial. Occasional drinkers and heavy drinkers also tend to report more burns.

---

[1] See Chapter 11 for an explanation of SALSA.

Domestic accidents

Exposure to home accidents

Body weight/obesity

Although body weight is not obviously associated with the risk of accidents, it appears to be strongly correlated with this risk. A body mass index (BMI) has been computed for those aged 20–80 years old and banded into four categories: 'underweight', 'normal', 'overweight' and 'obese'. For cuts, burns and collisions, the accident rate decreases progressively as relative body weight increases. The frequency of accidents amongst adults who are obese is under a half or, in the case of collisions, under a quarter that of the rate for those who are underweight. In contrast, for falls, there is relatively little difference in the accident rate between the four weight categories (Figure 16.3).

One possible explanation is that those overweight and obese are generally more inactive and, consequently, less exposed to the risk of cuts, burns and collisions, whereas they are less likely to avoid the normal risk of falls, on stairs, etc. For all accidents, the decrease in accidents with increasing body weight applies generally to both males and females, although the decrease is significantly less pronounced with females.

Accidents and physical activity

Some support for the correlation between accident rates and body weight being related to activity levels is given by the picture that is produced when accident rates are cross-tabulated with answers on physical exercise. Individuals who frequently exercise appear to have significantly more accidents than individuals who never exercise, except again in the case of falls, where their rates are roughly equal. It is possible that occupants who are active in sport and physical exercise are also more likely to be generally active in the home and garden and, consequently, more at risk from domestic accidents.

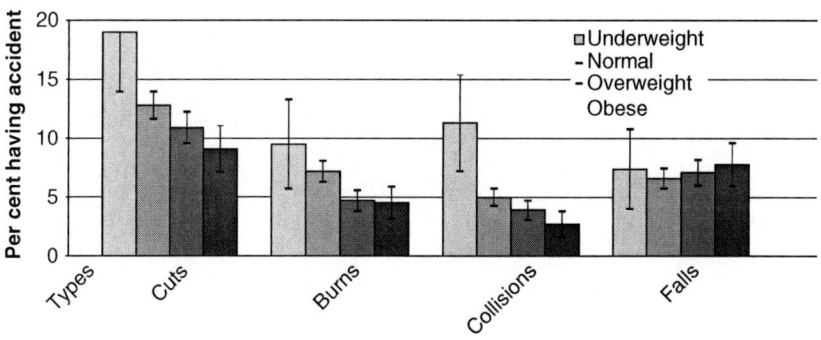

16.3 Main accident rates by body weight for persons aged 20–80 years old.

Domestic accidents

Do-it-yourself activity

DIY activity, with its frequent use of potentially dangerous hand and power tools, is known to increase the likelihood of accidents and this is largely confirmed by the LARES survey. Households were asked whether or not they had undertaken any DIY activities, or installed new furniture, within the last year.

There is a significantly greater proportion of accidents suffered by those both undertaking DIY work and installing new furniture than those doing no such work at all. The clearest and strongest correlation is for accidents resulting in cuts, where the former group suffer nearly twice as many accidents as the latter.

Hours spent at home

Compared with activity levels, the hours actually spent at home appear less important to the accident rate. In the survey, respondents recorded the average number of hours per day that they spent away from the dwelling, both on workdays and at weekends. From these data, the average total time per day spent out of the home has been calculated and cross-tabulated with each main type of accident. This analysis has been limited to 'adults' aged between 18 and 64 years old to avoid the influence of children, and senior citizens, both of whom tend to have higher accident rates and spend long periods of time at home.

There appears relatively little difference in the accident rates for individuals who spend most of their time at home and for individuals who on average are out of the home for long periods. As one might expect, the strongest correlation occurs with falls, but this is still not as strong as the correlations that generally occur with variables related to activity levels (Table 16.3).

The conclusion to be drawn is that, for adults, accident rates are much more strongly related to the lifestyle and activities of a person when at home, rather than the actual time that they spend in the home.

Housing factors

Space in the home

Lack of space in a home can increase the risk of accidents and the survey shows a general correlation between the proportion of residents reporting accidents and dissatisfaction with the size of the dwelling and the desire for more space.

For cuts, around 14% of respondents report accidents where dissatisfaction with the size of the dwelling or a desire for more rooms is reported, compared to under 12% where the household is satisfied with this aspect. However, the correlation is stronger for falls, the corresponding accident figures being some 12% and 9%, respectively. It is also strong for collision accidents, the accident rate

Domestic accidents

Table 16.3 Percentage of adults (18–64 years old) reporting accidents by hours in the home

Average time out	Cuts (%)	Falls (%)	Burns (%)	Collisions (%)	All accidents (%)	Sample (No.)
0–3 hours/day	14.6	8.9	7.7	4.4	25.2	481
4–6 hours/day	14.1	7.6	7.1	5.3	23.7	925
7–9 hours/day	14.8	5.7	7.5	6.8	24.1	1,862
10–12 hours/day	12.8	5.4	5.8	5.9	21.6	1,146
≥13 hours	13.1	6.1	7.6	4.4	21.8	473
All adults (18–64)	**13.6**	**6.5**	**7.0**	**5.6**	**23.0**	**5,605**

Table 16.4 Percentage of persons reporting accidents by satisfaction with dwelling size

Satisfaction with	Cuts (%)	Falls (%)	Burns (%)	Collisions (%)	All accidents (%)	Sample (No.)
1. Dwelling size						
Highly/dissatisfied	13.9	12.8	6.4	6.7	27.0	**1,369**
Neutral	13.7	10.1	7.1	7.2	25.2	**1,565**
Highly/satisfied	11.9	9.7	6.1	5.3	23.4	**5,559**
2. Preferences						
More rooms needed	14.0	11.9	6.8	7.6	27.1	**3,649**
Less rooms needed	12.2	10.3	6.8	3.8	23.5	**370**
Sufficient rooms	11.5	9.3	6.0	4.8	22.5	**4,413**
Don't know					nil	**32**
Total	**12.5**	**10.4**	**6.3**	**5.9**	**24.4**	**8,519**

Excludes non-response.

being around 8% where more rooms are desired, some 5% where sufficient space is perceived and under 4% where the dwelling is considered too large. By comparison, there appears less of a relationship in the case of burns (Table 16.4).

Dwelling layout

Poor arrangements in a dwelling can also increase the accident risk. For cuts, falls, burns and collisions, the accident rate is generally higher where the household is dissatisfied or highly dissatisfied with the dwelling layout than where they are satisfied or highly satisfied. For all accidents, only some 23% of respondents report cases where the household is satisfied with the dwelling layout compared with nearly 28% where there is dissatisfaction – an increase of nearly 20%.

Domestic accidents

Kitchen workspace

Other surveys covering accidents indicate that a large proportion of accidents occur in the kitchen. Table 16.5 shows the percentage of the population reporting accidents of each main type by whether the household reports having enough workspace in the kitchen for the preparation of food. Overall, nearly 30% of occupiers have accidents where not enough workspace is reported, compared to 23% where the household is satisfied with this facility. For all main accident types, the rates are higher where not enough workspace is reported, and for cuts, falls and burns the differences appear particularly significant.

Overcrowding

More accidents might be expected where dwellings are overcrowded and the LARES data largely confirms this. For nearly all types of accident, there is a very strong correlation between their frequency and the maximum number of children and/or adults sharing a bedroom. The correlation tends to be stronger for children than for adults, probably reflecting the high accident rate amongst children generally.

For cuts, the accident rate where 1–3 children share a bedroom (14%) is higher than where there are no children (10%), but higher still (17%) where ≥4 children share. For the same number of adults sharing, it is twice as high (20%) as for only 1 adult per bedroom (10%). For children sharing, there is a similar pattern for falls and burns, but the correlation is particularly consistent for collision accidents.

Home temperatures

It is known that, as well as the increased risk caused by ice on outdoor steps and paths, cold home temperatures can also affect the frequency of accidents. For all four main accident types, the rate is between 25 and 35% higher in cold homes than in homes not reported as cold.

Table 16.5 Percentage of persons reporting accidents by satisfaction with kitchen

Enough workspace	Cuts (%)	Falls (%)	Burns (%)	Collisions (%)	All accidents (%)	Sample (No.)
No	14.9	14.1	8.2	7.2	29.6	**1,593**
Yes	11.9	9.4	5.9	5.6	23.0	**6,857**
Don't know	19.1	14.6	7.9	6.7	37.1	**21**
Totals	**12.5**	**10.4**	**6.3**	**5.9**	**24.4**	**8,519**

Excludes non-response.

There are also a significantly larger proportion of cuts reported where the home is too warm or too cold (14%) than where temperatures are reported as satisfactory (11%). For falls, however, the incidence is greatest (13%) where the home is perceived as too cold, with only 9% of falls being reported in satisfactorily heated homes. The frequency of burns also increases with temperature problems, particularly where dwellings are too warm, and these also show more collision accidents.

Additional heating

Poor heating, as well as increasing the accident risk generally by making the dwelling cold, can also lead to particular types of accidents. For example, the use of supplementary heaters where the main system is inadequate, particularly the use of portable heaters, can increase the risks of burns as well as falls. Apart from collisions, all main accident rates are higher where portable heaters are likely, but the increases in falls (13.8% compared to 10.2%) and burns (9.6% compared to 6.1%) appear particularly significant.

Natural lighting

Good lighting is known to be important in the prevention of accidents. The frequency of accidents resulting in cuts or puncture wounds is significantly higher in dwellings where the interviewee reports the natural lighting as insufficient or 'misses the daylight' (both 15%) than where the daylight is reported as satisfactory (11%). The same is true for falls, although here accidents are highest where the main problem is glare. The incidence of collision accidents is also higher where there is 'too much light' (9%) than where the daylight is satisfactory (6%). By comparison, the correlation between burns and poor lighting is less pronounced.

Noise

The previous section on psycho-social factors showed that accidents were strongly correlated to tiredness. A subsequent question in the survey asked whether the respondent's sleep had been disturbed by noise during the past 4 weeks. For all types of accident, with the exception of choking, the accident rate in homes where sleep disturbance by noise is reported is significantly higher than where this is not the case. This is particularly so for cuts, burns and collisions (Figure 16.4).

Persons whose sleep is disturbed by noise are also more likely to suffer a greater number of different types of accident than those not so disturbed.

Domestic accidents

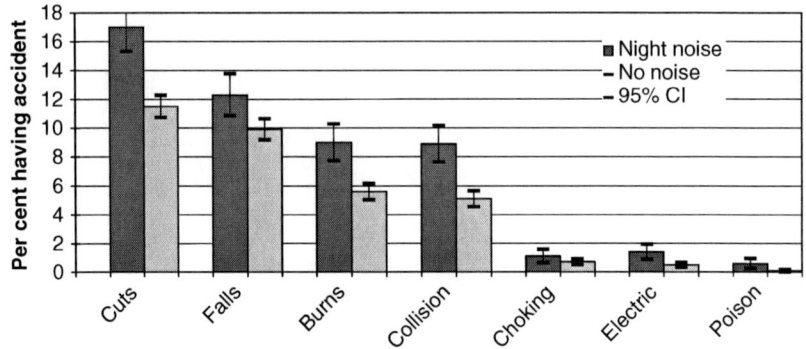

16.4 Accident rate by sleep disturbance from noise.

Around 14% of those whose sleep is disturbed report having more than one type of accident, compared to under 8% of those not affected by noise, whereas nearly twice as many have three or more types of accident, compared to those not affected (Table 16.6).

With no question in the LARES survey on the time of an accident, it is not immediately clear to what extent sleep disturbance from noise results in accidents at the time of the disturbance, that is generally at night, or subsequently due to the effects of sleep deprivation. However, a three-way cross-tabulation of accident rates by tiredness and sleep disturbance by noise provides some indication of the relationship.

As might be expected, a significantly higher proportion of individuals who report their sleep to be disturbed by noise also report feeling tired all, most or a good bit of the time (41%), than individuals who report no such disturbance (25%). However, for different degrees of tiredness, the accident rate is generally higher where sleep has been disturbed by noise, the difference in the two rates being generally higher the greater the degree of tiredness reported. For example, amongst respondents who feel tired all or most of the time, those who also report sleep disturbance by noise suffer nearly twice as many cuts as those who report no such disturbance.

Table 16.6 Number of types of accident reported by whether or not sleep was disturbed by noise

Disturbed by noise	Number of types of accident reported				Person sample
	0	1	2	≥3	
Yes	69.5	16.6	8.6	5.3	**1,937**
No	77.0	15.2	5.0	2.7	**6,390**
Total	75.3	15.6	5.8	3.3	**8,326**

Excludes non-response.

The notable exception to this general trends occurs with falls, where amongst the 'most tired' group there is no difference in the accident rate between those reporting and not reporting noise disturbance (both 16%). This finding and the fact that the accident types where there is the greatest divergence in rates (cuts and burns) are less likely to occur at the actual time of the disturbance (e.g. during the night) suggests consequent sleep deprivation to be the main causal factor – rather than just general tiredness.

As well as tiredness, the survey shows noise disturbance to sleep to be associated with other psycho-social problems that are strongly correlated to accidents. For example, for the same degree of tiredness, respondents reporting noise disturbance are significantly more likely to also report feeling nervous all or most of the time, than respondents reporting no such disturbance (e.g. 50% compared to 39% in the case of the 'most tired' group). Similarly, amongst people tired a good bit or some of the time, 25% of those reporting noise disturbance to sleep are also assessed as depressed, compared to 14% of the same group not disturbed by noise.

Of all respondents reporting noise disturbance to sleep, over a half suffer from tiredness, nervousness and/or depression, 11% recording all three conditions. By comparison, under a third of respondents reporting no noise disturbance have such psycho-social problems. However, the accident rate increases with the number of problems recorded: 35% of those with all three conditions suffer accidents compared to some 22% of those with no problems of tiredness, nervousness or depression. Similarly, the number of types of accident recorded is greater, nearly 7% of those suffering all conditions reporting three or more accident types compared with under 3% of those with none of these psycho-social problems.

In short, it appears that the sleep deprivation caused by noise may lead not just to tiredness but to a combination of tiredness, nervousness and depression, which together increase the risk of an accident or multiple accidents. Moreover, it seems probable that many of these accidents will occur during the subsequent day or days, rather than at the actual time of the disturbance, usually at night.

Detailed analyses of falls

Falls in general

Although falls are only the second most frequent accident type after cuts, they are clearly the most important after health outcomes are considered. The main accident questions in the Housing and Health Questionnaire do not distinguish between different types of falls: for example, between falls on the level, falls on stairs, falls between levels and falls associated with baths and showers. However, it is known that a large proportion of falls are falls on the level and that

Domestic accidents

a proportion of these arise due to faulty floors. In the Housing Inspection Survey, the surveyor noted the extent of faults or deterioration of the floors in up to eight rooms or spaces in the dwelling and, from these data, a simple numerical index has been constructed to indicate the severity and/or extent of any floor faults.

Where there are floor faults but the index is under 5, the proportion of persons reporting falls is slightly higher (11.3%) than when no floor fault is present (9.9%), and where the index is between 5 and 9, the proportion of falls is slightly higher still. However, where the index score is ≥10, indicating extensive floor faults and/or deterioration, nearly 22% of the population report falls – over double the number where there are no floor faults (Table 16.7).

Doorsteps are also known to present a potential accident point. In the Housing Inspection Survey, the surveyor was asked to record whether there were any doorsteps: (1) at the dwelling entrance door, (2) between rooms, (3) to the bathroom, (4) to a balcony, terrace or garden or (5) at some other location. Where there are doorsteps at one, two or three locations, the rate of falls is generally just under 11%, compared with a rate of under 9% where there are no doorsteps. However, where doorsteps are found at four or more locations, the rate increases to nearly 13%.

Falls on stairs

While the Housing and Health Questionnaire does not distinguish falls associated with stairs and steps from other falls, this distinction is possible from the accident questions in the Inhabitant Questionnaire. The question on 'items involved' includes an additional category 'stairs, staircase', whereas a subsequent question records the location of multiple accidents.

Compared with the Housing and Health Questionnaire of individuals, however, the Inhabitant Questionnaire underestimates the number of households where falls are reported. Because of this and because it is household rather than person based, the Inhabitant Questionnaire provides only a small sample of 130 stair falls. To overcome this problem, the health and inhabitant results have been used in combination to increase the sample for stair falls to 164 or nearly 5% of the total of just under 3,390 households. From the Inhabitant Questionnaire, it is

Table 16.7 Percentage of persons reporting falls by floor fault index

Floor fault index	No. of falls	Fall	Sample
No faults (score = 0)	90.1	9.9	6,400
Fault score < 5	88.7	11.3	1,720
Fault score of 5–9	88.0	12.0	359
Fault score of ≥10	78.3	21.7	60
	89.6	10.4	8,539

Domestic accidents

estimated that around 38% of these involve children, 40% adults and 22% persons aged ≥65 years old.

There is a very strong correlation between the occurrence of a fall associated with the staircase or stairs/steps and whether the respondent thought the staircase or the stairs or steps in the dwelling to be dangerous. However, this is hardly surprising as respondents are more likely to regard their stairs as dangerous if they or a household member has had a stair fall. Over 73% thought the stairs or steps dangerous where more than one fall had occurred, compared to less than 13% where there was no stair fall.

A more objective test of the correlation between falls and dangerous stairs is provided by the assessment of the stairs from the Housing Inspection Survey Sheet. For stairs and steps inside the dwelling, there is a strong correlation between the number of falls and the presence of loose and broken steps. Where stairs are judged to be slightly damaged or loose, the proportion of households reporting stair falls (over 17%) is significantly more than that of households where the stairs are perfectly safe (under 10%). Where stairs are assessed as heavily damaged and unsafe, as many as 1 in 2 households report multiple stair accidents, although the sample here is extremely small.

A higher proportion of stair falls (over 12%) is also reported where the surveyor notes a height difference in the steps, some 9% being reported where no difference is recorded. The presence of stairs/steps in front of the dwelling shows a similar increase in the accident rate. In contrast, the absence of handrails shows little or no correlation with the number of stair falls.

For steps and staircases in buildings housing multi-family units, the majority of which will be flats on one level, accident rates are generally lower. Rates are again relatively higher where the surveyor records broken or loose steps, but not to the same extent as with stairs inside the dwelling (some 5.3% compared to 3.6% for 'safe' stairs). Here, height differences in steps as well as the absence of handrails also show a similar correlation with the accident rate.

In multi-family buildings, the standard of lighting appears even more influential. There is only a slight increase in the fall rate with insufficient lighting, but a greater increase with non-operational lighting, albeit this may be a temporary problem. However, the frequency of falls increases significantly (to nearly 9% of households) for no lighting, although the sample here is small.

Housing hazards and accidents

Hazards identified by the surveyor

The LARES survey contains a number of questions aimed at determining particular hazards in the home. In the Inhabitant Questionnaire, respondents were asked 'Which places or equipment items do you assess as dangerous for the

Domestic accidents

residents in general?' and 'Is there a place/item in the dwelling which is especially dangerous for children?'. However, as shown above, coming immediately after the accident questions, the answers to these questions appear heavily biased by the frequency of actual accidents.

In the Housing Inspection Survey Sheet, however, the surveyor was asked a similar question (Are there any installations/locations in the dwelling that you see as potentially harmful?) and this is likely to provide more objective answers. For all main types of accident, a significantly higher accident rate is reported in dwellings where hazards are independently recorded by the surveyor than in those dwellings where no hazards are recorded. Moreover, for most accident types, the frequency progressively increases with the number of hazards recorded. This is particularly true for falls and collisions, where the accident rate doubles or more than doubles between dwellings recording no hazards and those having three hazards (see Figure 16.5).

There is a strong correlation between dwellings where the surveyor identified potentially relevant hazards and where accidents have occurred. For cuts, compared with an accident rate of below 12% where no hazards were recorded, 30% of residents report cuts where the surveyor judged the kitchen utensils or equipment to be hazardous, whereas 20% report cuts in the few dwellings considered to have insufficient lighting. For falls, the highest accident rate (25%) occurs in dwellings judged to have hazardous bathrooms, including 'slippery wet tiles', but hazardous floors and carpets, staircases and doorsteps, and furniture also correlate with fall rates of nearly 16%. By comparison, there are just 9% of falls where no hazards are reported.

Excluding the 'washing machine' category due to its small sample, burns like cuts are most likely to occur where the surveyor cites the kitchen (including the

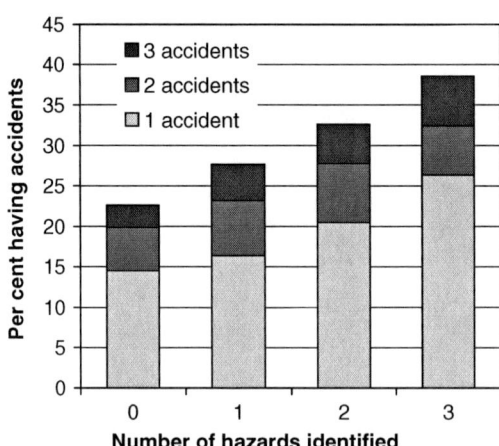

16.5 Number of accidents reported where hazard(s) were identified, by surveyor.

stove, cooker or oven) as hazardous, the accident rate here (11.4%) being double that in dwellings judged to be 'hazard free' (5.8%). Collision accidents also show a strong correlation with these same 'kitchen' hazards (14.3%) and also with dwellings where there is the potential for falling elements (12.8%). Both of these represent over twice the accident rate than for cases where no hazards are recorded (5.7%).

Because of the way both different types of hazard and types of accident are combined, the correlation between all accidents and the various hazard groups shows a somewhat different picture. The overall accident rate is again highest where kitchen hazards are mentioned; here 43% of residents report an accident of at least one type. However, some 35% of occupants report an accident in dwellings where the surveyor judges the heating, fireplace or chimney to be hazardous, whereas over a third report an accident where the furniture or doors are considered hazardous. These rates can be compared with an overall accident rate of under 23% in dwellings where no hazards are reported.

Items involved in accidents

Where accidents were reported, a supplementary question was asked about the actual items involved in these accidents, and this also provides an angle on the hazards in the home. To determine which particular items are most frequently involved with each type of accident, the analysis has been confined to those cases where only one accident type is reported. As might be expected, knives (75%) and kitchen equipment (18%) are most commonly associated with cuts, with only 4% involving construction features such as glazing. In contrast, 51% of falls relate to construction features, with furniture/furnishings and toys being reported in only 13% and 9% of cases, respectively. Nearly 16% involve other items.

With burns there is a wider spread of items involved, kitchen and electric equipment being implicated in 44% and 20% of cases and heating equipment and water in some 14% and 8%, respectively. Collision accidents involve construction features (41%) and furniture (43%) in almost equal measure.

A comparison between the list of items most commonly involved with each type of accident, and the potential hazards identified in the home, shows that the items actually involved are frequently similar to the items judged by the surveyor to be potential hazards.

Influence of each factor

Analyses using logistical regression

The correlations shown in the previous sections are useful in indicating the importance of psycho-social and housing factors on the risk of accidents but, due

Domestic accidents

to the interdependence of many of these factors, are of limited value in determining the independent influence of each factor. For example, in the survey sample, tiredness and physical constraints and handicaps can both be shown to be strongly associated with age. To gain a better understanding of which particular factors have the most influence in increasing the risk of an accident of each type, the data have been further analysed using a staged model for logistic regression.

Table 16.8 shows the odds ratios (ORs) generated by the logistic regression model for the significant psycho-social and housing variables for each of the main accident types. For each type, the highest five ratios are numbered in rank order to show the most important for predicting an accident of that type. In the age variable, those who are generally most vulnerable to accidents being younger (<25 years old) or older (≥65 years old) are contrasted with the remainder who are not most vulnerable (being aged between 25 and 64 years old). Where significant, DIY work is listed under social/behavioural factors, but may also relate to housing variables, being possibly prompted by the nature or condition of the property.

Table 16.8 Odds ratios for psycho-social and housing variable for each accident type

	Cuts		Falls		Burns		Collisions		All accidents	
Psycho-social										
Young/old	1.23		2.60	[1]	1.19		1.91	[1]	1.72	[1]
Nervous	1.88	[1]			1.93	[2]	1.60	[4]	1.46	[3]
Female	1.33		1.52	[5]	2.12	[1]	1.23		1.43	[4]
Active	1.45	[5]	1.28		1.24		1.53	[5]	1.36	[7]
DIY work	1.57	[4]	1.23		1.25				1.31	[9]
'Handicap'			1.73	[2]					1.29	[10]
Tired			1.32		1.30		1.47		1.19	
Depressed			1.48						1.18	
Obese			1.60	[4]						
In all day			1.28							
Housing										
Night noise	1.63	[2]	1.44		1.77	[4]	1.72	[3]	1.50	[2]
Stairs	1.28		1.62	[3]			1.28		1.38	[5]
Additional heater	1.61	[3]			1.92	[3]	1.81	[2]	1.38	[6]
Workspace	1.23		1.51		1.41	[5]	1.44		1.33	[8]
Room space			1.38				1.39		1.24	
Hazards							1.22		1.16	
Lighting	1.33								1.16	
Crowded	1.34						1.37			
Accidents	**1,023**		**823**		**516**		**487**		**from 7,885**	

All missing data omitted.
For each type of accident, the highest five ratios are numbered in rank order [square brackets] to show the importance for predicting an accident of that type.

Domestic accidents

Sleep disturbance caused by noise is shown as the best housing predictor for accidental cuts and indicates that the odds of such an accident are around 63% higher for individuals suffering such disturbance than for individuals with no such problem, other factors being equal. The presence of supplementary heaters is the second most important housing predictor. However, a psycho-social factor, i.e. nervousness, is an even stronger predictor, with an OR of 1.88.

Table 16.8 also indicates that the probability of a fall by those in the most vulnerable age groups is over two and a half times greater than for those in other age groups, while for those with physical constraints and handicaps the probability is 73% higher than for those with no such problems. Whereas not significant for most accidents, being overweight appears the fourth highest influence for falls, after accounting for the confounding factors. The three most important housing predictors for falls are, in reverse order, noise disturbance to sleep, too little workspace and the presence of private stairs in the dwelling.

The gender of a person is the main psycho-social predictor for burns, with an OR of 1.91, which implies that as you move from male to female the odds of such an accident almost doubles. Nervousness is the second best psycho-social variable for burns, followed by tiredness. As with other accident types, noise disturbance is an important housing predictor, with an OR of nearly 1.77, whereas the lack of kitchen workspace is also important to burns, increasing the risk by over 40%. However, the best housing predictor is the presence of supplementary heaters in the home, which nearly doubles the odds of a burns accident.

As with falls, age is the most important independent variable for collisions, with younger and older people being nearly twice as likely to have such an accident as adults of intermediate ages when faced with the same conditions. However, nervousness and an active lifestyle are also strong psycho-social predictors, showing ORs of 1.60 and 1.53, respectively. As with burns, the presence of supplementary (often portable) heating appears one of the best predictors in the case of collisions, with increased odds of some 81%, whereas noise disturbance is third in overall importance, with an OR of 1.72.

The final two figures in this section show the ORs for the significant psycho-social and housing predictors for an accident of any type. These main psycho-social and housing predictors are shown on separate graphs (Figures 16.6 and 16.7) but, for comparison, the most important psycho-social predictor (excluding age) is also shown alongside the housing predictors.

As with many of the individual accident types, age is the factor that is most likely to predispose a person to having an accident generally; the young and the more elderly are >70% more likely to be involved in a home accident of some sort than people of other age groups, other factors being equal. After age, being of a nervous disposition, female and physically active are the next best psycho-social predictors, these three factors being estimated to increase the odds of an accident

Domestic accidents

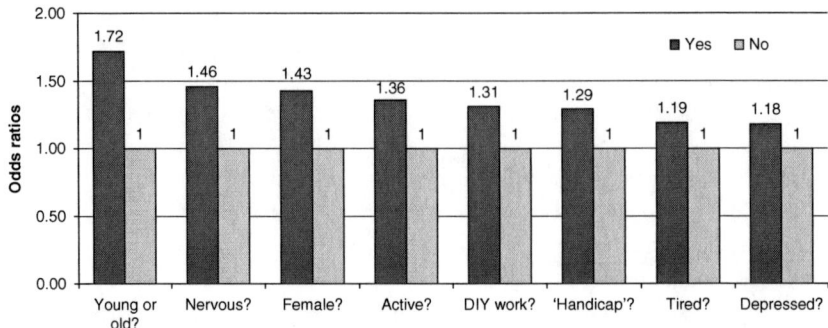

16.6 Odds ratios for significant psycho-social predictors for an accident of any type.

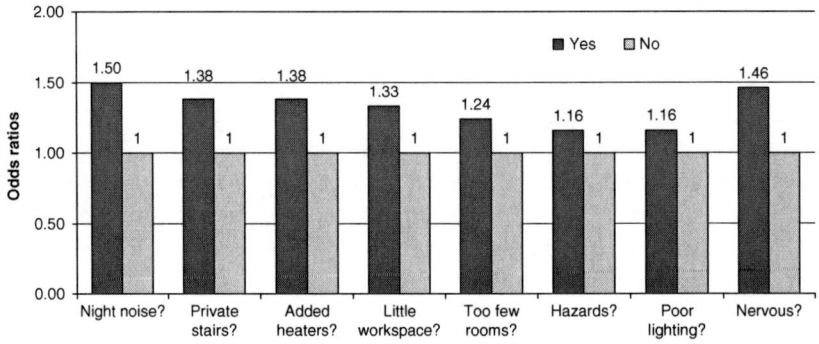

16.7 Odds ratios for significant housing predictors for an accident of any type.

by around 40% or more. After that, undertaking DIY work or having a physical constraint or handicap appear to provide the next strongest influence, both having ORs of some 1.30. Finally, being tired or depressed increases the odds of an accident by nearly 20%.

Noise disturbance at night is the most importance housing predictor; this problem alone is estimated to increase the incidence of an accident of any type by 50%. After noise disturbance, three housing predictors – the presence in the dwelling of stairs, supplementary heaters and inadequate workspace – all appear to increase the odds of an accident by around one-third or more. For the final three housing variables – the identification of hazards, poor lighting and too few rooms – the overall increase in the accident rate is from 16 to 24%.

Conclusions

The earlier sections of this chapter, particularly those on psycho-social factors and exposure to accidents, highlighted the strong correlation between the prevalence of accidents in the home and psycho-social and behavioural characteristics. Similarly, later sections, particularly those dealing with housing factors, with the more detailed analyses and hazards in the home, showed that the correlation between accidents and housing characteristics and housing conditions was equally strong in many cases.

By controlling for the confounding factors, the regression analyses in the last section further suggest that both behavioural and housing factors exert an independent influence on accident rates. Although dependent on the way age is categorised, these regression analyses are fairly conclusive in showing the age of the person to be the strongest overall predictor of accidents in the home. However, this is perhaps not surprising given the substantial differences in accident rates between different age groups, albeit before any confounding factors are accounted for.

After controlling for age, however, there appears little difference in the relative importance of psycho-social and housing factors in influencing the overall accident rate. As shown in the previous section, the main housing predictors, such as noise disturbance at night and the presence of additional (usually portable) heaters, are generally just as important and influential as any of the main psychosocial predictors, apart from age.

After controlling for confounding factors including age, the relative importance of psycho-social and housing factors is also similar for the main individual types of accident (cuts, falls and burns). However, in the case of collisions, it appears that housing problems are generally more important than psycho-social ones in influencing the probability of an accident. Although, as for the other main types of accident, behaviour is influential in collisions, external constraints imposed by the dwelling appear relatively more important in this type of accident.

In conclusion, it is clear from the analyses that there is a very strong correlation between accidents in the home and housing conditions. Moreover, after controlling for the confounding psycho-social factors, the strong relationship between accidents and housing conditions largely holds true. However, whether there is a direct causal relationship between accident rates and housing conditions is less clear-cut. Nevertheless, the comprehensive body of evidence provided by the LARES survey, as outlined in this chapter, points to this being the case. In short, we may conclude that, for each age group, accidents in the home are often caused by a combination of behavioural and housing factors, acting frequently in more or less equal measure.

References

Department of Trade and Industry (DTI) (2002) HASS 23rd Annual Report. London: DTI.

European Home and Leisure Accident Surveillance System (EHLASS) (1998) subsequently the Injury Surveillance System (part of the European Public Health Information Network). Post 2004, part of the New Public Health Programme.

Zaloshnja E., Miller T.R., Lawtence B.A., Romano E. (2005) The costs of unintentional home injuries. *Am J Prev Med* 28(1): 88–94.

17 A brief résumé of recommendations
David Ormandy

Introduction

The contributions here do not represent the complete picture. As well as papers by the experts directly involved in the LARES study, WHO has made the datasets publicly available and this has resulted in other analyses and reports, including papers on residential lighting and risk for depression and falls (Brown and Jacobs submitted) on dampness and mold in the home and depression (Shenassa *et al* 2007), noise-induced annoyance and morbidity (Neimann *et al* 2006), and home safety (Moore and Ormandy 2004; Ormandy 2004; LARES study 2008). What the contributions in this work show are some of the possibilities presented by the data generated by the LARES study. It is also worth noting that the LARES instruments have been adopted and adapted for other projects, including studies in Portugal and Australia, and are the basis of a proposal for a collaborative study in the United States and the UK.

As well as raising new insights and areas for further investigation, the contributions presented here provide suggestions and recommendations that can inform decisions and actions of policymakers and practitioners. These suggestions and recommendations are discussed below.

What do we expect from a house?

First, a house should provide a refuge and shelter from the outdoor world. It should provide for everyday life for the household and the individuals. Whereas the optimum indoor housing environment for human beings will be virtually the same, different households will have different lifestyles. This will reflect individual preferences, and will be influenced by the characteristics of the members of the household, by culture, and by socio-economic status. In addition, lifestyles, expectations, domestic activities and personal habits change. Houses need to be

A brief résumé of recommendations

able to cope with the normal spectrum of lifestyles, although what is 'normal' does not seem to have been defined and, anyway, it will change over the lifetime of a house. Although this may be true of all houses – providing that optimum indoor environment for a spectrum of lifestyles – how that can be achieved will vary, depending on local climate, geography, building traditions, economics, and cultural and political influences. Nonetheless, houses are, or should be, designed, constructed and maintained to cope with the normal biological and domestic activities that can be expected from households.

Houses should also provide a link with the outside world – a visual link through windows. Thus, the condition and nature of the immediate housing environment is important to the mental health and general well-being of residents, as is being able to use that space freely and without fear.

Potential housing hazards

While there is a growing body of evidence, much of it cited in this work, there remain areas where the evidence is weak. In addition, there are many difficulties in obtaining that evidence. One obvious difficulty is that, as this is about people and their homes, it is not possible to strictly control conditions or to have proper control groups. What amounts to recognised and acceptable evidence is often made difficult because the approach tends to concentrate on the medical research model, and reviews of literature concentrate on that in medical and health libraries, overlooking evidence from other disciplines, evidence often necessary to determine housing solutions.

The cause or causes of the threat to health and/or safety will usually be one or a combination of three factors – human behaviour, the state and condition of the dwelling, and goods (furniture, equipment and appliances) brought into the dwelling. The contributions here discuss the relevance and importance of these factors in respect of the subjects investigated. A comprehensive review of risks, causes and preventative actions can be found in *Review of Healthy and Safety Risk Drivers* (CLG 2008), which includes evidence from a wide range of sources.

Surveys

To determine the extent and range of problems in the housing stock, and so inform policies, sample house condition surveys should be carried out. The data to be collected should include information on the state and condition of the housing to determine what policies and actions are necessary to ensure dwellings are maintained as both personal and national assets. But, importantly, it should include data directed to the identification of potential threats to health and/or safety based on information from reported research on the links between housing conditions and health, including the findings from the LARES study.

A brief résumé of recommendations

While such surveys provide a 'snap-shot' of conditions, repeating them after a period, say 5 years, will monitor the impact of housing interventions and policies.

Reducing exposure

As noted above, threats to health and safety may be universal but remedial action is likely to be specific to the locality. Nonetheless, there are some general practical steps that can be recommended.

Guidance

Advice and guidance should be directed at all those involved in housing – planners, architects, builders, owners and occupiers. This should cover designing and constructing dwellings to avoid problems, maintaining dwellings and identifying problems before they become serious and actions by occupiers to minimise the likelihood of threats to health. Guidance should emphasise the need for energy efficiency, sound insulation, ventilation and the avoidance of potential risks of physical injury. It should also deal with the design and layout of estates and neighbourhoods and the provision of community facilities.

Codes and regulations

Standards and requirements controlling the design and construction of new dwellings should be directed at preventing threats to health developing. Such codes should ensure high levels of energy efficiency, effective sound insulation, adequate and effective means of ventilation and the avoidance of potential dangerous features. As new dwellings form only a very small percentage of the housing stock, there should be similar provisions to control and improve standards in existing houses.

Financial assistance

The cost of remedying problems in existing housing can be expensive, and may be beyond the reach of owners with limited resources. Financial assistance (grants and subsidies) should be made available towards the cost of remedial and improvement works. The cost of this assistance should be balanced against the savings from a reduction in the demands placed on the health services.

Management

Effective management of apartment blocks and of neighbourhoods will increase the quality of life of the residents, remove perceived threats to personal safety and promote a community spirit and pride.

A brief résumé of recommendations

Protecting and promoting health

Reducing exposure to potential threats to health will result in avoiding negative health outcomes. How to remove or minimise the threat from that condition or situation, and so reduce exposure, depends on what the threat is and also on the nature of the dwelling (how it is constructed). While threats to health and safety may be universal (e.g. mould and other allergens, noise and extremes of temperature), as most contributors point out, the solutions are more likely to be specific to the city or even the locality.

As well as avoiding negative outcomes by removing threats to health, improvements in housing and the immediate housing environment can give positive health gains that enhance well-being and the quality of life.

Housing should be recognised for the important social determinant of health that it is, and, as stated in the Declaration adopted at the Fourth Ministerial Conference on Environment and Health (2005), health should be at the core of housing policies.

References

Brown M., Jacobs J.E. (submitted) Residential Lighting and Risk for Depression and Falls.
Communities and Local Government (CLG) (2008) Review of Healthy and Safety Risk Drive B http//www.communities.gov.uk/ publications/planningandbuilding/reviewhealthsafety (accessed 30 September 2008).
Moore R., Ormandy D. (2004) Home safety in the U.K.: review of the influence of human and housing factors. *Rev Environ Health* 19(3–4): 253–70.
Neimann H., Bonnefoy X., Braubach M., Hecht K., Maschke C., Rodrigues C., Röbbel N. (2006) Noise induced annoyance and morbidity. *Noise & Health* 8(31): 63–79.
Ormandy D. (2007) Home: haven or accident blackspot? A review of the causes of home accidents. *Int J Environment and Pollution* 30(3–4): 404–10.
Shenassa E.D., Daskalakis C., Liebhaber A., Braubach M., Brown M. (2007) Dampness and mold in the home and depression: an examination of mold-related illness and perceived control of one's home as possible depression pathways. *Am J Public Health* 97(10): 1893–9.
WHO Europe (2005) Fourth Ministerial Conference on Environment and Health. Final Conference Report, January: pp 16–17.
WHO Europe, The LARES Project (2008) For all other publications and papers from the LARES study see: http//www.euro.who.int/Housing/lares/20080403_1 (accessed 30 September 2008).

Index

A
adults 150–52
age 147
age bands 107–8
air pollution 111–23, 289, 292
aircraft 277
alcohol 302
allergens 111, 123, 126, 322
allergic rhinitis 114
allergies 107, 277, 279, 286, 290–1
Alzheimer's disease 184
Angers (France)
   description 80–1
   heating systems 162
   sampling 8, 14
anthracosis 155
anti-social behaviour *see* crime
Armstrong, B. 143
arthritis 151–3, 277, 284, 286, 289
asthma
   and noise 276, 278, 280, 286, 291
   and residential energy systems 158, 164
   damp, mould and health 126
   indoor air pollution 111, 113–15, 118, 122–3
atopic/non atopic individuals 126

B
Bad Godesberg 81
Bartlett, P. 169
bathrooms 312
Berlin 81
Beuel 81
biomass 111, 113, 155
bivariate logistic regression 128
body mass index (BMI) 108, 149, 303
Bonn (Germany)
   age/gender/neighbourhood distribution 13
   description 81–2
   domestic accidents 298–9
   fear of crime 180
   respiratory health problems 147
   ventilation 161
Boumendil, A. 144
Bratislava (Slovakia)
   age/gender/neighbourhood distribution 13
   arthritic health problems 147
   description 83
   domestic accidents 298–9
   fear of crime 172
   heating systems 162
   problems of dampness 129
   socio-economic characteristics of households 160–1
British Crime Survey (BCS) 168–9, 172
bronchitis 276–80, 283–4, 289, 291
Budapest (Hungary)
   cardiovascular problems 147
   description 85–6
   domestic accidents 299
   fear of crime 172
   heating systems 162
   sampling 9, 13–14
   socio-economic characteristics of households 160–1
   ventilation 161
burns 299–303, 305–7, 312–13, 315, 317

C
carbon monoxide (CO) 113
cardiovascular problems 151–3, 263, 266–9, 275, 280, 282–4, 286, 289–90, 292
carpets 312
CHAID modelling 129
challenge examples
   a broken shoulder 101

Index

detention of an innocent dwelling 99
the burned house 95–6
the cut-off electricity 98
the drunken man 100
the mystery of the boxes 97
the rescuing taxi driver 97
wrong questionnaire 99
children
  cold homes 150–2
  damp/mould and health 127
  domestic accidents 295–6, 299–300, 304, 306, 311, 315
  health 263, 265
  indoor air pollution 123
  mental health 188
  noise 278–9, 283, 286, 290–1
  residential energy systems 155–6
  safety/crime 180
chimneys 313
choking 307
cigarettes *see* tobacco
cities 145–6, 149–50, 158, 180, 249
climate 145
cockroaches 115–16, 122
codes/regulations 321
cold/throat illnesses 164
collisions 301–7, 312–13, 317
combustion products 111
community 4
crime 168–82
Cronbach alpha curve (SCAC) 206, 208–9
cuts 299–303, 305, 307, 309, 312–13, 317

D
damp 125–9, 132, 134, 137–40, 143, 153, 158, 163, 181
depression 262–9, 277–8, 280, 282, 289, 292, 302, 315
diabetes 286
diarrhoeal diseases 164–5
Diogenes syndrome 196
do-it-yourself activities 304, 314, 316
dog excrement 179
domestic accidents 295–313, 315–17
doorsteps 310
'dose effect' 197
double-glazed windows 163
draughts 150, 152–3
drinking *see* alcohol
Dubravka 85
Duisdorf 81
dwelling 3–4

E
eczema 114–16, 122, 138
education level/occupational status 108–9
Edwards, D. 207
Eits, M. 290
electric equipment 313
Epidemiology of Mental Disorders project 2004 184
Evans, G. W. 184, 264

F
falls 299, 304–7, 309–10, 312, 315, 317
Fanger, P. O. 143
Ferreira do Alentejo (Portugal)
  cardiovascular problems 147
  cold in winter problems 149
  deaths in winter months 142
  description 87–9
  domestic accidents 299
  extreme mould 147, 149, 150
  heating systems 162
  problems of dampness 129
  sampling 8–9, 13
  socio-economic characteristics of households 160–1
  ventilation 161
  village houses 5
  warmest city 149
financial assistance 321
fireplaces 313
floors 312
Forlì (Italy)
  dampness 129
  description 89–90
  domestic accidents 299
  heating systems 162
  sampling 13–14
  socio-economic characteristics of households 160–1
  ventilation 161
Fourth Ministerial Conference on Environment and Health (2005) 322
furniture 312–13

G
gas appliances 116–18, 122
gastric/duodenal ulcers 164, 165, 283, 286
gender bias 13
Geneva (Switzerland)
  dampness 129
  description 90–2
  domestic accidents 299

Index

energy systems 165
  sampling 13–14
  socio-economic characteristics of households 160–1
glazing 313
graffiti 179, 262
graphical modelling 207
guidance 321

H
Harz study 291
health
  effects 247–9, 251, 255, 262–7
  indices 109
  self-rated health 256, 264, 268–9
Health Questionnaires 97
hearing 290
heat 144
heating 307, 315–17
Hecht, K. 266
Heiderhof 83
home
  definition 3
  temperatures 306
House Condition Survey (England) 179
Housing and Health Questionnaire (HH) 6, 9, 17–44, 108–10, 156, 187–9, 200–3, 249, 296–7, 309
Housing Health and Safety Rating System (HHSRS) 127
Housing Inspection Survey Sheet (HI) 6, 11, 98, 109, 114, 127–8, 156–9, 187, 200–3, 249, 310–12
housing quality score (HQS) 109
hypertension 164, 277, 283, 289–90

I
income 109
Inhabitant Questionnaire 6, 11, 14–72, 114, 127–8, 156, 187–9, 249, 310–11
insulation 166
International Crime Victim Survey (ICVS) 168, 172
internationality 94
Ising, H. 290

K
Kantrowitz, E. 264
Karlova Ves 85
kitchens 306, 312–13, 315
knives 313
Korea 113

L
Landon, M. 143
Lange-Asschenfeldt, H. 290
LARES project
  challenges 94
  cities involved 79
  cold homes 142–53
  conclusions 101
  crime 170–82
  domestic accidents 296–313, 315–17
  health effects 249, 251, 255, 262–7
  implementation of surveys 99–101
  indoor air pollution 111–23
  introduction 3–5
  local base set-up 98
  mental health 187–9, 194–8
  noise 276–80, 282–6, 289–93
  opportunity to study housing/health conditions 127–9, 132, 134–7, 139
  quality of life 200–1, 203–4, 208–12, 214
  residential energy systems 155–67
  results of the analyses 105–6
  résumé of recommendations 319–21
  scores and conventions 107–10
  training 98–9
Lauritzen, S. L. 207
Leitmann, T. 290
Lieber, G. F. 290
lighting 177, 180, 307, 311, 316
Likert scales 7
litter 179, 262, 264, 268

M
management 321
marginal model (Liang/Zeger) 115
Maschke, C. 266, 290
Matheson, M. P. 266
'mean healthy people' 203
men 116, 300, 303, 315
Mendelberg, R.C. 142
mental health 108, 139, 152–3, 181, 184–9, 194–8, 265–7
Meteonorm 4 program 145
migraine/headaches 164, 277–8, 280, 286
mites 125–7
mould 113–14, 118, 122, 125–9, 132, 134, 137–40, 143–7, 149–50, 153, 158, 322
mould/dampness score 109, 163
musculoskeletal systems 275–6, 284, 290, 292
myotoxins 126

Index

N
nasal allergies 115–16, 122
neighbours 277
nervousness 301–2, 315
neuroendocrine system 275
Niemann, H. 266
nitrogen monoxide (NO) 113
noise 110, 265–70, 275–80, 282–6, 289–93, 307–8, 315–17, 322
Noise and Risk of Myocardial Infarction Study (Willich et al) 291–2

O
obesity 248, 303, 315
open space 177
Outcome of Depression International Network (ODIN) study 2001 184
overcrowding 306

P
particulate matter (PM) 113
Pascoe, T. 169
pests *see* cockroaches; rats/mice
Petrzalka 85
pets 115–16
physical exercise 303

Q
question A (HI) 201–2
question B (HH) 201–3

R
railways 276
Rasch model 207–9
rats/mice 122
recreational facilities 179
residential energy systems 155–67
respiratory conditions 150, 152, 165, 275, 284, 289–92
Review of Healthy and Safety Risk Drivers (CLG 2008) 320
Ruzinov 85

S
sampling 7–8, 95
senior citizens
    and domestic accidents 295, 299–300, 304, 311, 314–15
    and indoor air pollution 116, 118, 123
    and health 151–3, 267, 277, 286, 289–90, 292
    and residential energy systems 157, 162

Serra, H. A. 142
Shaping the Future (World Health Report 2003) 155
sick building syndrome (SBS) 164–5
SINUS database 8
skin diseases 286, 291
sleep 262, 265–7, 269, 275–7, 279, 285–6, 289, 292–3, 307–8, 315
smoking *see* tobacco
socio-economic status (SES) 110, 163, 165
space 304
Spandau Health Survey 290, 291
Spearman-Brown formula 205–6, 249
staffing 96
stairs 310–11, 315–16
Stansfeld, S. A. 266
Statview program 147
strokes 283, 286
Strusberg, I. 142
surveyor training 9–12

T
Tannenbusch 83
thermal comfort 143
tiredness 301, 307–9, 314–15
tobacco
    cardiovascular/smoking connection 149
    environmental tobacco smoke (ETS) 113
    passive smoking 113
    smokers/active smoking 115, 122, 138
toys 313
traffic 262–4, 266–7, 277, 282–3, 289–92, 301
training 9–12, 98–9
tumours 283, 286

V
Valleron, A. J. 144
vandalism 178 *see also* crime
vegetation 262
ventilation 158–9, 161, 163, 166, 321
Venusberg 83
Vilnius (Lithuania)
    cold in winter problems 149
    coldest city 149
    crime 172
    description 92–3
    domestic accidents 299
    heating systems 162
    multi-family houses 5
    respiratory/arthritic/cardiovascular problems 147

sampling 13
socio-economic characteristics of households 160–1
volatile organic compounds (VOCs) 111, 113–14, 116, 122–3
Vrakuna 85

W
water 313
weather-tightness 161, 163, 166
Weinhold, H. 290
Wermuth, N. 207
wheezing 115–16, 118, 126
Whittaker, J. 207
Wilkinson, P. 143
Wolf, U. 290
women 116, 300, 303, 315
workspace 315–16
World Health Organisation (WHO) vii, 3, 5–7, 9, 11, 96–7, 319
'worst healthy people' 203